PSYCHOPHYSIOLOGIC APPROACH
IN
MEDICAL PRACTICE

PSYCHOPHYSIOLOGIC APPROACH
IN
MEDICAL PRACTICE

WILLIAM W. SCHOTTSTAEDT, M.D.

*Associate Professor, Department of Preventive Medicine
and Public Health, Department of Medicine, and Department of
Psychiatry, Neurology and the Behavioral Sciences
The University of Oklahoma Medical Center*

THE YEAR BOOK PUBLISHERS · INC.
200 EAST ILLINOIS STREET · CHICAGO

Preface

THE following pages were written primarily for medical students, interns, residents, and practicing physicians who are interested in psychophysiologic phenomena but who do not expect to have formal psychiatric training. I have had two aims in writing. The first of these was to provide a framework of concepts into which additional facts and ideas could subsequently be placed as understanding of human behavior and its relation to health and disease increases. The second aim was to develop from these concepts and ideas a sound basis for treating ailments associated with emotional disturbances. These form a large segment of medical practice. Many of them would not require psychiatric care if the internist or general practitioner felt at ease in using a few basically simple psychotherapeutic techniques.

In pursuit of the first of these aims, half of this book is devoted to a presentation of background material essential for a comprehensive understanding of human behavior and psychophysiologic interrelationships. The diseases commonly called psychosomatic are not dealt with as such. In none of them has a clear-cut emotional or psychogenic etiology been firmly established. These diseases can be characterized only as being conspicuously responsive to emotional disturbances, with exacerbations and remissions often associated with alterations in the emotional state of the patient. This is a difference in degree only, for, to a lesser extent, the same can be said of most diseases. The mechanisms which account for fluctuations in the course of "psychosomatic diseases" are the same as those which are associated with fluctuations in the course of diseases in general and are again the same mechanisms as those resulting in the whole gamut of "functional" complaints. Consequently, the material of the first half of this book is presented in terms of the mechanisms involved rather than in terms of disease processes.

The second half of the book discusses the practical implications of

5

this material for treatment. It is not a manual of practical psychiatry nor is it expected that what is presented will be adequate for the handling of psychiatric entities. Here, as in every other field of medicine, the practicing physician must be able to evaluate the patient and decide what is appropriate therapy. If the proper treatment is formal psychiatric care, referral should be made to a psychiatrist. Many patients seen in a medical setting have emotional or situational problems which affect their health and require professional attention if the physician is to give good medical care. Many of these patients neither want nor need psychiatric care. The physician who feels secure in questioning patients about their feeling states and who has some understanding of basically simple psychotherapeutic procedures can do much to help them. Indeed, many of them respond rapidly and easily once their problems have been clarified in their own minds so that they are able to attack them directly. The second portion of the book is written to help nonpsychiatrists attain some proficiency in this process.

This book makes no pretense of covering the field of psychosomatic medicine comprehensively. Its aim is to set the stage so that current and future work in this field can be read intelligently and the many reference works available can be used with profit. A complete bibliography has not been attempted. References from the psychosomatic literature have been chosen to illustrate a point rather than to present a detailed account of the work of investigators in this field. Fairly complete bibliographies are available and should be consulted by those wishing to pursue a point further.

It should be evident that the aims of this book are limited; yet no book now available meets the needs noted. If these pages arouse the interest of medical students and physicians in psychophysiologic phenomena and give them the courage to try to deal with some of the common emotional and situational difficulties which affect the health of their patients, this book will have served its purpose.

WILLIAM W. SCHOTTSTAEDT

Table of Contents

Chapter 1

Stress

PHYSICIANS spend much of their time evaluating and treating symptoms which have arisen in settings of stress. In doing so they are practicing psychosomatic medicine and, by necessity, must concern themselves with all those phenomena in which attitudes, emotions, behavior, and their associated physiologic changes affect the well-being of patients. Such physiologic reactions in healthy persons may give rise to symptoms and in the ill may result in exacerbation or amelioration of disease. They are frequently associated with stressful situations in the environment. But the stressful stimulus may be an internal one or may be illness itself. To give adequate care to patients, we must concern ourselves with their personal lives, trying to understand what is stressful to them while standing ready to help in any way we can.

When we say that a stimulus is stressful, we are expressing our evaluation that it has threatening significance. Much confusion arises from our tendency to view all events through our own eyes rather than through the eyes of the person to whom they are happening. Stress is subjective and personal. What is threatening to us may not threaten the patient who seeks our help. To project our own reactions into him can only confuse the issue. We must try, instead, to learn what the event or stimulus has meant to him.

This is true even when we are dealing with a situation which would be considered stressful to most people. The death of a relative or a close friend, the loss of one's income, a catastrophe which suddenly ends the ability to continue one's lifework are events which most people consider threatening and with which physicians must deal frequently. The fact that these situations are stressful to most people, however, should not blind us to the individual character of stress. The meaning of such situations is different for different persons; the attitudes toward them differ, and even these extreme situations are not stressful to everyone.

It is not only the tragic in life which may be stressful. A methodical draftsman accustomed to doing his work precisely, always using one pencil until it is too short for further use before starting a new one, may be tremendously disturbed by the "sloppy" habits of a partner who keeps several pencils at his drawing board and uses whichever one he happens to pick up first. Similarly, a meticulous housewife may be greatly distressed when her child walks across a clean floor with muddy feet. Why should a stimulus so trivial in the life of one person be a major stress in the life of another?

Not only is there variation from one person to another in what is considered stressful but the same person may find a situation threatening under one set of circumstances and not under another. Thus one who ordinarily enjoys eating between meals may find eating between meals stressful during Lent, if it is contrary to his religious practices. Another person may find it stressful to argue with his wife but a delight to argue with his friends. Why should an act be pleasurable in one situation and painful in another?

Repetition of an act may alter its meaning. Talking with a patient may be quite stressful to a medical student the first time he takes a history. With constant repetition, this becomes an accepted part of the day's work and, under ordinary circumstances, is no longer viewed as a stress. Clearly, stress is not objective nor is it a quality inherent in an event or a situation. This is plainly seen in clinical medicine in patients' reactions to their symptoms. A patient's belief that he has cancer is stressful to him even though he may not have cancer. Contrariwise, a patient who believes that his lesion is benign is not under stress even though the lesion is malignant and incurable.

A consideration of facts such as these makes it apparent that the stressful nature of a situation or event depends on the person's perception of it, his evaluation of its relation to him, and his feelings about it. It is an evaluation in which the situation or event is perceived as a personal threat. Viewing stress as an evaluation makes it understandable that a situation may be stressful to one person and not to another, or stressful at one time and not at another. We cannot assume that a situation is stressful to someone else because it would be to us. Neither can we assume that it is not stressful to another person because it would not be so to us. You must view the situation through the eyes of the patient you are trying to help. If you are trying to help a man who is angered when his partner uses a long pencil when a short one is at hand, your concern is with the question "Why is this stimulus so threatening?" An objective and impersonal outlook can be most helpful. Stressful situations are seldom unique. No matter how distressing a situation may seem to the person involved in it, similar situations have been met and solved by others. Keeping this in mind helps avoid becoming so entangled emotionally in the patient's difficulties as to be unable to think clearly or to help solve his problems. It fosters an optimistic attitude toward the patient's problems—a helpful attitude for the person who feels trapped in an impossible situation.

When a person interprets a situation or event as threatening, his evaluation depends upon his ideas of himself and of his capacity to meet such situations. The medical student about to take his first history may be uncertain of his ability to handle this situation smoothly. With little previous experience to draw on, an evaluation of this ability is not a part of his concept of himself. This is the basis of his uncertainty. After a few successful experiences, he finds that he can take an adequate history and can handle the interpersonal relationship easily. His concept of himself then includes this self-evaluation, and the situation is no longer stressful. Until this self-concept is formed, however, the experience will continue to be stressful. Thus a person's concept of himself becomes of central importance to an understanding of what is stressful to him.

SELF-CONCEPT

How does one develop a concept of himself? A complete picture of this process can be obtained only by a fusion of many lines of work and thought. It must include the cultural, social, and physical environment

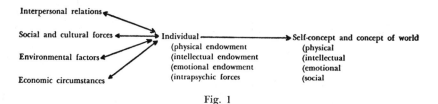

Fig. 1

and the constitutional endowment. It must include personal development, both physical and psychologic. It must include interpersonal relations, emotional needs, and conscious and unconscious motivations. (See Fig. 1.)

PHYSICAL

It is obvious that people differ in body build and physical capacities. Each person must come to terms with his own physical limitations and form some concept of how his physical capacities and limitations compare with those of other people. This process is seen most clearly in people in the lowest or highest percentile in height and weight, but everyone must form some concept of his physical self, even if it is only that he is like the majority of others. Physical development follows a definite sequence and everyone must adjust to this sequence as it progresses. The problems of adjustment are increased for those who have an early or a late puberty; but everyone goes through these changes, and self-concept must change accordingly. In addition, each person must develop some concept of how he compares with others in regard to his speed of movement, his dexterity, his strength, and his endurance. This concept of physical self depends in part on physical constitution and development. It depends also on the contacts one has with adults, brothers and sisters, and friends and on what expectations one is led to have of his body from what is said to him by them. Thus a man's concept of himself, even physically, may not accord with what another person would consider appropriate for him. The man who is stronger than most of his fellows may feel physically inferior if he has been raised among people who are stronger than he or by parents who expect him to display greater strength than he has. In such a case, the stress of competitive sports may well be out of proportion to his actual physical ability.

INTELLECTUAL

The same is true of intellectual endowment. In addition to the general level of intelligence, as measured by intelligence tests, a person may have special gifts in one particular intellectual line or another. People are born with different intellectual endowments and one's concept of his own intellectual ability is formulated in much the same way as his concept of his physical capacities. Thus a person of superior intellectual gifts may consider himself dull and lacking in talents if he is raised among people who are superior to him or by parents who consider him intellectually inferior. Similarly a person of modest endowment may consider himself to be superior if raised among people of lesser endowment or by parents who consider him to be superior.

EMOTIONAL

People have different emotional constitutions as well. Some are highly sensitive and emotionally labile by nature; others are not. The basic emotional tone may be so altered by specific conflicts during life, by the demands made to control the expression of emotions, and by the emotional outlets discovered that it is sometimes difficult to sort out the basic endowment from the subsequent elaborations. However, Gesell's work with children[1] leaves little doubt of a basic difference in this realm. It also shows a difference in the sociability of people, that is, in their ability to relate to other people and their enjoyment of such relations. He states that these differences are clearly evident by 16 weeks, if not before.

COMPARISON WITH OTHERS

FAMILY.—In all of this, there is much comparing of oneself with others. This process begins within the family. Harry Stack Sullivan has described this phase of interpersonal relations beautifully in his interpersonal theory of psychiatry.[2] Here, the child learns new things about himself and formulates concepts of himself and of others. All subsequent learning must occur against the background of what is learned during this early phase. If the concepts formed of figures in authority (originally the father and mother) and of colleagues (originally brothers, sisters, and friends) are incorrect, subsequent learning requires correction of wrong concepts as well as learning new ones. This is much more difficult and less lasting than the original learning process itself. It is for this reason that so much emphasis has been placed upon early family relationships, particularly with the mother and father.

The family is the basic social unit. Its functions are procreation, the transmission of cultural ideas and beliefs, and the teaching of social mores. It poses standards of performance which must be met. It forms the context in which affective relationships are first formed, thereby establishing the pattern of such relationships for later life. It trains the child for future roles even though much of this training is by imitation involving no conscious, premeditated educational effort on the part of the parents. A person's orientation to society in later life is determined in part by how his parents played their roles within the family.

In a person's assessment of his own capacities the importance of early relationships and the judgments of other family members is sometimes striking. The warping effect on subsequent development can be extreme and at times tragic. A good example of this was Mrs. Winn, a middle-aged woman who felt she was inferior to everyone she knew. She was the eighth of 11 children. Her parents had left her upbringing to two older sisters, who had considered her dull-witted and unattractive. Because of her dark complexion, they taunted her about her racial background, insisting she was not really one of the family. They used every opportunity to point out their superior knowledge and ability. They made her feel unwanted by their friends. She grew up a lonely and unhappy person. She received a master's degree and was the only member of her family to complete college. She became a certified public accountant and earned a very adequate personal income. She married and had a child. Despite her record of achievement and the friends she had made, she felt intellectually inadequate, socially rejected, and inferior to all with whom she associated. Many of the stresses in her life were determined to a large degree by her distorted evaluation of herself.

Discipline is an important part of family living. Since the early affective relationships are concentrated around a few people, largely the mother and father, the giving of affection or of punishment is a potent weapon in education of the child. The child has no one else to turn to. If he desires approval, he must conform. Thus authority, discipline, and affection become closely intertwined.

Sibling relationships are extremely important in a family group. Brothers and sisters vie with each other for the affection and approval of their parents, whether this is recognized within the family or not. In many families, competition cannot be carried on openly without evoking disapproval. A conflict is therefore engendered which must be faced if competitive relationships later in life are to be handled adequately.

THOSE OUTSIDE THE FAMILY.—The importance of relationships outside the family is to leaven adverse influences within the family and to broaden concepts to make them more generally applicable. If the parents have led a child to consider himself more gifted intellectually than he is, school associations may correct this appraisal. If a child has formed the impression that all adults are harsh and punitive because his parents are, association with teachers or other adults may reduce the fear and rebellion engendered at home. This function is particularly important when the family group is unusual. Only by broadening his concepts to include the community at large can one adequately place himself in the community and see his function there.

Later in life the concept of one's place in the community becomes closely associated with the idea of social class and community status. It is not only the actual level at which one lives—upper, middle, or lower class—that is important but the direction of change and the orientation of the person to his status. If he is content as he is, less stress and strain is put on him than if he is dissatisfied and feels he must strive to better his position. Striving to attain higher status can produce great stresses and strains and result in illness and disability.

Environment

But relations with other people are not the only things important in determining a person's concept of himself. His experiences with the environment at large are also important. His ability to cope with problems and to solve them adequately may make an important contribution to his feelings about what is threatening to him and what is not. Acts of fate, death, separations, illnesses, catastrophies, and unexpected occurrences form the basis for his feelings about his relation to the universe at large and to religion. Impersonal social forces, acting through people to be sure, also have their part to play. Economic forces, industrialization, unemployment, depression—these all are significant in helping form a self-concept.

The ability to meet new and unexpected situations is an important aspect of life. A man's ability to meet the unexpected depends on his previous experiences with unexpected events and how well he handled them. It also depends on the type of event, whether it demands physical capacity, intellectual activity, or social ability, and on his evaluation of his abilities in this area.

None of these statements imply that an evaluation is necessarily conscious or easily verbalized. Certain aspects of it are close to awareness, but much of it is not. The emotional needs of a person and his unconscious drives and conflicts have much to do with his concept of himself. Some of these conflicts arise from ideologic contradictions in our culture of which the individual may be quite unaware, despite having assimilated both sides of the contradiction into his make-up. The masculine ideal of aggressive competition and success by excelling others exists beside the Christian doctrine that the meek shall inherit the earth. The democratic ideal of assertive individualism, with each person making his own decisions and coping with problems actively and effectively as they arise, exists beside an authoritarian family relationship wherein children are rewarded for obedience to parental decision.

In adolescence, these conflicts are accentuated; then a person is told one moment to accept his responsibilities like the adult he is soon to be and told the next moment that he may not share in certain privileges because he is still a child. We live among contradictions. Hostilities and frustrations are bound to be engendered. Yet much educational effort is expended in teaching the young that they are not to express anger. From sources such as these and from many others spring conflicts. Feelings of guilt may arise at the vague awareness of unacceptable impulses within oneself; situations which arouse these feelings will then be stressful.

There are several possible reactions to the culture in which one is raised, and the relationship of parent and child is an important determinant. He may accept the culture passively, trying merely to be "a good boy" and get into no trouble but having no deep convictions about what the culture represents. He may, on the other hand, try to be a model of cultural virtues, living as a lesson to others and trying to inculcate his associates and his children with similar virtues. He may try to modify customs and introduce new ideas in an attempt to create new values within his culture. He may expend his energies in manipulating his environment and cultural value systems to his own advantage. He may also react with rebellion and defiance. These attitudes toward life and the culture in which one lives help determine what is stressful and are important to mental and physical health.

A fascinating aspect of self-concept is its influence on what happens to people. If they see themselves as inadequate and hence feel threatened they will avoid situations in which inadequacy is made evident. The inadequacy, which may have been very real in childhood, may be far from real later in life; yet they never permit themselves to be in a situation where their concept of themselves can be corrected and continue to feel inadequate. In his book *Creative Evolution*[3] Henri Bergson wrote "It is then right to say that what we do depends on what we are; but it is necessary to add also that we are, to a certain extent, what we do, and that we are creating ourselves continually." This creation of oneself is an important part of life. Though it depends on past experience and one's ability to integrate experiences with what one considers to be true about oneself, it is nonetheless a potent force in determining what one will become.

In the course of normal development people meet a large enough, or a "normal" enough, sample of the population to formulate a generally applicable concept of themselves. Ordinarily this concept undergoes changes consistent with the developmental patterns through which they progress physically, intellectually, emotionally, and socially. They therefore enter adult life with a concept of themselves as adults rather than as children and with a realistic evaluation of their capacities and limitations consistent with their level of development. When some aspect of a person's concept of himself is consistent with his childhood state but not with his adult state, he may seem "immature" or "neurotic." Such a concept has not undergone normal evolutionary development.

An example may clarify the process and its effects. Mrs. Winters went to her physician complaining of diarrhea, that was only partially relieved by the usual medications. She was a fairly large woman who considered herself unattractive because she was "big-boned." Her father had been a janitor and she grew up considering herself socially inferior to her playmates and colleagues. She did well in school but was never outstanding. In adolescence she met a dashing young man from an upper middle-class family who quite swept her off her feet. They were married, but his family never accepted her and considered her unworthy of them. Within a few weeks of the marriage, her husband also rejected her. From then on he always referred to her as "the janitor." He was very successful financially and traveled a great deal. He lived freely and openly with other women. He even showed his wife the letters he received from other women to prove to her that he was very attractive and to make her aware of what a prize she had got when she married him. He told her repeatedly how stupid she was, how inept in all of the household duties, and how utterly incapable she was in anything of practical importance. They had three children. Neither he nor the children helped her with any of the household duties. Whenever one of the sons offered to help, the father would say, "Oh, let the janitor do it." She resented his attitude greatly but felt that it was justified and that she was indeed unworthy. When she was first seen, the older son was spending a long weekend with his girl friend in another city. She was unhappy about the relation which she knew existed between them. Her younger son was about to be married. He was very disturbed, and a short time later he had an acute paranoid breakdown. Her teen-age daughter was making a very poor social adjustment and she did not know how to help her. Her husband had established a monthly budget for household expenses early in their married life, and he had never changed it, despite the increase in the cost of living and the birth of three children. When she asked for an increase in the allowance, he refused. Feeling completely inadequate to cope with the situation, she had considered separation but was so convinced of her own inferiority and her inability to do anything satisfactorily that she did not have the courage to consider divorce seriously.

Mrs. Winters was a person whose self-concept had not undergone normal evolutionary development. It was distorted and disabling. Because of her feeling that she was incapable of solving problems or meeting life adequately, she never allowed herself to learn that she was capable and adequate. As she began testing herself in the course of treatment and finding that she could do some things well, she became a very different person. And though she did not leave her husband or try to establish an independent existence, she found that she was able to cope with the situation without symptoms. Since her concept of herself had undergone a major change, her evaluation of the stressful circumstances in her life was altered.

EVALUATIONS

ATTITUDES

The evaluation which we call stress may be expressed in terms of attitudes. These attitudes have a number of basic forms which vary widely in their detailed manifestations. In one attitude the threat is viewed as one which can be met adequately and efficiently, provided one exerts control, is alert, and is ready to respond. Another attitude is expressed in a sense of futility and complete inability to meet the threat. Yet another attitude may be aroused when a situation is seen as uncertain or the person is unsure of his ability to meet the threat adequately. The situation may prevent the attainment of some goal and arouse an aggressive or hostile attitude. Many other attitudes may be aroused in stressful situations.

The evaluation may be expressed as an attitude and as an emotion simultaneously. *An attitude* is a state of readiness for a particular type of response, which may be verbalized in terms of what one would like to do. *An emotion* is an intimate fusion of psychic and somatic components into an integrated affective experience accompanying the attitude. It is not necessary that a person be able to verbalize this experience or even be conscious of its presence, for an emotion, like an evaluation, may lie outside awareness.

EMOTIONS

Emotions, like attitudes, have considerable variety. They may fall into the fight-or-flight type of reaction, made so familiar by Cannon[4] —that is, the response to a situation may be anger or fear, aggression or withdrawal. Situations may also be met with more chronic emotional responses which are described by such words as "tension" or "depression." Excitement and apprehension may be manifest as part of an evaluation of a stressful situation. Emotions or feeling states are closely associated with attitudes. Thus the attitude described as involving control, alertness, and readiness to respond is ordinarily associated with the feeling of tension. The attitude of complete inability to cope with a situation is associated with an emotion of fear, dejection, or depression. The attitude of uncertainty about one's ability to cope may be associated with emotions such as excitement or apprehension. And the attitude that the stimulus is preventing one from reaching his goal may be associated with an emotional response of anger or resentment.

PHYSIOLOGIC CHANGES

Attitudes and emotions are associated with physiologic changes. Anger may be associated with certain vascular and muscular responses visible as a reddening or blanching of the face and as an increased tonus of muscles. Depression may be manifested by pallor and tears and is often associated with gastrointestinal disturbances or with headaches. An apprehensive person may break into a cold sweat or have altered respirations and tachycardia. Tension is associated with muscular tenseness.

These physiologic changes, which are a normal accompaniment of attitudes and emotions, may become the basis for symptoms if the reaction is intense or prolonged. Thus, an apprehensive patient may complain primarily of tachycardia and make no comment about his anxieties or fears. Similarly, a depressed patient may be concerned entirely with his gastrointestinal complaints and not at all with his feelings of depression. The physiologic components of the evaluation have then become stressful of themselves and are a more immediate stress than the situation which evoked the response.

Grace and Graham[5] studied the association of physiologic manifestations with attitudes. They reported that many patients with urticaria were in situations in which they saw themselves as being beaten or hammered upon but, at the same time, felt there was no way of getting back. They described Raynaud's phenomenon as occurring when a person was angered and wanted to strike out at someone. Diarrhea was observed when a person was impatiently anxious to be rid of a situation, whereas constipation was present when he felt that he must hang on grimly, come what may. All of these were the patients' evaluations of their relation to situations. They depended on their concept of themselves and their feelings about their role in the situations. They depended ultimately on basic endowment and past experiences. That further study may modify the specific associations does not destroy the underlying concept. It is important to understand that attitudes and emotions are associated with physiologic changes which may give rise to symptoms in many parts of the body.

BEHAVIOR AND SOCIAL RELATIONSHIPS

Evaluations are not only expressed in terms of attitudes, emotions, and physiologic changes, but in behavior and social relationships as well. The behavioral responses may be "normal" or "maladaptive." People may be aggressive, may withdraw completely from the situation, may indulge in delinquent behavior, may be prim and proper, or may be free and uninhibited. These behavioral responses likewise depend on a person's concept of himself and on his concept of his role.

Psychologists and psychiatrists have described a number of mental defense mechanisms which operate to determine behavioral response. The mechanisms used depend in part on the strength of a person's basic drives, that is, on constitutional endowment; in part on events and interpersonal relations, that is, on experience; and in part on his concept of himself and of his role in life, both of which act as a guide for behavior. All of these affect his evaluation of the way in which a threat may best be handled. The most direct and obvious mechanism is simple gratification of a desire. One can gratify a desire freely if he knows that gratification will be successful and will not run counter to his concept of himself and his role in the world. If attempts at gratification will meet with punishment or failure, direct gratification is deterred. If a person's concept of himself does not permit direct gratification, some other mechanism will have to be sought. Gratification, however, is the natural course for drives to take unless something makes one utilize other mechanisms.

When simple gratification is not possible or desirable, sublimation may be an appropriate and successful solution. Through sublimation the basic desires can achieve gratification in a socially and personally acceptable fashion. Thus gratification is actually achieved, though indirectly. Other defense mechanisms are (1) withdrawal from an unpleasant situation; (2) denial that the situation exists; (3) suppression or repression of the undesirable stimulus or situation; (4) indulgence in fantasy. Symptoms themselves may sometimes be defenses against unpleasant situations since they may keep one from having to recognize an undesirable or unacceptable situation. The list is incomplete but indicates the variety of defenses available. These defense mechanisms are the basic components of which behavioral responses are. made. Whether the response is normal or maladaptive behavior, a psychoneurotic or a psychotic reaction, or symptom formation, it is an adaptive effort to deal with stressful stimuli.

These mechanisms are directly related to the idea of stress. When a desire can be gratified, energy is expended only in carrying out the movements necessary to achieve gratification. With sublimation or displacement, some additional energy may be needed to divert the drive into the new channel. The stress or strain imposed then depends on how closely related the new goal is to the original one and how readily the substitution can be made. Suppression or inhibition imposes its own stress; the drive is not permitted either direct or sublimated expression but is held in check. The forces inhibiting a response are sometimes very considerable and can be associated with a good deal of internal strain.

Emphasizing the importance of an evaluation to the concept of stress does not in any way imply that this evaluation is verbalized or conscious. People are making evaluations throughout waking life without conscious awareness of them, and the process continues through sleep. A person may dream of some catastrophic event as a threat to himself, perhaps awakening in fright. He may dream of the same event as an uninvolved spectator. The difference lies in an evaluation of his relation to the event. External stimuli are evaluated similarly. The housewife may awaken to the faint cry of an infant in the next room and sleep through the ringing of an alarm clock next to her bed. Again, it is the evaluation of the stimulus and its relation to her which determines the response. In both instances, the evaluation has been made at some other level than that of conscious awareness.

The intensity of stress is again determined by an evaluation. In this case it is an evaluation of the balance between the expenditure of energy required to meet the threat and the supply of energy available. If the energy available is great in proportion to that needed to meet the threat adequately, the stress is considered mild. If the two are approximately equal, the stress is great. When more energy is required than is available, the possibility of withdrawal and avoiding the threatening situation makes a new evaluation possible and may result in reduction of stress. When avoidance seems impossible despair or panic may result. The fact that the intensity of stress is a personal evaluation accounts for the greater intensity of stress for similar stimuli during times of fatigue or chronic illness. The energy reserves available for meeting a threatening situation are then depleted, and the balance of the energy available to the energy required is disturbed.

STRESSFUL STIMULI

A word should also be said about the nature of stressful stimuli and situations. In defining stress as an evaluation of the relation between a stimulus and a person in which the stimulus is perceived as a threat, we are apt to think of the stimulus as external to the person. This is often true. External stressful stimuli may be threatening physical acts. They may equally well be social patterns and ideas about role playing which the person has learned. Thus the culturally accepted pattern of male dominance may be a source of considerable stress to a man who knows that the pattern specifies that the male should be dominant but who finds himself in a marital relationship in which he is totally unable to assume the dominant role. The goal of individual independence may likewise be a personal stress when others expect a man to be independent in a situation in which he cannot.

Many stresses are not external but arise from characteristics of the person himself. Prominent among internal threats are goals and ambitions. A goal becomes a stress when one faces the possibility of failure to attain it. Considerable energy expenditure may be necessary to meet this threat of failure; the stress is then very intense. When we see a person bending all his energies toward attaining some goal he has set, the potency of these goals is obvious enough. A common mistake, however, is to overlook ambitions and goals as a source of stress in a patient who complains of chronic fatigue, is depressed, or appears apathetic.

In addition to goals and ambitions, emotions may be threatening. Some people conceive of anger as bad, dangerous, or sinful. Anger then must be met by suppression or repression. It is an emotion which should not be felt and the need to prevent awareness of it is answered by suppressing or repressing the feeling altogether. Any arousal of anger in such a person must then be met by energy spent to overcome the anger rather than by energy directed at the stimulus arousing the anger. The anger has become the greater threat and the greater stress. This is seen repeatedly in the course of working with patients.

The physiologic changes which accompany attitudes and emotions may also be stressful. This is evident in the person who complains of tachycardia when the tachycardia is actually a part of a reaction of fear and in the person who complains of gastrointestinal symptoms when his basic problem is depression.

The threat may also lie in the interaction between stimulus and person or in some specific behavior pattern. The man who wishes to strangle another may be threatened little or not at all by the other man. He may accept his anger as "righteous indignation." Yet he may restrain himself from the act because the act itself is a threat because of strong conditioning by social forces against violent acts of this nature. In this case the contemplated action is the greatest threat and energy is expended in meeting it.

It should be emphasized that all these separate aspects of evaluation —behavior, attitudes, emotions, unconscious motivations, and physiologic changes—form a single integrated response of the person as a whole. The specific evaluation made depends on social forces and past experiences, on basic emotional needs and unconscious conflicts, on all those factors which form a part of one's self-concept and his perception of the world about him. The response, however, is a unitary response. Perhaps this can best be illustrated in terms of infantile behavior. When the infant is hungry, his whole body responds. He is hungry, he is frustrated, he cries, he moves his arms and legs violently. The infant who wants to be fondled expresses this desire through his behavior. Attitudes and behavior are not isolated phenomena. The desire for attention and the cry are part of one response.

As the child grows, he learns other ways of satisfying his needs or getting other people to satisfy them. He can inhibit certain parts of the total reaction, the voluntary behavior more readily than the autonomic reaction. Darwin, in his book *Expression of the Emotions in Man and Animals*,[6] describes this well: "A man when moderately angry, or even when enraged, may command the movements of his body, but he cannot prevent his heart from beating rapidly. His chest will perhaps give a few heaves, and his nostrils just quiver, for the movements of respiration are only in part voluntary. In like manner those muscles of the face which are least obedient to the will, will sometimes alone betray a slight and passing emotion. The glands again are wholly independent of the will, and a man suffering from grief may command his features, but cannot always prevent the tears from coming into his eyes."

New types of experience may arouse feelings of frustration, but when these feelings arise they are accompanied by old types of behavior, emotions, and physiologic changes. In addition, attitudes develop toward various forms of emotional expression. Habits of reacting are formed not only for overt behavior but also for attitudes and emotions and therefore, obviously, for physiologic fluctuations. These habits in reaction patterns are important for an understanding of response to stress and of symptom formation in a setting of stress.

To illustrate how all these diverse elements combine to mold personality and result in symptoms let us consider the life story of Mrs. Bertrand.* At the age of 31 she was referred to a New York City clinic because of headaches, obesity, hypertension and angina. Her background was complex but fascinating and it was certainly pertinent to her complaints. Since she spent most of her early childhood with her maternal grandmother it is appropriate to start with a few comments about the grandmother's background and personality.

Her grandmother, half Negro and half Indian, married, at an early age, a man whom she felt loved his mother more than he loved her. Shortly after this marriage ended in divorce she married a stevedore. She was a devout Baptist who felt deeply guilty about the failure of her first marriage and her rapid second marriage. She knew she would be punished for the rest of her life for these sins. Her husband was a chronic and abusive alcoholic who beat her and the children freely and frequently, but she devoted her life to trying to make him happy, without success. They had two daughters, the patient's mother and her aunt.

At an early age Mrs. Bertrand's mother developed an intense hatred for her parents and rebelled against everything either of them represented. She followed no religion. She refused to accept either her Negro background or her deprived economic status. She was openly looking for happiness in the form of money and fun.

Mrs. Bertrand's father was the son of an aggressive, competent, and successful Jewish lawyer, who had high hopes for his son and expected him to excel in all things and to become a lawyer. However, the boy felt

---

*Mrs. Bertrand's history is given in detail because it will be referred to often in following chapters.

overpowered by his father, stammered in his presence, and could not imagine being a lawyer as his father wished. The father felt contempt for his son and his stammering. He punished him for it, made harsh comments about his work in school, and was cutting in his comments about his companions. This boy also rebelled against his parents and what they represented.

These two maladjusted people met when she began working as an elevator operator in the fashionable New York apartment where the lawyer and his family lived. The two young people fell in love and, despite violent protestations from both families, finally married. The marriage was unsuccessful from the start. She wanted money, clothes, and plenty of fun. He wanted a quiet home where he could settle down and have no demands made upon him. When Mrs. Bertrand was born, her mother resented her, saying she wanted to have a little fun in life before she settled down to being a housewife. So Mrs. Bertrand was sent off to live with her grandmother. Her mother complained constantly about not having enough money. Her father complained that his wife was never at home to prepare his meals or clean the house. The marriage ended one night when the father came home and found another man in bed with his wife. When he started to object, the other man told him to leave or he would shoot. He left. Mrs. Bertrand was 4 at this time.

The patient was brought up largely by her grandmother. She was expected to be quiet and not disturb her grandparents. Her grandmother often reminded her that were it not for her she would be living in an orphan's home. When her mother remarried, she lived briefly with her. However, after one of the lodgers in the apartment made sexual advances toward her, it was decided to find another home for her.

When she was 8 she lived with three different families, in none of which was she accepted as an equal or given ordinary care and attention. Each of her moves was precipitated by a visit from her grandmother who found conditions below her standards. During this year she had frequent episodes of fainting, usually preceded by dizziness so she could reach a safe place but always continuing to loss of consciousness. When she regained consciousness she almost invariably vomited. This occurred once or twice a month for a year and then stopped spontaneously.

By the time she was 9 she was again living with her grandmother and continued to do so except for brief periods until she was 18. These brief periods were spent with her aunt when her grandfather got into one of his "ugly moods" or her grandmother became tired of having her around and told her to leave for a while. She was filled with anger and resentment during this period, but when she complained of not seeing her mother or that her mother never did any of the things for her that other mothers did for their children, her grandmother always came to the mother's defense with "Your mother can't do everything, you know." If she complained further, her grandmother turned her out of the house to stay with her aunt for a few days.

During this time, no one had taken an interest in her schooling. Consequently she was almost 9, and big for her age, when she entered the first grade. She remembered this experience with some horror, both for being older and larger than the other children and for the troubles her racial background provided. Her father took her to the school and enrolled her there. The principal seemed horrified and asked him why in the world he had waited so long to start his child in school. He gave a weak answer and left. Her address was in a Negro neighborhood. Consequently there was considerable discussion among the teachers as to whether she was Negro or white. The principal called her in several times to ask her. She did not know how to answer. She finally asked her grandmother who told her "Oh, say you're cosmopolitan," but this did not satisfy the principal of the school. In addition to this, she had a great deal of trouble with the other children at school. The Negro children taunted her with being half white. The white children called her "nigger." Thus she was faced with a serious social problem at the start. She did not belong to the minority or the majority group but lived on the fringe of both, accepted by neither. She felt completely alone and disliked school intensely.

The years from 10 to 13 were unhappy ones. She was not accepted by her family, at school, or in any neighborhood group. She did not even have a racial tie to give her "roots." She knew what other mothers did for their children; her mother did none of these things for her. She knew of friendships among her schoolmates; no one would be her friend. Her resentment against the world only brought disapproval from her grandmother. Her desire for activity provoked anger from her grandfather. She felt insecure and fearful of being alone, yet none of her associations with others brought any real satisfaction. Her evaluation of herself was that she was "bad," so bad that no one would have anything to do with her, and that she was helpless, a small girl pitted against the world.

She had always been somewhat obese, weighing 100 pounds at the age of 10; during the years from 10 to 13, she gained weight rapidly. She developed an ungovernable craving for sweets, particularly when she was feeling sorry for herself or when transiently happy over something that had gone right in her life. By the age of 13, she weighed 170 pounds.

An important change occurred in her life when she was 13. On one occasion when her grandmother punished her for some minor offense, she objected violently to being punished and was told it had been for her own good. If she felt so strongly about it she must be crazy. With this remark the grandmother washed her hands of her, having little to do with her thereafter, though allowing her to live in the house. Rejected completely by her grandmother as well as by both parents, with hostility and insecurity at their peak, she began to have frequent severe headaches, spontaneous crying spells, intense craving for foods, particularly sweet things, and severe hay fever. Her aunt took her to a doctor because of her headaches. When he took her blood pressure, he exclaimed "It can't be that high!" He did not tell her what her pressure was, however, nor did he prescribe any medication. Her hay fever, which began when she was 13, usually appeared in the middle of August and lasted until the first frost. It was so severe that she was never able to start school until October. This always put her at a disadvantage but, despite this, she completed high school when she was 18.

During the years from 13 to 18 her only social contacts were through the church. She sang in the choir and taught Sunday School. It seemed to be the only social outlet which was acceptable to her grandmother and satisfying to herself. The church became a source of deep satisfaction to her, took up three or four evenings of each week as well as Sunday, and was the only source of pleasure she managed to find during these adolescent years.

When she was 18 she went to live with her aunt and was surprised to find that with constant association the aunt was as surly and disagreeable as the grandfather had been. The aunt was unmarried but looking for a husband. She did most of her looking in beer taverns about town and would frequently take the patient with her on these excursions. The evenings always lasted until the small hours of the morning. Consequently, though they gave her a small amount of companionship, they left her unable to stay awake the following day at school. In addition to this, she found little pleasure in the drinking and companionship to be found in bars. She therefore soon learned to avoid these contacts as much as possible even though she thought they represented a friendly gesture from her aunt.

When she was 20, she married a man who was half Negro and half white. Her husband was a quiet and understanding man with whom she felt perfectly at ease. With him, for the first time, she felt she could be herself. She could pour out her troubles freely to him and know that she was accepted. He had planned to be an accountant but had been unable to complete his plans because of failing eyesight due to retinitis pigmentosa. Despite impaired vision he got a job as gateman at a railway station and continued to work there, though fearful that some day his employers would learn of his handicap and discharge him. He was very reserved, confided in no one, and seemed much depressed by his coming blindness.

A year or so after their marriage they had a daughter. The pregnancy was extremely traumatic to Mrs. Bertrand. She felt well, yet every time she saw a doctor there was talk about her blood pressure and the possible need for hospitalization. The doctors seemed so worried that she also began to worry. During the eighth month, her blood pressure began rising. It was decided to deliver the baby prematurely rather than risk toxemia. Labor was induced and she delivered after 3 frightening days in the hospital. She was then told she should never have another child. While still in the hospital, she began having severe migraine headaches. She continued to have these periodically during the next 2 years.

The 2 years after the birth of her daughter were very difficult. The child seemed never to sleep through a night. She didn't sleep either, but sat with the child as long as she was awake, determined that her daughter would not feel alone or unwanted as she herself had felt. Also during these first 2 years, her husband worked the evening shift, coming home after midnight. She began to overeat again, "just to be doing something," while sitting up with her daughter. Then she would eat again when her husband came home from work. She had gained weight during pregnancy and continued to gain until she weighed 210 pounds. As she watched the neighbor children, she noted the adverse effects of over-protective rearing practices on one of them. She decided that she was not going to fall into that extreme. As a result, she made a determined effort to take a more normal attitude toward her daughter. She felt she succeeded, and her daughter seemed to develop into a fairly well adjusted child.

Her husband went to a clinic for a time to see if something could be done about his eyesight. There was nothing that could be offered and he felt more depressed when he left than when he came, so he soon stopped going. He did not make use of the Aid-for-the-Blind Program since this would have required a note from his employer and he did not want his employer to know about his failing eyesight lest he lose his job. With his wife's cooperation they organized a personal campaign against his failing vision, agreeing that they would live as though he could see as well as anyone else. Though this plan had some immediate advantages, in the long run it raised more problems than it solved.

During the following years she continued to have hay fever, hypertension, occasional mild headaches, and obesity. The event which precipitated more serious trouble was a simple one but devastating in its meanings. She had become aware that her husband's blindness was increasing, though neither of them spoke about it. One evening he was preparing to write a note and asked her where the ink bottle was. She told him it was on the table directly in front of him. Then, with a terrible sinking feeling within her, she watched his hands groping over the top of the table trying to find it by touch. At that moment the tragedy of his blindness seemed to flood over her and she allowed him to become aware of a tremendous pity for him. This, she felt later, was the worst thing she could have done. It caused him to withdraw into himself and she became aware of a barrier between them.

It was at this time that she first noted a recurring, dull, pressing sensation under the sternum which sometimes radiated up toward the left shoulder. This pain came whenever she exerted herself unduly and disappeared promptly with rest, but it also occurred when she was emotionally upset. Because of this pain, she had to restrict her activities more and more. During the following 2 years, the severity of chest pain increased so that she was unable to keep up with her daily housework.

At the age of 31 a slight intermenstrual bleeding developed, and she went to a clinic to have this evaluated. No cause was found, but her blood pressure on this visit was 230/140. Because of this, she was given an appointment for a medical evaluation. The elevated blood pressure was confirmed, with a higher pressure in the legs than the arms. She had mild hypertensive changes in the eyegrounds, an enlarged heart, a systolic murmur over the entire precordium and electrocardiographic evidences of left ventricular hypertrophy. There was no evidence to support a pheochromocytoma, and urinary function was good. She was referred to the neurologic service to be evaluated for sympathectomy.

The physician who saw her in the neurologic clinic was brusque. He thought she was a good candidate for sympathectomy and advised it strongly, telling her she could not live more than 2 years if she did not have surgery. However, he would not promise her more than 2 years if she did have surgery and, furthermore, told her that it was a major operation which would make her an invalid for several months. The entire discussion threw her into a panic. She was unable to think or speak. He misunderstood her hesitancy and abruptly dismissed surgery with the comment that, since she refused surgery, she would have to "diet or die." She was given a rigid reduction diet with severe restriction of salt intake. She found it most difficult to adhere to this diet.

Her mother suggested she see a chiropractor, and Mrs. Bertrand went to him. He spent a little time manipulating her back but much time discussing her problems with her, and she felt better after these visits. He suggested she set aside 1 day each month on which to eat what she wanted so she could stay on her diet the rest of the month. On this plan, she managed to lose 50 pounds. Though each day of free diet resulted in a 5-pound gain, indulging herself once a month seemed to make the diet tolerable for the rest of the month. She continued seeing the chiropractor for the next 6 months and kept her weight well under control.

Some months after her visit to the neurologic clinic, she was referred to a psychosomatic clinic. The relation established with her physician there seemed to have great sustaining value for her. She was able to discuss her problems freely with him without fear of censure or of making the situation worse. To discuss with her husband the feelings of insecurity aroused by his increasing blindness would only burden him with further worries and might easily widen the gulf which seemed to be developing between them. If this occurred, her own situation would be worse. She needed a third person with whom to talk, one who could help her find some adequate way to meet the difficulties in her life. Her physician fulfilled this need.

This account of the life of Mrs. Bertrand illustrates the close interrelation of the social, psychologic, and physiologic aspects of life. The social and cultural factors at work are perhaps more prominent because of the dramatic contrasts present. Certainly there is little need to point out the importance of racial, religious, and economic forces in her life. The contributions ordinarily made by the family in the development of personality—security, a sense of belonging, warm interpersonal relations—are emphasized by their very lack. The functions of the family in the transmission of cultural ideas and the teaching of social mores were vested almost entirely in the grandmother who taught one system of living in her words and another in her actions.

During her childhood, Mrs. Bertrand was rejected by both of her parents. What little affection she got came from her grandmother, in whom discipline and authority were also vested. She identified herself with the grandmother, though with some ambivalence. When both affection and authority come from the parent of the same sex and the child identifies with that parent, one expects a strong conscience to develop with inability to express aggressive feelings.[7] The predominant conflicts in such a situation should be those of dependence and aggression. This seemed to have been true for Mrs. Bertrand. She was dependent on her grandmother for security in childhood and felt panic-stricken when she had to depend on herself. She had tremendous hostility but found it impossible to express it in any adequate form. Her obesity seemed to have been related to these conflicts, for she stated that she could not curb her craving for sweets when she was overcome by self-pity.

Certainly many other things contributed to her feelings of insecurity. She was not only rejected by her family but also by those who should have been her playmates. She was moved from one household to another in a most arbitrary fashion. Economic security was always tenuous. It was not until adolescence that she found any stable force in life—religion. Her devotion to it lay partly in the emotional security it offered. The attitudes which made life endurable developed from her association with the church. It was interesting that, though the age of 13 seemed a landmark in her life because of her grandmother's total rejection of her, she considered the years which followed to be more pleasant than those preceding. All of the pleasant memories from these years were rooted in the church.

She had another problem to face, for she was born of two distinct cultures and classes. She found herself rejected by both of the groups from which she stemmed. Two solutions were possible. One would have been fight-or-flight, trying to avoid the problem, rebelling against it, or doing both alternately. Mrs. Bertrand instead chose the other way of dealing with the situation—a quiet acceptance of the rejection with no attempt at fighting. This solution came gradually during adolescence and was made possible by her acceptance in her church. In childhood her reaction had been one of rebellion and resentment. But by the time she reached physical maturity, she had accepted the fact that she was not really a part of either group. She developed a superficially pleasant and cheerful exterior which belied intense feelings lying dormant beneath it.

In marriage she was faced with another problem. Though only one-eighth Negro and fair of complexion, Mrs. Bertrand considered herself to be more Negro in origin than white. This was probably because she was raised by her Negro-Indian grandmother in a Negro neighborhood. She might, therefore, have been expected to find a Negro husband. Such a marriage could have been very successful since her fair skin would have given increased prestige; in her marriage she would have found a partial acceptance back into one of the groups from which she came. Her mother had married three times, always to white men. Mrs. Bertrand could have married a white man and tried to relate to the other group from which she came. She did neither and married a man who, like herself, had mixed origins. Though she felt accepted by him, the marriage did not bring her closer to either of her racial origins. It emphasized her marginal position and forced her to find all of her security in one person. The security-giving values of marriage were therefore heightened for her, and the threat arising from hostility or friction in the marriage was increased.

The interrelations are plain enough. But life experiences do not exist apart from behavior and physiology. In discussing physiology, we are not dealing with a totally separate body of data but are viewing the same body of data from a different point of view and therefore picking out a different set of facts as the focus of our attention. The attitudes, emotions, and behavior which arise as a part of life experiences have their physiologic counterparts. These may be the basis for symptoms or for disease when sufficiently intense or prolonged. Mrs. Bertrand's physiologic processes were not studied during the years detailed here, but her symptoms tell us that physiologic changes were associated with the stresses she met. Mrs. Bertrand gained weight when desire for food increased in a setting of feeling unloved and misunderstood. She ate less when she became afraid that excessive eating might lead to death. The relation of these physiologic changes to her psychologic state and of this to the social situation are evident. But this was not the only physiologic relationship made clear by her symptoms.

Many vascular changes were also associated with her life experiences. These will be discussed later in more detail but it should be noted here that migraine headaches, hay fever, and hypertension all involved vascular responses. Vascular headaches are usually a response to stress, associated with vasoconstriction during the stressful period and vasodilatation during the subsequent period of letdown. Vascular and glandular changes occur during hay fever, as well as the neural and muscular reactions necessary to produce sneezing. An allergic factor was suggested by the seasonal nature of her complaint, but it also seemed clear from her story that her response to allergens was heightened by the emotional turmoil of her life. Hypertension also represented a vascular reaction, with peripheral vasoconstriction. One of the factors important in its genesis was probably the threatening nature of her environment, her need to be on guard at all times, and her resentment of discrimination against her because of her mixed origins. Experimental evidence later accumulated demonstrated that threats of this nature in her environment could induce marked elevations of blood pressure. Finally, the angina, which led to so much change in her way of life and was so stressful, was also related to stresses in her life: the stress of exertion on the job or while doing housework and the stress of watching her husband's blindness progress. She found that brooding over any of the problems which threatened her security could lead to an attack of angina.

Her life can be viewed in terms of the racial and cultural problems she faced and their impact on her emotional development and on her health. It can be viewed in terms of her struggle to find social acceptance and economic security and the repercussions of this struggle on her physical being. It can be viewed psychologically in terms of her personality conflicts and continual striving to find emotional security and the development of illness in close association with these strivings. It can be viewed in terms of continuing physiologic adaptations to an unfriendly environment, with progression of these adaptations into irreversible disease processes. A dynamic pattern of interrelations is present here, as in every life. It should be emphasized that it is only the point of view which changes. The facts remain the same; the focus of attention changes. But an understanding of any one facet of the problems offered by this patient is increased by an awareness of the total picture and of the dynamic nature of the interrelations of all the problems.

Chapter 2

Physiologic Mechanisms

Events in people's lives are reflected in physiologic changes. The mechanisms involved in these interrelations are extremely complex and not fully understood. However, much current research should increase our information on this subject. No attempt is made here to present in detail present knowledge of these mechanisms. Rather, a framework within which the information can be viewed meaningfully is presented.

The importance of a subjective evaluation in determining what types of situations will be stressful has been emphasized. This evaluation is complex, involving stressful stimuli on one hand and personal resources on the other. Basically the evaluation concerns relations between a person and his environment. Sometimes the perception of the stressful stimulus, the awareness of the field within which it occurs, the evaluation of its relation to the person, and the decision as to the appropriate response can all be performed momentarily, as when one is crossing a street and sees a car approaching rapidly. This is particularly true when the situation is a familiar one for which there is a large backlog of experience. With unfamiliar situations, considerable scrutiny may be necessary, accompanied, perhaps, by tentative responses which serve to test the situation and help form an appropriate evaluation.

The problem of evaluating one's resources to meet a situation adequately is of equal importance and again may be accomplished without being aware that an evaluation is being made. A situation requiring the expenditure of physical energy would be judged differently by a young athlete than by a middle-aged clerk or a man crippled with arthritis. Each would evaluate it differently if he felt exhausted from prior exertions than if he were rested and ready for action. The evaluation of resources, therefore, requires at least a gross estimate of the amount of energy needed, based largely on previous experiences with similar situations, and an evaluation of the energy available at the moment. This evaluation may be grossly distorted by one's self-concept—whether the stress be physical, intellectual, emotional, or social.

RECEPTIVE AND INTEGRATIVE MECHANISMS

Mrs. Bertrand (p. 26) had had a very unhappy childhood during which she often felt that no one cared for her at all. When her own daughter was born, she was determined from the outset that her child would feel loved and wanted regardless of whether or not she ever had the material comforts of life. During the first 2 years of this child's life, therefore, Mrs. Bertrand devoted herself to meeting the needs of her daughter as she saw them. She was with her constantly. She kept her in the room with her at night so that no cry would go unanswered. The cry of her child was an acute stress to her and required excessive expenditure of physical energy. She was up frequently at night, sometimes all night. At such times, thoughts of her own childhood ran through her head again and again. Thus she relived past stresses; these increased the intensity of current ones. She seemed to remain alert despite physical exhaustion and often had trouble going back to sleep when the opportunity was afforded. Many times she was unable to meet other demands made upon her. She let the housework go and neglected her husband's needs in order to assure herself that her daughter should never feel unloved as she herself had felt as a child. The need to meet this stress adequately was so great that she exhausted herself physically. Maintaining the house became stressful in its turn, but her evaluation of her energy resources for this demand often made her turn aside and leave it undone. That evaluations were being made is plain. This process obviously continued during the night. The street noises of Manhattan did not disturb her sleep; the cry of her child awakened her at once. These evaluations were intensely personal. They involved perception of the cry, an evaluation of it in terms of past experience and present aims, an evaluation of her physical reserves, and translation of this into action. One can question whether these evaluations were "right." They were made, however, and some understanding of the mechanisms involved is helpful to the person interested in psychosomatic correlations.

In recent years, Magoun and his associates[8] have been studying an area of the central nervous system which functions as an alerting center, the reticular activating system. Sensory impulses pass the reticular formation on their way to more central areas, some passing directly into it. Intimate connections exist between this formation and other areas of the brain, and impulses pass in both directions between cortex and subcortical areas and the reticular formation. Connections also exist with the cerebellum.

The reticular formation seems to be of primary importance in arousal and alerting. Arousal occurs before the impulses achieve awareness. Thus a person may be aroused from sleep without knowing what has awakened him. Arousal is not entirely dependent on the intensity of stimuli. Mrs. Bertrand's ability to sleep through the noise of an elevated train but waken to the cry of her child illustrates that an evaluation is involved in arousal.

Stimulation of the reticular formation in animals increases the alertness of the animal so that all degrees of wakefulness can be seen. The scale of alertness passes from deep to light sleep, through drowsiness, relaxed wakefulness, alertness, to intense excitement. The degree of alertness achieved by Mrs. Bertrand as she sat with her child at night seemed to be related to ruminations about her own childhood. This would suggest that cortical connections are important in alerting.

A person may become habituated to sounds of one frequency so that these are not associated with alerting, while other sound frequencies are. Alerting may also be associated with inhibition of sensory impulses. Thus in experiments performed on cats[9] it was demonstrated that sensory impulses evoked by a sound signal were reduced if mice in a jar were shown to the cat. Selective visual attention to the mice apparently altered the auditory impulses reaching the brain. These various observations suggest that past experiences are integrated with sensory stimuli to determine whether alerting occurs and that alerting influences the sensory stimuli which reach the brain to be perceived.

In addition, the reticular formation and the autonomic system are intimately connected. With stimulation of the reticular formation and alerting of the animal, there are changes in respiration and pulse rate as well as in attentiveness. These changes are accompanied by decreased reaction time and increased accuracy of response. The ability of the animal to make fine discriminations seems to be improved.

Perhaps this is significant for human behavior. Certainly it is generally accepted that alertness improves performance. An increased capacity for making fine discriminations and an increased accuracy in response must both be important in determining what an individual learns and how quickly he learns it. Much of learning is a matter of making appropriate discriminations, and the rapidity of learning is markedly affected by success and failure, which are themselves determined by accuracy of response.

The capacity to inhibit passage of neuronal impulses is, of course, essential to human behavior. However, the process by which this might be accomplished has proved difficult to unravel. When Lorente de No[10] described multiple and closed circuits within the internuncial system of neurons, it became possible to construct a model which could explain central inhibition. But this model did not seem entirely adequate to account for many of the facts known about the process of inhibition. In recent years a direct inhibitory pathway has been traced through the nervous system.[11] This pathway includes intermediate neurons which liberate a specific inhibitory substance quite different from the activating substance liberated by other neurons. Thus a mechanism exists by which response may be directly inhibited.

The integrative functions of the nervous system are not localized. On the contrary, they are sufficiently diffuse that destruction of cerebral tissue in widely separated areas of the brain may result in comparable deficit of these functions. The amount of tissue destroyed seems to be more important than the precise location of the damage.[12] Even small lesions may result in deficit of such functions as abstraction, imagery, creativity, and spontaneity. Only with large lesions is there loss of the ability to comprehend social situations. Of particular interest is the observation that the most vulnerable function, the one most frequently impaired even with small cerebral lesions, is the ability to sustain organized behavior during and after situations of failure or frustration.

The reflex arc is often considered the functional unit of the nervous system. Classically, it is diagrammed as a sensory, or receptor, nerve synapsing with a motor, or effector, nerve. Though many internuncial neurons may be interposed between these two, they do not alter the functioning of the two ends of the circuit as a unit. With stimulation of the sensory end of the reflex arc, the motor end responds automatically unless some inhibitory influence is present.

The conditioned reflex is merely a modification of this simple reflex arc. Pavlov[13] demonstrated that if a tone was sounded each time food was presented to a dog, the sound would soon be followed by salivation whether or not food was simultaneously presented. This is a conditioned reflex. The effect of conditioning on human physiology was shown by an experiment in which a bell was sounded coincident with plunging the hand into cold water, as in the cold-pressor test.[14] Eventually, the sound of the bell was associated with vasoconstriction even in the absence of cold water as a stimulus. The intensity of this response was increased by allowing several weeks to intervene between the conditioning experiments and presentation of the sound without the cold water. It was also discovered that vasomotor responses conditioned to verbal stimuli were more lasting than those to nonverbal stimuli. This fact emphasizes the importance of speech in human experience. These experiments also demonstrate the validity of conditioning in humans and the significance of simultaneous events.

Perhaps a similar process is involved in giving rewards for desired behavior. When one is trying to establish a new behavior pattern in animals, this technique is common. In teaching a rat to distinguish white and black boxes in favor of white ones, food may be placed in the white one. After a few random trials, the rat comes to associate white with food and will thenceforth choose the white boxes. The same sort of thing is done in the training of household pets. And, in fact, we do something similar in child rearing, though it is usually done less methodically. With consistent reinforcement, one finds that a habit is readily established, but when reinforcement is omitted the habit is easily lost. With irregular reward systems, the learning is much more stable—it takes longer to extinguish the response when the reward is no longer given. Thus an animal which is irregularly rewarded with food when he chooses the white box will learn much more slowly that the food is not there when it has been removed permanently.

We can illustrate the stability of such a pattern by telling briefly about Mrs. Brown, a patient with frequent vascular headaches usually occurring late in the evening. She described a typical day as one of endless housework although she had a small house and a 16 year old daughter who was well able to assist in the housework. She said she dusted every object in the house every day, washed the dishes immediately after each meal, and picked up anything which was out of place to put it where it belonged immediately. She seemed never to be through with the day-to-day tasks that had to be done. She admitted that the duties tired her and left her feeling exhausted when the day was over, yet she never asked her daughter to help with any of the duties at home nor did she suggest that her husband keep his things in order.

It did not take much discussion with this patient to find out that what she wanted was approval and affection from her husband and her daughter. She got little of this. She felt, in fact, that despite doing everything she could to please her husband she more often irritated than pleased him. Her way of seeking approval was to keep things orderly, always having each thing in its place and at its appointed time.

How had such a pattern developed? She was one of several children and during childhood had obtained little recognition in the family. She was much more conscientious around the house than any of her brothers or sisters and what little praise she received was for these traits. She sought approval from others by being neat and orderly and helping with the housework. In the new situation these traits were not prized. Her husband cared little about having the dishes done immediately after supper each evening or about having his slippers picked up the moment he took them off. He would have liked a more relaxed schedule than she was able to give. She recognized that he did not respond as she wanted but did not realize that what she was really seeking was his approval and affection. Her way of seeking attention had become habitual, and she had not re-examined its value or its aim. She expected people to give approval for such actions, as she approved of herself for being neat and orderly. Though obviously many factors contributed to this situation, one of the important elements in it was the habit of neatness, which, in a setting in which it was never rewarded, could still not be dropped. This is one instance of the force of learning and the difficulty of extinguishing a habit which has been established by an irregular reward system.

Some learning is by association of events, as in the conditioned reflex experiments or in teaching rats to choose white boxes rather than black. Such learning may be completely outside awareness, and much of psychotherapy is helping patients see such associations in their own experience. Making the association often gives the patient a new perspective for understanding his behavior.

Another type of learning is the plodding, prosaic learning by practice and repetition. Skills of all sorts must be learned in this way. There is no difficulty in recognizing the importance of practice in learning some highly skilled physical act, such as playing a piano. One does not learn this simply by gaining insight into the fact that striking a key results in a tone. Social skills must be learned in the same way. If, from repeated experiences in childhood, one has learned poor habits in interpersonal relations, it is not enough to gain insight, to be able to say "This is the way I should act." One must also learn these new habits of communication, both of ideas and emotions, by practicing them under appropriate circumstances. A good deal of the interplay between physician and patient in psychotherapy is reeducation, helping the patient learn by doing.

The meaning of an event is derived not only from past experiences with similar events but also from one's current state. A secretary may warn someone not to approach her boss with a certain question that day because of his irritability. This is a recognition that the state of a person influences his reaction to similar stimuli presented on different occasions. One's response to stimuli is also affected by physical fatigue and degree of alertness. A person who is tired and worn out will not respond to stresses in the same way as one who is rested and ready for action. A person who is ill and weak will not respond to physical or mental stresses with the vigor that he would when feeling well. The awareness of fatigue is built up of many incoming stimuli of which proprioceptive sensations are an important part. Just how stimuli are integrated with past and present experience to determine the final response is still not certain. It is certain, however, that past experience and proprioceptive stimuli are somehow integrated into the perception of sensory stimuli to give these stimuli meaning in relation to the current state of the organism.

An integral part of most stressful situations is an emotional response. This arises within the organism and is integrated into the total experience of external and internal sensory impulses and memories of previous ones. The emotion may arise as a side effect of frustration, but it may also be capable of activation in its own right and powerfully influence the behavior pattern which results. Cannon[4] speaks of the strong emotions of fear and rage as energizing in their effects. They seem to impart a drive to behavior which is absent when they are absent. Not all emotions have this quality, however. Depression is often associated with a decrease in activity and a loss of energy.

The limbic system in the brain seems to be of primary importance in emotional behavior. In emotional states it plays a role similar to that of the reticular formation in arousal and alerting. Stimulation of the limbic system results in frontal lobe activation and in a number of motor and autonomic responses. A common response is inhibition of respiration; gastrointestinal motility and vascular tone also change.[15]

Investigators who implanted electrodes into this area of the brain have reported a variety of emotional responses following electrode stimulation. Delgado and his associates[16] reported a fear-like response which seemed to have all of the drive properties of a true emotion. The reaction could be used to establish conditioned responses; it could be used to motivate trial-and-error learning; and it could serve as punishment. They also found that stimulation in closely related areas could produce aggressive behavior. In their experiments stimulation of this area of the brain in a cat caused it to start fighting immediately with another cat which had been sitting next to it in a friendly way. These investigators were therefore interested in the effects that the limbic system might have on social interaction.

Olds[17] used similar techniques in the same general area of the brain. He found that stimulations of electrodes implanted in closely related areas seemed to have a reward value. He placed mice in a box containing a lever which they could manipulate. With no reward for pressing the lever, the animal might do so 5 to 10 times in an hour. With a small pellet of food as the reward, the rate would rise to 100 times per hour. When electrodes were implanted into the hippocampus and the experiment was arranged so that pressing the bar would stimulate the electrode, the animals would press the bar 500 to more than 5,000 times an hour. If levers were put at either end of the box and the animal permitted only three stimulations from one and then required to go to the opposite end of the box to get more it was found that he would run back and forth in the box pressing the bar at either end to stimulate the implanted electrodes. Mice would run across an electrified grid even when it contained a considerable amount of current. On one occasion a mouse was actually knocked out by the strength of the electric current, but this did not prevent him from trying to cross the grid in order to get stimulation to his hippocampal region by pressing a bar at the opposite end of the box. The reward from electrical stimulation of this area of the brain was sufficient to outweigh the sexual drive, hunger, the need for sleep, or the pain inflicted by an electrified grid.

Brady[18] seemingly produced a conditioned anxiety in animals. When a clicker sounded a sufficient number of times before an electric shock, the animals responded to the clicker by immobility, crouching, and defecation. Brady considered this to indicate that anxiety had been aroused by the clicker in anticipation of the shock which was to come. If these animals had been taught to press a bar to get food as a reward, the clicker interfered with their seeking food, illustrating the effect of anxiety on hunger. Stimulation in the area Olds had reported as a "reward" center caused the anxiety response to disappear completely. It seems clear, therefore, that the limbic system is important to emotional life and related in some way to anxiety and motivation.

The many connecting pathways between these parts of the nervous system give a neural basis for the influence of emotions on thought and the effect of emotions on degree of alertness. Everyday experience demonstrates that a train of thought can evoke an emotional response associated with it and that alertness affects the emotional state. All these aspects of experience are closely interwoven. In some way the activities of these areas of the brain are integrated so that stimuli are perceived and evaluated, and the evaluation has an emotional component.

EFFECTOR MECHANISMS

Neural and humoral mechanisms may alter behavior and physiology associated with evaluations. These mechanisms may be the source of new sensations which may affect evaluation of a situation. They are used in the process of adapting to the environment or meeting its challenges. Symptoms resulting from their use are not evidence of "neurosis" but may appear in anyone under appropriate circumstances.

NEUROMUSCULAR SYSTEM

The neural pathways involved in the neuromuscular system are fairly well known. Through this system a person is able to carry out various physical acts which alter his relation to his environment. Under the impact of violent emotions, amazing feats of physical strength and endurance have been performed. Most such muscular exertion involves alternating contraction and relaxation. Muscles can continue this alternation over long periods without difficulty. With sustained muscular effort, however, fatigue and muscular pains are not uncommon. It should be remembered that a person may be exerting sustained muscular effort without movement. When a movement is desired but inhibited, muscles producing the movement and those opposing it may both be called into play, and no visible movement results. A continuous, sustained contraction giving rise to fresh sensations of fatigue and pain may alter the total situation and thereby alter the evaluation made. A change of behavior may follow, such as relaxing the contracted muscles or going to see a doctor.

These effects are of considerable importance to a physician. In addition to generalized aches and pains they may cause localized muscular spasm accompanied by localized pain. Thus, if the muscles of the back are chronically contracted, a patient may have back pain. When muscular contraction is limited to muscles about the head, a tension headache may result. Similarly, pain in a contracted pectoral muscle may give rise to precordial pain. Abdominal pain may result from spasm of the muscles of the abdominal wall. Pains in the extremities are perhaps the commonest manifestation of muscular tension.

When muscular contractions occur in a person with a disease of the muscles, bones, or joints, symptoms may be intensified and, in some cases, the disease process may be exacerbated. For instance, muscle tension may aggravate rheumatoid arthritis, for antagonistic contractions of muscles impair joint function and result in increased friction within the joint. Efforts directed at muscle relaxation, either by measures applied directly to the muscles or by treatment designed to relieve the emotional conflict which has resulted in antagonistic muscle contraction, may then be an important part of treatment.

Autonomic Nervous System

Another neural and humoral mechanism is the autonomic nervous system. This system has both cortical and subcortical representation. The two divisions of the autonomic system are the sympathetic nervous system, including the adrenal medulla, and the parasympathetic system. Sympathetic stimulation is followed by many changes throughout the body which often, though by no means invariably, are opposite to those seen after parasympathetic stimulation. As a general statement, heart rate and cardiac output are apt to be increased by sympathetic stimulation and decreased by parasympathetic stimulation; coronary vessels tend to be dilated and cutaneous vessels constricted by sympathetic activity, with the reverse occurring under parasympathetic action. Sympathetic activity usually results in bronchial dilatation, decreased gastrointestinal motility, and increased glycogenolysis in the liver; parasympathetic activity may result in bronchial constriction and in an increased gastrointestinal activity and secretion. This antagonism of response is not clear-cut. Sweat glands and vessels in the muscles may react similarly to sympathetic and parasympathetic stimulation. Sympathetic response is further complicated by two humoral mediators which differ particularly in their cardiovascular effects. These are epinephrine and norepinephrine. Though both increase blood pressure, with epinephrine the rise is primarily systolic; norepinephrine affects both systolic and diastolic levels. Whereas epinephrine increases both heart rate and cardiac output, norepinephrine may have no effect or even cause a slight decrease. Epinephrine has little effect on peripheral resistance; norepinephrine increases it markedly. Epinephrine produces a marked rise in blood sugar, norepinephrine a very modest increase.

Activity of either division of the autonomic nervous system may be associated with changes which give rise to new sensations. Thus a person may be aware of a rapid heart rate and may complain of this to the physician. Or he may be aware of flushing or blanching of the skin. These changes may increase the severity of symptoms due to other influences, as in dermatitis. They may likewise heighten the severity of physiologic changes not perceived as a symptom, as when sympathetic activity raises the blood sugar level of a diabetic.

HYPOTHALAMUS

Much interest has been focused upon hypothalamic activity because of its great importance to emotional behavior. With the development of electrode emplacement, which permits studies of intracerebral stimulation in the unanesthetized animal, it has been possible to study the effects of electrical stimulation of this area. French[19] and his associates have reported that stimulation of the hypothalamus may result in peptic ulceration. They showed that hypothalamic stimulation resulted in (1) release of ACTH by the pituitary, giving a delayed increase in gastric hydrochloric acid; (2) vagal stimulation, resulting in immediate increase in gastric hydrochloric acid; and (3) splanchnic stimulation, resulting in increased gastric motility and vasomotor changes. Hypersecretion, hypermotility, and vasodilatation are the pertinent physiologic changes in the production of peptic ulcer, and it is of more than passing interest that stimulation of the hypothalamus produces these changes and eventually leads to ulceration.

These studies also indicate the close relation between the hypothalamus and the autonomic nervous system. Much research is being done in this field. One aspect of this research deserves emphasis here; this is the relation between the sympathetic nervous system, the adrenal medulla, and anger and anxiety. Cannon[4] found little difference in physiologic reactions during anger and fear. He considered both to be associated with the release of adrenalin. It was later found that adrenalin consisted of a mixture of epinephrine and norepinephrine and that the two could be liberated independently. Recently Funkenstein[20] reported that anger directed outward is associated with a physiologic change similar to that produced by norepinephrine and that anger directed inward and anxiety are associated with a physiologic change similar to that produced by epinephrine. The mechanism by which a differential secretion of these two hormones might be mediated is not known.

ENDOCRINE SYSTEM

The secretions of each endocrine organ and their effects could also be listed, since they are mediators of response in the body. The relation of these secretions to emotional stress is not clearly delineated, however. A large body of knowledge has been brought together by Selye,[21] who has studied what he terms "nonspecific" reactions to stressor agents. The stressors studied have been ones which affected the entire body, such as extensive burns, exposure to cold, severe trauma, hemorrhage, anaphylaxis, infection, and irradiation. He has described in some detail a syndrome which occurs in response to all these diverse agents. The pattern of reaction has been divided into three phases: (1) the alarm reaction, (2) the stage of resistance, and (3) the stage of exhaustion. These three form Selye's general adaptation syndrome.

The alarm reaction is the immediate response to intense stressor agents, beginning with a "shock" reaction of hypothermia, hypotension, hypoglycemia, leukopenia, and central nervous system depression. These reactions evoke an outpouring of epinephrine and norepinephrine, ACTH, and adrenocortical hormones, which tend to reverse the changes and may result in hyperthermia, hypertension, hyperglycemia, alkalosis, and diuresis. He has called this the phase of countershock. With repetition of the stress, a stage of resistance develops, in which the organism has increased resistance to this particular stressor but, interestingly enough, shows decreased resistance to other stressors. The changes noted during the phase of countershock disappear; yet, if the stressor has been cold, for example, the animal can be exposed to temperatures which would ordinarily be lethal and survive. The stage of resistance is often of considerable duration but eventually exhaustion occurs, and the animal can no longer adapt to the stressor agent.

It is interesting to note that the same external stressor agent may elicit opposite types of response—may on one occasion be resisted readily and on another cause the animal to succumb, depending upon the past history of the animal. The observation that development of resistance to one type of stressor is associated with a change in reaction to others is a very interesting one. The reaction, therefore, is nonspecific only in that it occurs in response to a wide variety of stimuli. It is specifically related to the animal's previous experience with the same or similar stresses. The specificity of response is also noted in the fact that pneumococci, for example, may elicit the adaptation syndrome when growing in the lung but do not do so when in the pharynx or on the skin. The syndrome seems specifically related to general systemic threats. Here, as with emotional stresses, exposure to a stressful stimulus is given meaning by past experience and the response can be understood only in a broad framework which includes genetic and environmental factors.

The endocrine organs respond to impulses related to emotional states and attitudes aroused by environmental circumstances. The occurrence of pseudocyesis, apparently associated with the wish to be pregnant, is a striking example. Acute rises in protein-bound iodine shortly after stress interviews[22] indicate that thyroid activity is affected by situations perceived as threatening. It is probable that pancreatic secretions are also affected by stressful life situations, particularly in view of the occurrence of hypoglycemic episodes in association with stress.[23] Indeed, all endocrine secretions so far studied have shown a high degree of sensitivity to stressful situations.

HYPERVENTILATION

Hyperventilation deserves special emphasis because of its importance in giving rise to symptoms. As has been noted, stimulation of the limbic system is associated with irregular respirations. Many emotional responses are likewise associated with respiratory alterations. Though the patient is often unaware of the change in breathing, marked changes throughout the body may result. When sighing respirations occur, an excessive amount of carbon dioxide is blown off. This process ultimately results in a state of respiratory alkalosis with effects throughout the body. Many sensations result from this chemical derangement: numbness and tingling of the extremities and about the mouth, nausea, blurring of vision, ringing in the ears, dizziness, weakness, and a strange sense of being remote from the immediate surroundings. Precordial pain may develop, and the electrocardiogram may change. If hyperventilation continues long enough, spasms of the hands and feet (tetany), a feeling of being paralyzed, and actual loss of consciousness may occur. Electroencephalographic alterations may appear, and convulsive seizures may be precipitated. Any of these manifestations may arouse fear; the more dramatic ones ordinarily do. Recognition of the underlying mechanism is essential for both diagnosis and treatment.

EFFECT OF EMOTIONS

The expression of emotions involves all of these mechanisms and therefore can produce a multitude of sensations, any of which may, on occasion, provide a symptom which brings a patient to a physician. Activity of the neuromuscular system results in behavioral changes which are readily observed. Since this system is under voluntary control it is possible to inhibit the behavioral changes or to alter them according to circumstances. They are the least stable but the most readily observed and described. Behaviorists have been most concerned with this aspect of emotion and quite correctly point out its dependence on learning and environment. A hypothetical sequence of events has been described wherein the child learns from his parents and others about him what is meant by the word anger and the appropriate way to express this. From such a learning process may arise many variations in the expression of anger, even to complete inhibition of motor behavior so that a casual observer may be quite unaware that anger is being experienced.

The humoral mediators of anger and fear are chemically closely related. The difference is that of a methyl group. Overt expression of these emotions is dramatic and may be quite violent. They arise in similar types of situations, the difference being, again, one of relationship and degree of threat rather than of kind. Thus a remark made by a brother may arouse anger while the same words said in the same tone of voice by a father may evoke fear. Both emotions prepare the animal for violent activity of the fight-or-flight type. The physiologic changes associated with epinephrine or norepinephrine secretion have this effect whether through the production of hyperglycemia or increased cardiac output. Gellhorn[24] has stated that mild neural stimulation is associated with secretion of norepinephrine; intense stimulation, with epinephrine. This would be consistent with the apparent facts that severe threats evoke fear and that anger appears usually when there is some hope of mastering the situation. This is not incompatible with the fact that either anger or fear may be experienced as a violent emotion.

The proportionate secretion of epinephrine and norepinephrine seems to differ among people. There also seems to be an innate difference in autonomic lability.[25, 26] Such observations form a groundwork for understanding individual variations in the physiologic expression of emotions. Nonetheless, the fact that an epinephrine-like response is commonly associated with anxiety and a norepinephrine-like more commonly with anger gives us a physiologic basis for predicating some basic similarities in these emotions in different people. That individual variation exists does not mean that there are no similarities nor that the situation is chaotic.

In fact, expression of the intense emotions of anger and fear is sufficiently uniform from one person to another and from one time to another to allow the emotion to be recognized by an observer and to allow a fairly reliable description of it to be offered. Darwin[6] draws the following picture of anger: "Under this powerful emotion the action of the heart is much accelerated, or it may be much disturbed. The face reddens, or it becomes purple from the impeded return of the blood, or may turn deadly pale. The respiration is laboured, the chest heaves, and the dilated nostrils quiver. The whole body often trembles. The voice is affected. The teeth are clenched or ground together, and the muscular system is commonly stimulated to violent, almost frantic action. But the gestures of a man in this state usually differ from the purposeless writhings and struggles of one suffering from an agony of pain; for they represent more or less plainly the act of striking or fighting with an enemy."

Anger has been described in association with opposite types of vascular changes, both dilatation and constriction of the peripheral vessels. It has been described with a pressor response or without it, with tachycardia or bradycardia. The difficulties in precise definition of what occurs during anger are partially clarified by Funkenstein's distinction between anger directed outward and anger directed inward against the self. Another differentiation which would seem to be important is the degree and type of control exerted over expression of anger. A person who is controlling anger is more apt to have a vasoconstrictor response than one who is expressing anger freely. Thus someone who reddens with anger may be in a different state than someone else who turns pale with anger.

The vascular responses associated with anger account for the pertinence of this emotion to such clinical states as Raynaud's phenomenon, essential hypertension, angina pectoris, peptic ulcer, and urticaria. Despite the striking differences in these conditions, in all the state of the vessels is of primary importance. A localized vasoconstriction is responsible for Raynaud's phenomenon. A generalized vasoconstriction with an overall increase in peripheral resistance is an important mechanism in essential hypertension. A localized vasoconstriction may precipitate angina pectoris. Dilatation of vessels in the stomach affects the course of peptic ulcer, and vasodilatation is one of the mechanisms responsible for urticaria.

Not only the vascular system participates in the emotion anger. Alterations in other organ systems have not been clearly defined in terms of the direction of anger and the control or lack of it, but anger has been described as associated with gastric hyperfunction, with increased blood flow, increased motility, and increased secretion.[27] Anger is also said to be associated with colonic hyperfunction, including increased motility and vascularity.[28] A decrease in clotting time of the blood[29] and urinary changes, especially increased sodium excretion[30] have been described. Hyperglycemia[31] and intense muscular contraction[32] have been reported. Many organs and systems participate in this emotion.

The physiologic expressions of anxiety are like the changes seen with infusions of epinephrine. These include tachycardia, systolic hypertension, constriction of the vessels of the skin with dilatation of the vessels in muscles, and similar changes. In addition, an anxious person often has irregular respirations, which may become sufficiently severe to produce all of the manifestations of hyperventilation. The overt behavior is usually avoidance, ranging from a readiness or desire for flight to actual running away. Many physiologic changes which accompany stressful life situations have been summarized by H. G. Wolff in his book *Stress and Disease*.[33]

The effects of anger and of anxiety are well illustrated by an experiment in which Mrs. Bertrand (p. 26) was the subject. While she was lying on a ballistocardiographic table, the highly charged topic of sympathectomy was raised and she was asked to recount in detail what had occurred the day this procedure had been advised and "refused." This was an event she recalled vividly and with great resentment toward the physician giving the advice, since she thought he had been unduly brusque and lacking in understanding. As she told about the event, her old feelings were reawakened forcefully. The results of this stress interview are given in Table 1.

During the initial baseline period, while she lay quietly on the table, blood pressure, pulse, stroke volume, cardiac output, and pe-

TABLE 1.—BALLISTOCARDIOGRAPHIC FINDINGS ON MRS. BERTRAND DURING STRESS INTERVIEW

TIME	REMARKS	BLOOD PRESSURE	PULSE	STROKE VOL. cc./min.	CARDIAC OUTPUT L./min.	PERIPHERAL RESISTANCE
10:40	Baseline	192/122	76	70	5.3	46
10:44	Discussion begun	224/154	86	79	6.8	45
10:57	Operation?	250/146	88	71	6.2	57
11:02	"Diet or die"	266/180	86	85	7.3	44
11:05	Tears	262/150	129	92	11.9	28
11:11	Reassurance	222/138	81	68	5.5	51

ripheral resistance were recorded. The discussion was begun with a few comments about hypertension in general and its treatment by sympathectomy, without reference to herself. During these preliminary minutes, her blood pressure rose from 192/122 to 224/154 with slight increases in pulse rate, stroke volume, and cardiac output. Her attention was then focused on her decision against sympathectomy and she was asked to describe the episode in which this decision had been made. She did this, maintaining a factual account with minimal indications of her feelings of resentment. But as she came to the physician's dramatic pronouncement "Diet or die!" her anger at his brusqueness was clearly evidenced. At this time her blood pressure had risen to 266/180 without significant change in pulse rate or stroke volume. This suggests norepinephrine release, since peripheral resistance had risen to 57 as the blood pressure increased. At the peak blood pressure, resistance was 44. At this point she became overwhelmed with thoughts of her illness, the imminence of death, and worries about what would happen to her husband and child when she finally did die. She broke into tears. Her anxiety was expressed in a fall of diastolic pressure to 150 and in a sudden sharp increase in heart rate from 86 to 129, accompanied by a slight increase in stroke volume from 85 to 92 cc., a major increase in cardiac output from 6.8 to 11.9 L./min., and a sharp decrease in peripheral resistance. These changes are consistent with liberation of epinephrine into the circulation. Reassurance promptly turned the abnormal values back toward baseline levels. Less than ten minutes elapsed from the display of resentment at being told to "diet or die" to restabilization following her tears.

Though Mrs. Bertrand had developed a remarkable philosophy of life which allowed her to accept what came with at least a superficial calmness and with compassion and understanding for others, she was by no means immune to racial discrimination. She considered herself to be a Negro and had felt rejected by others for both her Negro and Jewish backgrounds. With the Christmas holidays, extra help was needed at many New York stores. She applied for work as a sales clerk, stating clearly on the form that she was Negro. She was telephoned and asked to appear the following day, since a sales clerk was needed. But when she appeared at the store, they took one look at her application and told her they were very sorry but a mistake had been made. They had no sales position open but they did need someone to help in the stock room. She knew that a sales job was open and felt certain that it was her Negro origin which made the sudden change in attitude. She worked the one day, so angry she was afraid to say anything and was unable to eat any lunch. She did not return to work after this.

Arrangements had been made to perform an experiment the next week. When she came to the laboratory, she sat quietly while a baseline was established. She was relaxed and idly looking at pictures in a magazine. She chanced upon several pages picturing deplorable living conditions among the Negroes. She was obviously upset and the period of stress interview began with a discussion of this problem and racial discrimination. This led promptly to a full account of the day of work, as well as more remote episodes of discrimination affecting herself and her family. She also told with feeling about hearing Georgia's Governor Talmadge discuss the horrors of allowing Negroes to appear on television programs which could be viewed in the South. Feelings of resentment and humiliation were strong during this discussion, though the blood pressure rose only moderately from a baseline of 184/116 to

234/136 during the interview and back to 178/118 subsequently. Urinary excretion showed dramatic variations in sodium output, as shown in Table 2.

Anger and fear are not the only emotional states, of course. Grief and depression are emotions and also have striking physiologic and behavioral manifestations. Maternal and filial love are also emotions,

TABLE 2.—RENAL EXCRETION DURING DISCUSSION OF
RACIAL DISCRIMINATION

PERIOD	REMARKS	VOLUME cc./min.	SODIUM µEq./min.	POTASSIUM µEq./min.	CHLORIDE µEq./min.
1	Baseline	1.9	244	47	163
2	Stress interview	2.3	464	51	260
3	Post-interview	0.9	174	38	89

but neither an exciting nor a depressing effect on bodily processes has been described; they lend a sense of security and contentment. Intense relief following a stressful experience may be described as an emotion. The range of emotions is wide and the physiologic changes associated with them are varied.

SYMPTOM FORMATION

The physiologic processes described do not of themselves constitute symptoms. A symptom is a subjective experience based on a person's evaluation of a sensation or bodily change as representing a deviation from health. Someone who has engaged in hard physical labor and becomes aware of mild muscular soreness is apt to consider the soreness a normal aftermath of hard work and not a symptom of illness or disease. However, if the soreness is still present 2 weeks later with no additional work to account for it, he may very well complain of it as a symptom. If the pain is more intense or more prolonged than he considers appropriate under the circumstances or if he cannot understand it in terms of mechanisms operative in health, the pain (or other bodily change) may become a symptom. Thus symptom formation involves an evaluation as well as a change in physiology or metabolism and is therefore dependent on past experience and on attitudes toward health and illness. As an evaluation it is subject to error, and an actual deviation from health may be considered inconsequential and within the limits of normal or normal patterns of change may be misinterpreted as illness.

Do psychosomatic symptoms arise only as a part of the physiologic patterns of emotional states? A consideration of the functional complaints with which patients present themselves suggests that more than this is involved. Three major relationships exist: (1) emotions may be associated with physiologic changes which, if misinterpreted or if sufficiently intense or prolonged, may be perceived as symptoms; (2) emotions may permit extraneous bodily sensations to be perceived as symptoms; and (3) emotions may lead to behavioral changes which give rise to symptoms.

That symptoms may be associated with the physiologic changes which are a part of an emotional reaction is a commonplace observation. Increased rapidity of the heart is a part of the experience of anxiety but it does not become a symptom until a patient notes its presence and is disturbed by it. Similarly, constipation is a common accompaniment of a simple depression. It is not a symptom, however, until it disturbs the patient who is depressed.

Symptoms may also result from a heightened reactivity to bodily sensations during emotional states. Again using the example of anxiety, it has been shown that people react more to pain when anxious than when tranquil.[34] A slight discomfort which might otherwise go unremarked may then be perceived as distinctly painful. A symptom thus arises that is not related to the usual physiologic pattern of anxiety. Also, a person may find it easier to tolerate anxiety if he can rationalize it in some way. He will therefore look for reasons for the anxiety. If any unusual bodily sensation arises at such a time, he may consider this the reason for anxiety. It becomes a symptom and the patient then seeks the physician's help in removing it, hoping thereby to be rid of the anxiety.

The origin of symptoms through changes in behavioral patterns is illustrated by obesity. It will be recalled that Mrs. Bertrand had an "ungovernable" craving for sweets when she was feeling sorry for herself or lonely. The altered eating habits led to obesity. Though this type of relation between an emotion and the development of a symptom seems quite simple, it involves rather complex readjustments in the mechanisms regulating food intake and the deposition of fat. Another common behavioral change associated with emotions has already been described in hyperventilation. Here the respiratory patterns of behavior are altered, and the symptoms may be marked. Attitudes and goals may lead to intense and prolonged muscular exertion or to considerable muscle tension during quiet activity. In either case, muscular aches and pains may appear and the period of increased activity may be accompanied by or followed by headache. Here again a change in the behavioral patterns is responsible for the development of symptoms.

CLINICAL APPLICATIONS

The associated physiologic changes in emotional states are much more significant than has been indicated by the discussion thus far. Though they are important factors in the development of symptoms in otherwise healthy people, they may become far more serious in people with preexisting illness. At such times these changes may lead to serious disability or threaten life. The effects are then far more dramatic, but they are of the same nature and quality. The case of Fred will help to clarify this.

Fred was 19 when he was first seen in the clinic. He had been born in New York into a lower-class family. His father was an odd-job man and his mother worked as a hostess in a restaurant. He was told that he had been a plump, happy baby. When he was 4, his father deserted the family and did not return for 3 years. During the months following his father's disappearance, Fred changed markedly. He lost weight, became nervous, a facial tic developed, he bit his nails frequently, and developed a peculiar, hopping gait which became so ludicrous and conspicuous that he later forced himself to give it up.

At 6 he started school but did only fairly well because his teachers were "too strict." He had already become a very independent little boy who got up early in the morning and prepared his own breakfast, left home for the day either to go to school or roam the streets according to his desire, and returned home when he felt like it. He was not at all affectionate, he said, and therefore his mother gave all of her affection to his brother, who was 2 years younger.

When Fred was 7, the father returned home briefly, but his stay in the household caused continual arguments. After only a few months, he left again and remained away for another 3 years. On his return, he was promptly inducted into the Army and again was absent from the home. During these years Fred was afraid of his father, though he never knew why. When he was about 14, his father returned from the Army and they became "buddies," drinking together as though they were old Army pals.

The patient entered the Army when 16, in the summer of 1950. During his first few months of Army life, his attitude toward his

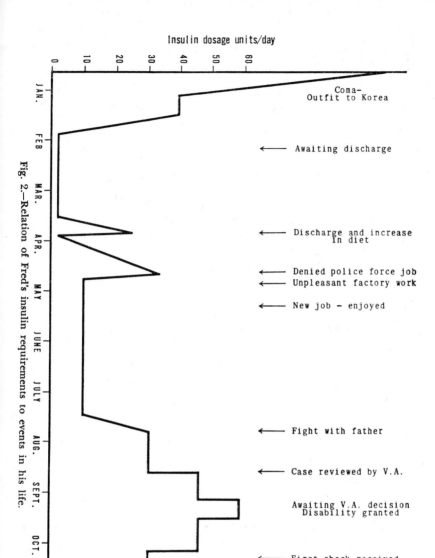

Fig. 2.—Relation of Fred's insulin requirements to events in his life.

Insulin dosage units/day

Coma—
Outfit to Korea

←— Awaiting discharge

←— Discharge and increase
     in diet

←— Denied police force job
←— Unpleasant factory work

←— New job – enjoyed

←— Fight with father

←— Case reviewed by V.A.

Awaiting V.A. decision
Disability granted

←— First check received

father changed. He resented his father's complete irresponsibility and failure to support the family. During the fall months of this year, he began gaining weight, and early in December he noted that his appetite had increased and that he was drinking more water. Despite the increased appetite, he was losing weight. He reported to sick call, complaining also of being easily fatigued; the doctor told him there was nothing wrong with him and sent him back to duty. At about this time, word began to spread through the outfit that they were going to be shipped overseas, probably to Korea.

On Christmas Eve he and some of his friends drank a good deal of beer. The next day he was discovered in coma and was taken to a hospital where a diagnosis of diabetes mellitus was made. He was given 160 units of insulin that day and an equal amount the next. On December 27 his unit left for front line duty in Korea, leaving him behind. His diabetes was regulated on a 1300-calorie diet with 40 units of insulin. This continued through February, and during this time he learned he was to be discharged from the service. With this information he relaxed and his insulin requirement gradually fell so that by the end of March he was taking 5 units of insulin twice a week.

He was discharged about April 1 and returned to civilian life. He began to eat more, since he felt that he had been placed on a starvation diet. With a marked increase of intake, his insulin requirement became 5 units a day. He decided he would like to get on the police force or become a fireman; but he was turned down for both jobs because of diabetes. This aroused considerable insecurity, and his insulin requirement jumped to 25 units a day. He got a factory job and his insulin requirement fell almost immediately. However, he soon intensely disliked the job, since it was heavy physical work and not at all what he was interested in doing. Despite the increase in activity, insulin requirement rose to 35 units a day. He finally decided to quit completely and left the job. He found a new job in which he sat most of the day. This was much more to his liking, and his insulin dosage dropped back to 5 units a day.

During the next few months things went fairly smoothly for him. He spent his weekends making the rounds of night clubs and drinking beer. He sometimes drank 20 or 30 beers in an evening. He often got into two or three fights during such a weekend. But even after a weekend of beer drinking and fighting, his urine sugar never ran more than 2 or 3 plus and reverted to 1 plus, without additional insulin, early in the week.

Things changed abruptly the first of August. While in the service he had saved some of his money and on discharge from the Army had bought a television set for his mother. Early in August his father sold the television set without telling anyone he was going to do so, in order to get money for another drinking spree. Fred was furious, ordered his father to leave the house, and told his mother that he would go if his father did not. His father packed up his things and left. For several weeks after this Fred was very irritable, nervous, and unsociable. He got into fights easily, even with his best friends and over things which he knew were wholly inconsequential. His insulin requirement jumped quite suddenly to 30 units a day.

He then received word that his case was to be reviewed by the Veterans Administration to determine whether he would receive compensation. While waiting for the day of examination to come, he noted increased urine output and a series of 4 plus sugar reactions. On the day of his examination, blood sugar was 488 mg./100 ml., and he had 4 plus glycosuria. Insulin dosage was increased to 45 units a day. During the following 2 weeks he was anxious and nervous, wondering what the outcome would be. Every day on returning home from work, his first gesture was to look in the mailbox to see if a check had arrived. He was increasingly upset that none came. On 45 units a day, he continued to spill sugar and had marked polyuria. Insulin dosage was gradually increased to 60 units a day. Then he received notification that the disability had been granted and he would receive a monthly check. He began having minor insulin reactions and cut the amount back to 45 units a day. Early in October his first check arrived, an accumulative check amounting to 425 dollars. He was delighted, gave some of it to his mother, some to his brother, and spent 200 dollars on new clothes for himself. It was a time of good feelings, relief and relaxation. He again had several insulin reactions and reduced his dosage to 35 units a day. At about this same time he was promoted at work, becoming manager of his department with a small increase in pay. He felt quite at ease with the world, though his friends still commented on his moodiness, which had begun when his father left home and continued, though he was not aware of being disturbed.

The dramatic fluctuations in insulin requirement can be readily understood when we recall that anger and anxiety are associated with the release of norepinephrine and epinephrine. It is known that these agents evoke an outpouring of sugar from the liver, resulting in hyperglycemia. Normally, hyperglycemia calls forth compensatory mechanisms to keep the fluctuations within broadly physiologic limits. In the diabetic, these compensatory mechanisms may not be available. In addition to the effect on glucose, anxiety and anger have been shown also to be associated with polyuria and a loss of fixed base in the urine, quite apart from whether sugar is excreted or not.[30] The loss of fixed base and of water result in dehydration and acidosis. The combination of all of these factors can lead to diabetic coma and, if untreated, to death.

With easing of the stresses in Fred's life, the circulating blood sugar fell and the insulin dosage had to be decreased to avoid severe reactions. Thus the decreasing insulin requirement was as expressive of the importance of emotional states to the health of the diabetic as was the increasing requirement under stress. The diabetic, particularly the labile diabetic, graphically illustrates the potential seriousness of the physiologic changes associated with emotions when disease interferes with the compensatory mechanisms of the body.

Similar examples can be given for many other diseases. Rheumatoid arthritis may be reactivated, intensified, or greatly prolonged by emotional reactions. Controlled anger is one of the most adverse emotional states for arthritic patients. The vasodilatation associated with anger may cause increased redness, heat and exudation into the joint. The effort to control anger is associated with muscle tension. Many of these patients are restless, and muscle tension leads to mechanical disadvantage, with increased friction and increased wear and tear at the joint. All these changes tend to increase the disability.

The importance of the physiologic changes which accompany emotional states to disease processes can be stated fairly simply. When the changes accentuate a lesion already present or are altered in the direction of a disease process, they aggravate the illness and may endanger life. The opposite statement is also true. When the direction of physiologic changes is opposite to the changes accompanying the disease process, they may help to ameliorate the condition.

In these pages on physiologic mechanisms, only the broad outlines have been sketched in. But even the broad outlines indicate the importance of these mechanisms to health and disease. Many of the details are still not known, but a knowledge of physiologic mechanisms can increase our understanding of patients and their symptoms. Increased understanding affords a firm and rational basis for treatment.

Chapter 3

Mental Mechanisms

A<small>N</small> understanding of mental mechanisms is as important to a clear comprehension of physical symptoms as is an understanding of physiologic mechanisms. When physiologic changes are intense or prolonged or are not comprehended as being related to stress, they become sources of anxiety and cause the person to seek help for them. In this process the intensification and prolongation of the physiologic changes and the inability to see the relation to stressful circumstances are closely related to mental mechanisms. To understand symptoms arising in response to stress, one must understand these mental mechanisms and their associated changes in physiology.

The common mental mechanisms are listed variously by different writers. A useful list for our purposes is: gratification, suppression or inhibition, avoidance, displacement (including sublimation), reaction-formation, denial and repression, and identification. These mechanisms are the chief ways people deal with the stresses in life. They are not abnormal. They are used by everyone. Some people make use of many of them, suiting the defense used to the circumstances. Others early in life select one or two as most suitable and come to use them habitually, whether appropriate to the situation or not. It would seem obvious that a person with numerous defensive maneuvers at his command would be more adaptable and better able to meet life stresses than one who limits himself to one or two. The person with many resources, when confronted with a situation which cannot be solved by the first defense he uses, turns from one mechanism to another until a solution is discovered. The person with a single defense at his command, when confronted with a situation which does not resolve by the use of that mechanism, finds the situation intolerable, feels trapped in it, and may become ill as a result. It is beneficial, therefore, to have more than one mechanism to meet stresses, though a few people who rigidly use the same mechanism over and over again may find that this works satisfactorily.

Mental mechanisms are usually discussed in psychology courses or introductory psychiatric lectures as though they existed apart from body physiology. Their relevance to the psychic life of the individual is usually explored, sometimes quite thoroughly.[35, 36] Their possible origin in central nervous system chemistry and physiology is sometimes commented upon.[37] Their pertinence to physical health and disease is usually ignored. Yet a constant awareness of them as you talk to patients can speed your formulation of what is going on within the patient and contribute significantly to an understanding of human behavior in health or illness.

GRATIFICATION

Simple gratification is considered to be the "normal" way of meeting stressful circumstances. When a man is hungry, it is expected that he will eat. This is goal-directed behavior expressed in an obvious way. When a man is angry the normal response is attack. Viewing the man in isolation and considering only the fact that he is angered by the situation in which he finds himself, the response of attack is goal directed and normal. But no one is completely isolated, and direct gratification is often not a socially desirable solution to a problem. In fact, gratification on occasion may indicate serious emotional problems. This must be remembered not only in getting the patient's history but in therapy as well.

Marian Hays was a single woman 33 years old who came to the clinic because of uncontrollable attacks of rage. Studies were done to determine whether or not the rage attacks from which she suffered were a manifestation of premenstrual tension. As a part of a diagnostic and research study, she was asked to collect urine specimens at regular intervals throughout the day over a period of several weeks while she was going about her regular activities. Though the studies showed no relation between the attacks of anger and her menses, they did reveal some very interesting information.

Early in the course of the study she invited a friend, Ken, to her apartment one evening. He brought along a friend of his named Bill. Bill worked in the same office with Marian, but they had not become well acquainted there. The two men got into a philosophic discussion of the meanings of medieval art. Marian had no interest whatever in medieval art and was bored by the conversation. She asked them to discuss something of more interest to her. However, they were deeply engrossed in their own thoughts and continued to discuss the meaning of art. She became furious with them and, after a heated argument, threw them out of her apartment and followed them angrily down the stairway, kicking at them to get them out faster. At the bottom of the stairway she found the landlord waiting to see what all the commotion was about. He complained that she was creating an undue disturbance, so she kicked him in the shins as well and returned to her room. A day or two later she returned to the clinic, and during the course of her interview the entire episode was recounted with renewed expressions of anger as well as with a certain amount of anxiety lest the physician to whom she was talking reprimand her for her loss of control. About 10 days after this, she had to see the landlord to pay her rent. This was the first occasion on which she had seen him since kicking him the night of the argument, and she was quite depressed, feeling that she had been "a bad girl" and wondering whether he would mention the occasion to her.

Renal excretion rates on these three occasions were of considerable interest. During the evening of her fight with the two young men and her landlord excretion of water and sodium was slightly above her average evening rates. The difference was not particularly striking, however. Either the excretory changes associated with this outburst of anger were too brief to make a significant change in the five-hour excretion rate, which the specimen represented, or the free expression of anger was not associated with marked changes in renal excretion. From other data, it would seem more likely that it was the brevity of the episode rather than a lack of change which accounted for the almost normal excretion rates. However, during her interview concerning the argument, excretion rates were considerably higher than the average afternoon excretion rates during the rest of the study. Volume, sodium, potassium, and chloride were all increased. Both anger and anxiety were aroused during this interview, and these feelings were maintained for the greater part of an hour while the episode was being discussed. On the third occasion, when she was feeling depressed at her actions and wondering how her landlord would view the entire episode, the excretion rates for water, sodium, potassium, and chloride were all well below average for afternoon specimens during the remainder of the study.

Here, then, we have an episode of anger which caused less disturbance in renal excretion during the actual period of anger than during an interview wherein the anger was reawakened and anxiety aroused because she was discussing it with a physician whose opinion she valued. We also have an episode wherein subsequent consideration of it, in the light of an anticipated visit to her landlord, resulted in decreased urinary excretion rates, quite the opposite of changes associated with the original episode or the discussion of it. It should be noted that in the first two episodes anger was turned outward toward the people about her, whereas in the third episode she felt depressed.

These data suggest that, though direct gratification of a desire may

TABLE 3.—SUCCESSIVE REACTIONS (RENAL EXCRETION) TO A SINGLE EPISODE

SITUATION	VOLUME cc./min.	SODIUM μ Eq./min.	POTASSIUM μ Eq./min.	CHLORIDE μ Eq./min.
Average excretion rates, evening	1.41	86	26	88
Fight with friends, evening	1.83	122	28	154
Average excretion rates, afternoon	1.44	106	34	119
Interview with physician, afternoon	2.26	175	56	215
Visit to landlord, afternoon	0.66	79	16	76

result in less intense and prolonged physiologic changes, it does so only if there is no subsequent brooding over the episode. Reconsidering events in discussing them with other people is associated with physiologic changes, and feelings of guilt at having gratified one's desire are also associated with physiologic changes, though these may differ from those during the original episode. Physiologic processes of the body, therefore, are not only affected by the events which arouse strong emotions but by anything which reawakens these feelings.

In the episode described, one could consider the outburst of anger as a direct gratification of emotions and a desire to attack. Gratification, however, was probably a defensive maneuver to prevent Marian from becoming aware of the anxiety she felt at being rejected, even in so mild a fashion as by having two friends continue to discuss a subject after she had asked them to stop. "It is more bearable to be hated for what one *does* than for what one *is*," it has been said.[38] Her reaction may be an expression of such a feeling.

SUPPRESSION

Direct and immediate gratification is often undesirable for personal reasons, quite apart from any social acceptance or disapproval. In the process of maturing, one is expected to learn to accept a certain number of frustrations in the course of attaining long-term goals. If every frustration resulted in a temper tantrum, the long-term goals would never be attained. In addition to social and cultural pressures which discourage frequent or violent expressions of anger when immediate gratification is denied, goals and aims may temper actions and result in giving up immediate gratification in the interests of some future goal.

A mechanism which may be used when gratification seems undesirable is suppression, or inhibition. With suppression, there is frequently a partial gratification. For example, a person who feels anger may not express the anger directly and openly, yet suppresses it only partially so that the person who has aroused the anger is very much aware that he is sulking or pouting even though the anger has been expressed in a less overt form. However, under other circumstances, suppression or inhibition may work so well that people around the person concerned are quite unaware that any emotion whatever has been evoked.

The importance of suppression and inhibition to physiology and symptom formation is that they prolong the emotional reaction and the physiologic changes accompanying it. For example, the day after Marian had kicked Ken and Bill out of her apartment in a fit of rage, Bill seemed a little distant, but they had never been very friendly so she was not sure what this meant. He seemed to be very busy at his work. She spent the morning at her own work, but periodically tried to decide whether he was really preoccupied with what he was doing or was trying to ignore her. She was rather tense during the morning, while trying to evaluate the situation, and her excretion rates were lower than her average morning rates. This is illustrated in Table 4.

TABLE 4.—Repercussions (Renal Excretion) of Fight
with Friends and Landlord

Situation	Volume cc./min.	Sodium μ Eq./min.	Potassium μ Eq./min.	Chloride μ Eq./min.
Average excretion rates, morning	1.56	134	47	161
Bill "distant", morning	1.00	74	33	170
Rejected by Bill, morning	2.56	311	56	299
Average excretion rates, afternoon	1.44	106	34	119
Brooding over Bill's rejection of her	2.53	156	49	185

On the following morning, however, she became quite certain that Bill was really avoiding her. She decided that the best way to find out was to put it to a test; so she asked him if he would have coffee with her during the morning coffee break. He refused rather coldly. She was furious at him for refusing but turned on her heel and went off to coffee with other girls in the office without making any comment to him. In this case, she suppressed her anger and desire to react with bodily violence, but the anger bubbled up inside of her for the rest of the morning. It will be noted that excretion rates for this morning were several times as great as on the previous morning. Nor did this stop at lunch time. She continued to brood over this affair all afternoon, feeling angry and humiliated by his refusal to have coffee with her in the morning. And it will be noted in Table 4 that excretion rates during the afternoon remained significantly elevated, the volume being higher than it was when she had the fight with the young men or when she discussed it with her physician. Thus it is seen that suppressing the overt action and brooding over the event prolonged the physiologic changes so that they continued to exist throughout the entire day at work rather than being over briefly with an initial expression of anger.

From the discussion of the importance of controlling mechanisms in arousing feelings of tension, you would expect inhibition or suppression to be associated with tension. This is commonly but not necessarily true. Thus, when Marian discovered Bill was openly rejecting her, she inhibited any overt expression of her anger but removed herself immediately from the situation in which expression of anger would be pertinent. Thereafter her anger as such represented no threat to her and required little or no control. She could allow it to bubble up inside of herself freely, reliving repeatedly in the succeeding hours the actions she would have liked to take to express her anger. Little tension was present at this time, if we can judge from her statements about her feelings or the physiologic data. Tension may have been present at the moment during which the outburst of anger was inhibited. It did not last long enough to be recognized as such or to be evident in the data collected.

Many systems of the body respond during periods of this sort when anger is experienced freely but inhibited from adequate physical expression. A young patient who suffered from periodic attacks of urticaria had worked on the night shift in a bakery for a number of years without difficulty. In discussing with him the circumstances under which the urticaria appeared it was discovered that he had been working under a new supervisor for a few months and that the episodes of urticaria occurred 15-45 minutes after a visit by this man. He was on the night shift and the job was not supervised closely. However, when the supervisor came he was almost invariably critical and accepted no arguments or explanations. The patient accepted these criticisms with no strong feelings of anger at the time. However, after the supervisor left he was quite resentful though in no position to do anything about it. This is the attitude Grace and Graham[5] considered pertinent to urticaria. In this instance tension was aroused to control the anger while the supervisor was criticizing him. This was recognized by the patient. Only when control was no longer being exercised did urticaria appear. To judge from other observations on peripheral vascular responses, it would appear that feelings of tension are commonly associated with vasoconstriction. After tension subsides vasodilatation occurs and urticaria may then develop.

One might well ask: Is anger inhibited or gratified when it is allowed free expression within the person but is not expressed in behavior? It would seem to be both simultaneously—a partial gratification and a partial inhibition. Certainly in this way the original anger may be fairly well dissipated over the course of hours or days, though with some people it may not finally subside for weeks or months. The important point in terms of the development of symptoms is that this state of partial gratification is associated with the physiologic concomitants of the emotion as long as it continues. Partial inhibition is therefore a potent force in prolonging physiologic changes. It may even intensify these changes while the person ruminates over all the related episodes in the past, each new thought arousing fresh anger. At such times symptoms are apt to develop.

The importance of inhibition and the tension which may on occasion be engendered in the process of inhibiting expression of anger is perhaps most clearly seen in the voluntary muscle system. A 42 year old legal secretary was troubled with generalized muscular aches and pains which prevented her from standing for more than a few minutes or walking more than a half a block. The symptoms had been present for 20 years, getting steadily worse. She had been thoroughly studied by numerous physicians and in several special clinics. No disease had ever been discovered and it was the general opinion that her aches and pains were related to muscle tension. Her complaints were so disabling that she took a taxi from her home three blocks to the subway and from the other end of the subway two blocks to her place of work. She took her lunch with her regularly since she found it too tiring to walk the half block from her office building to the nearest restaurant.

This patient had many emotional problems, some of them very severe. But the problems pertinent to her physical complaint concerned her job as a secretary. She had worked throughout these 20 years for a lawyer whom she considered crude and blustering, if not actually vicious. She was constantly irritated by his manner of speech and by his demands upon her. In 10 years she had received no raise in pay though every other secretary in the office had been given a raise during that time. She hated her boss and said so openly. She could scarcely bear to have him speak to her or ask her to do something for him. She said that when he did speak, she had a great desire to "hit him over the head with my notebook." Despite this she had been unable to leave his employ for fear that she could not get another job. She felt so inadequate that she was sure no one else would hire her. There were many other reasons why she did not leave his employ, but it is sufficient to note that the forces keeping her at her job were stronger than her dislike of her boss and her desire to get away from him. The symptoms from which she suffered could be understood in terms of her need to control her impulse to strike him or to run away. And this, of course, was also the key to treatment. To formulate this patient's problems entirely in terms of hostile impulses would be to miss the core of her personality problem. It seemed plain that most of her symptoms were associated with rigid control. The need for control was occasioned by the constant rearousal of anger and the need to be on guard against expressing it lest she lose her job. This emphasizes the importance of the controlling forces in symptomatology, though it should be equally evident that the exercise of control implies something that needs to be controlled.

The illustrations given have all dealt with control of anger. This is a very common phenomenon, since our society puts many restrictions upon the expression of anger and some religions denounce it in any form. Strict adherents to these sects wish to have no such feelings and certainly discourage any expression of them. Anger is not the only emotion which may arouse efforts of control. Almost any emotion may, on occasion, require suppression or inhibition.

An example of this, unrecognized by the physician handling the patient, was Mrs. Bertrand's intense anxiety when she was advised to have a sympathectomy. Her efforts to control her anxiety prevented free communication with her physician. The pertinence of these efforts at control to her subsequent course is indicated by her reaction to telling about them in an interview during which the physiologic responses were being recorded (Table 1, p. 52). In this phenomenon, we may have an indication of the value of expressive therapy. Expression allows at least a partial gratification of the feelings which have demanded control. Observations such as these also suggest that control itself plays some part in physiologic patterns.

Another of the patients mentioned was seen when feelings of depression and guilt needed control. Fred (p. 56) visited his physician one day in a state of agitation and was obviously depressed and self-accusatory. He had fallen in love with a model who for 4 years had been "going steady" with one of his friends. A week before this interview, the model had broken off her engagement to his friend, who had come to Fred to tell his troubles, not knowing who the "other fellow" was. Fred was unable to tell him that he was responsible for the broken engagement but felt intensely guilty and unworthy. He was uncertain of his ability to keep the model's affection. During the discussion of these events, he sighed occasionally and seemed ill at ease in talking. As the discussion became more uncomfortable, tears came to his eyes. At this point he tried to dismiss the entire subject, saying repeatedly that it didn't really make any difference to him at all. The denials were an attempt to control the feeling state, since he obviously cared a great deal. His feelings of guilt, a form of anxiety, and his feelings of depression at being unworthy both of his friend and the model were the emotions which seemed to be overpowering him, and his efforts were directed at inhibiting their free expression.

AVOIDANCE

When the cues in a situation suggest danger ahead, a person may detour or turn back. Many people develop this to a fine point, avoiding facing one problem after another. This is not necessarily an unsuccessful or pathologic mechanism. The child who does not learn to avoid touching a hot stove is seriously handicapped. The child who cannot see that he is arousing anger or disapproval in his parents by some action he is about to take is not going to become adequately socialized. Skillful avoidance of stressful situations may prevent intense or prolonged physiologic changes. Insofar as it succeeds, it is a useful mechanism.

Avoidance becomes a hazard when it is the only mechanism a person has at his command to handle problems he must face. If he then meets a problem he cannot avoid, he is not equipped to cope with it.

There is no solution available, since he has learned no other way to handle problems. He then feels trapped.

Avoidance may be associated with symptoms even when it is successful. Mr. Grant, a young man of about 30, went to his physician because of recurring episodes of abdominal pain. The characteristics of the pain suggested that it was related primarily to spasm of the abdominal muscles. The pain was never severe but was sufficient to prevent him from continuing whatever work he was doing at the time. He had gone from one job to another, usually getting along well during the first week or two. Between the third and sixth week on each job, he began to have attacks of abdominal pain and eventually quit work and sought employment elsewhere. He blamed most of the attacks on the work he was doing.

This patient had been raised in a household in which marital discord was almost constant. His parents argued on almost every subject. At one stage in his life he had reacted to this with intense anger and tried to stop their fighting by arguing with them. This had no effect except to make a good deal of trouble for him. Later in his life he burst into tears whenever his parents fought. They both expressed contempt and anger for his tears but continued their arguments. Nothing he did seemed to affect the arguing. He then tried to avoid listening to them, leaving the house, if necessary, whenever they began to argue. When 12 years old he decided to leave home permanently to get away from their constant fighting. He went to live with an aunt and uncle. His career following this was a succession of disagreeable situations which he tried to solve by leaving them. He became increasingly sensitive to arguments and bickering among other people. He turned away from any group when hostility began to be expressed. He was particularly sensitive to criticism from his superiors; this, it turned out, was the precipitating factor in most attacks of abdominal pain which he could remember in detail. He got along well on the job until the boss tried to tell him a different way to do something or criticized his work. At such times, abdominal pain appeared and became so disabling that he would have to seek another job.

With this patient, avoidance was the only mechanism which had proved satisfactory in handling the problem of parental arguments. Applied to difficulties arising at work, it could only result in a poor work record and increasing trouble finding work. He had to make a living in some way and was ultimately forced to face the fact that something was wrong with his way of meeting problems. He did not understand the mechanism he was using to solve problems nor why it failed, but there was no question in his mind about the poor work record and the fact that he had trouble finding jobs because of his many changes in occupation. He blamed this on recurrent abdominal pain and sought medical assistance for it. Yet he had enough insight into the relation between emotions and symptoms to be able to accept the possibility that his abdominal pain might be related to his adaptation to life and to be willing to consider this as part of his treatment.

The similarity between this patient and Brady's rats (p. 43) is rather striking. The rats had a conditioned anxiety to the clicker even when no shock followed. This patient reacted to critical remarks or a rising inflection in the voice as the rats did to the clicker. It was a warning signal of a painful argument to follow. Instead of reacting to this with crouching and defecation, as the rats did, he reacted with abdominal muscle spasm (crouching?) and pain. He also reacted with avoidant behavior, which would remove him from any possibility of witnessing or being a part of a painful argument. If this were entirely on the basis of a conditioned reflex, he would not necessarily have been aware of the stimulus to which he was reacting or its meaning to him. He was aware of this, however, and this made an understanding of his problem much easier for his physician.

Avoidance, though it may work in many situations and is a normal and desirable way to handle some problems, may contribute to the development of symptoms and illness. When this mechanism fails and the patient is unaware of his problem, it is frequently very difficult to get him to see what the trouble is. Even then, avoiding trouble before it arises is so obviously the right and logical way to go through life that changing to other mechanisms may be difficult indeed.

DISPLACEMENT

When a person can neither avoid stressful situations nor control the emotions aroused by them and will not permit direct gratification, another mechanism, displacement, is available. At such times the aim or object of the drive is changed but a discharge of the force present is permitted. The person who controls his anger toward his spouse but takes it out on the children or some family pet is displacing his anger. Thus scapegoats, whether cultural or personal, allow gratification of a drive which might not otherwise find socially acceptable expression.

Displacement can be a successful and desirable mechanism. When anger has been aroused in an argument with a friend or relative, it may be to everyone's advantage for this to be controlled temporarily. By allowing subsequent expression of anger by hammering angrily at a loose shingle on the roof or digging vigorously in the garden the anger may be fairly rapidly dissipated so that it does not get in the way of social relationships.

The importance of this mechanism to psychosomatic medicine lies not in the change in direction as such but in a by-product which is by no means inherent in displacement. People often utilize displacement as a habit without being aware of the origins of the feelings aroused or of the aims actually being pursued. At such times there is no way for them to check their actions or to ascertain that direct gratification might not actually be better. There is no way to guide actions by logic and common sense. At such times, displacement as a mechanism may solve no problem and may, on the contrary, contribute to illness.

The word "sublimation" is usually used to describe a type of displacement, though it is also used by some authors as a general term to describe any mechanism which is successful in allowing discharge of a drive.[36] When we try to categorize specific situations and responses, however, the matter of success may sometimes be difficult to determine with certainty. Freud, in *A General Introduction to Psychoanalysis*,[39] defined sublimation as the abandonment of direct gratification of an instinctual impulse and the adoption of a new aim which appears social, not instinctual, in nature. We will use this definition without any implication as to success, though Freud may have implied success when he added that the process served as a protection against illness.

Sublimation, despite its socially acceptable quality and its frequent description as a successful mechanism, can be the source of illness and of incapacity. Mrs. Brown (p. 40), the patient with frequent vascular headaches exemplified this well. She worked endlessly keeping her house in order and received no word of praise for doing so. The relation of this behavior pattern to an irregular reward system in her childhood has been discussed. The same behavior pattern, however, also represents sublimation. As a child she had had little affection from her parents except for being neat and orderly. In a large family, these traits became her own special "talents" for which she received approval. The basic need to be loved became sublimated into "doing for others," a socially approved way of asking for love and affection. This sublimation was successful through childhood and adolescence and became a way of life for her. After marriage it no longer brought the rewards which she had come to expect. The first failures resulted in redoubled efforts. The lack of thanks for this increased her intensive work about the house. This was her way of receiving affection and the only way she knew was to work harder and harder until somebody expressed approval for it. But the effort came to outweigh the compensation received and she became resentful of those for whom she did so much and from whom she got so little. This intensified her need for control; for now she needed not only to control her behavior in doing as much work as possible but to control her feeling of anger so that she would not express it to people from whom she wanted affection and approval. The effort and control must have been associated with vasoconstriction, if our understanding of the mechanism of vascular headache is correct; and in the evenings, when she was able to relax, the period of relaxation was accompanied by vasodilatation and vascular headaches.

In this example, the behavior pattern described arose as a socially acceptable displacement of the original drive. It was instinctual in origin and social in expression and was, therefore, sublimation. It became a part of her personality and a habitual way for her to handle certain kinds of situations. However, its basic origins and aims were lost to her. It had simply become the "right" way to do things. Consequently, when faced with a situation in which it no longer was successful in gratifying the needs from which it sprang, it continued to be used blindly but with mounting feelings of frustration. She was not able to examine what was happening in a logical manner though aware of her lack of satisfaction. She needed help in understanding what she was really striving to attain and help in finding more suitable means by which to do this.

Displacement from one person to another may be quite obvious, as when a woman angry at her husband spends the next few hours criticizing her children for their every act. It can easily be missed, however, if one is unaware of the original source of friction. Yet its recognition is crucial to an understanding of the person and it is essential before intelligent therapeutic help can be proffered.

A case in point was Charles, a 19 year old boy with ulcerative colitis. He came to the hospital complaining bitterly about his stepfather and correlating his exacerbations of colitis closely with episodes of anger toward him. He ordinarily worked in the house with his mother, not in the fields with his stepfather as did the other children. Diarrhea developed whenever he was angry at his stepfather, consequently colitis was worse whenever he tried to work with him. It would therefore seem appropriate to investigate this relationship closely to find out the sources of the anger, but whenever Charles was questioned for specific instances he had to admit that nothing had happened to justify anger of the intensity he felt. His stepfather was, in fact, an understanding person who made few demands on his stepchildren.

Charles's father had deserted the family when the patient was 2 months old. He had no recollection of his father and little knowledge about him. He and his mother lived together until she remarried when the patient was 2 years old. She married a man who was 48 years older than she and the marriage was for financial security only. The patient remained her favorite despite the birth of three other children; in fact, he was favored over the stepfather. The marriage was a very unhappy one with much marital discord. When the patient was 6 years old, his stepfather died. For a year he was the undisputed favorite in the family, with no rivals for the mother's affection.

When he was 7 years old, his mother married a third time. This time she was very much in love with the man she married, a chiropractor who had left his occupation to become a farmer. The boy's colitis began during his mother's honeymoon, on which, interestingly enough, he accompanied her. Following this marriage the mother was less affectionate to Charles, who thenceforth had a secondary position in the family. At the time of the marriage he liked his second stepfather very much; but he soon changed his mind, though he could never say exactly why.

This story suggests that the patient had a very strong attachment to his mother and was unable to tolerate being second in her love. The anger he felt toward her for not loving him more than others was apparently displaced to his stepfather. There are a number of important things to be noted in this story. First of all, though he felt a great deal of anger and hostility, its expression toward his stepfather was only an apparent gratification. Actually he was angry at his mother. He could express anger toward his stepfather indefinitely without getting any relief whatever and without solving the basic problem. Another point to be noted is that the symptoms arose in relation to this displaced object, since the patient had an exacerbation of colitis whenever he worked with his stepfather and whenever he was angry at him. The fact of displacement obscured the basic problem. It obscured it effectively from the patient himself and from people who were trying to treat him. The displacement prevented the patient from facing his real difficulty. It was also responsible for prolonging physiologic changes since it gave rise to more frequent feelings of anger. Thus displacement obscured the basic problem, prolonged the difficulty, and prevented an adequate discharge of the emotions aroused.

Emotional discharges of this sort can also be displaced upon oneself. Mr. Miller, a 40 year old man with neurodermatitis, illustrated this quite well. He had considerable conflict around his ability to handle a masculine role in the world and a good deal of conflict in trying to handle his hostility toward other people. He was married to a very domineering woman who wanted to run the household. His troubles began after the birth of their first child. At this time the wife was very occupied in taking care of the new baby and it fell to him to do the laundry, including washing the diapers, cook the meals, wash the dishes, and keep the house clean. This intensified his conflict about masculinity, and aroused a great deal of hostility toward his wife. However, this hostility was not directed toward her, but toward himself. While berating himself for what was happening, neurodermatitis developed.

The physician who undertook to treat this patient started out impersonally and rather coldly without establishing a favorable doctor-patient relationship first. He saw that the patient's problem was one of unexpressed hostility and his early attempts were to arouse hostility in their relationship in the hope that they could work it out on this level. Since the patient characteristically handled hostility by displacing it upon himself, it was not surprising that he did so in this situation. The hostility was certainly aroused; but the patient did not direct it at the doctor, he directed it at himself, becoming extremely depressed and feeling that he was a "bad" person for being angry at someone who was trying to help him. Neurodermatitis became unmanageable and the patient made an abortive suicide attempt. A change in therapy, whereby a good doctor-patient relationship was established before working with the problems, resulted in a successful outcome for the patient.

One can also displace gratification from one drive or instinct to another. Mrs. Bertrand clearly displaced a desire for affection to the hunger drive. What was basically wanted was companionship, love, and affection. Not receiving this, she gave herself gratification in another sphere to compensate for the loss in this one.

It is evident that displacement may manifest itself in many ways. It may be seen as an inhibition of response in one setting with discharge later in a more neutral situation. It may involve displacement of emotional discharge from one person to another, from another person to oneself, or from oneself to someone else. An instinctual drive may be displaced in some socially acceptable activity. And energy may be displaced from one drive to another. Displacement is a common mechanism which can have beneficial results or be disastrous depending on the circumstances and the way in which the displacement is handled. Accordingly it may contribute to the health and maturity of the individual or be a factor in producing or prolonging illness.

DENIAL AND REPRESSION

Another mechanism by which people try to handle stressful situations, one of great importance to both physical and mental health, is denial. It is not an unusual way of meeting the unpleasantness of life. The child or adolescent who finds his life unsatisfying and constructs a world of fantasy in which he has new parents, unlimited wealth, or capacities beyond what is human, is, in part, denying the realities with which he is faced. Fred, who almost in tears kept repeating "It makes no difference to me," was trying to deny his feelings in an attempt to control them. Because of his lack of success the mechanism used was obvious. Had he been more successful he might have convinced himself and his physician that his problem really was of no consequence to himself. Mr. Grant could in all sincerity deny that he had difficulties with interpersonal relations because he avoided difficult situations with other people before they reached a stage at which his feelings could no longer be denied.

Denial is also related to a mechanism called "undoing." This is seen in the person who, having performed some act or said something potentially harmful, proceeds to deny the act or word or to perform some ritual to render it harmless. This has many similarities to superstitions. Recently I heard someone comment that a certain patient would never have reached his present state of disability if the physicians who had seen him had given proper treatment earlier in the course of his disease. This statement was immediately followed by

"Of course this is no criticism of his doctor." But of course this was a criticism of his doctor. The statement quoted was simply a denial of something that had been said which might arouse a hostile reaction in someone else. In psychiatric patients, this mechanism may result in elaborate rituals to deny a previous act or its hostile intent.

Reaction-formation is also closely related to denial. A 16 year old boy whose relationship with both of his parents was highly sexualized and ambivalent learned that his mother was pregnant. His reaction during the pregnancy was one of anger that she had become pregnant, jealousy of the unborn child such that he could not tolerate discussion of plans for its arrival, and constant demands upon his mother for her attention and affection. He expressed hatred of the coming child on numerous occasions before delivery. But when a baby brother was born, he suddenly found himself filled with boundless love. His concern for his brother's welfare was constant and excessive; no sacrifice was too great. This was a reaction-formation in which hatred was not only denied but was transformed into its opposite, love.[40] The boy was saying, Not only do I not dislike you; I love you very much.

Denial therefore is related to avoidance, inhibition, fantasy formation, undoing and reaction-formation. But, psychiatrically, it is perhaps most closely linked with repression, a mechanism of great importance to psychiatric formulations. Repression is a dynamic inhibition of such strength that the person is quite unaware that the drive, thought, or affect has ever been present to need inhibition. When repression is not sufficiently strong to obliterate awareness of the undesirable impulse, the "return of the repressed" can cause considerable anxiety. Awareness that the controlling mechanisms are not sufficiently strong to hold a drive in bounds arouses fears of loss of control or of insanity and may be quite devastating.

The protective value of successful repression is perhaps well illustrated in a very frightening episode in the life of Mrs. Bertrand. She had been having anginal attacks upon minor emotional provocation and with any unusual physical activity. One day as she sat in her apartment, the door open, she was suddenly confronted by a horrifying spectacle. Her neighbor burst from her room, her clothes in flames, screaming for help. Mrs. Bertrand sprang into action, picked up a small rug from the floor and wrapped it quickly around her friend. Others came running from adjoining rooms and took over the duties of getting her to a hospital and to medical attention. During the actual emergency, Mrs. Bertrand had no angina and afterward could recall no emotional response whatever. A job obviously needed to be done and she acted without thinking. As soon as others took over, however, she was overwhelmed with horror at what had happened, sank trembling into a chair, and had severe, persistent anginal pain.

In this case, the repression of affect was brief and its return afterward came soon enough after the fire for the relationship to be obvious. The return of the repressed affect was associated with all the physiologic manifestations to be expected with fear and anxiety, and with severe angina as well. When a longer interval, months or years for example, intervenes between the time of the repression and the time at which the affect begins to become conscious, the relationship may be difficult to establish. The physiologic manifestations of anxiety or anger are present when these begin to break through the defenses erected around them, not before, so that their appearance is evidence that the defense mechanisms being used are no longer sufficiently strong to afford protection.

Denial and repression are extremely important in medicine since they form the background for hysterical symptoms—amnesia, fugue states, somnambulism, hysterical hypesthesia or anesthesia, conversion paralyses, hysterical blindness or deafness, and bizarre pains. This is an impressive list of rather dramatic difficulties which may issue from repression and denial. It should be remembered, however, that when the mechanisms are completely successful, the repressed material is present without awareness or manifestation of it.

IDENTIFICATION

Identification is perhaps less often a direct cause of illness, but it indirectly affects the health of many people. Identification with another person may intensify goals and ambitions until these constitute a stress. It may cause frequent stresses and result in illness; it may also arouse considerable anxiety.

One of our patients was a banker who was hospitalized on a metabolic ward where the patients ate together in a dining room. Another banker, in the hospital at the same time, was severely disabled by arthritis. Studies planned on the arthritic banker involved feedings through a gastric tube. A day or two before the studies were to begin, a tube was put into his stomach so that he could get used to it before the experimental procedures were started. He appeared one evening at dinner time with the tube in place but planning to eat his meal as usual. He complained throughout the meal about the discomfort of the tube, and because of it he drooled into his plate. Our patient was extremely distressed by this episode. Perhaps the fact that they were both bankers made identification easier. In any event, the patient reported that his feeling was one of intense pity combined with a feeling of "There, but for the grace of God, go I." Under these circumstances he developed considerable anxiety and had a profuse diuresis involving all substances being studied.

Identification can work in other ways as well. A 40-year old man was seen in our clinic with symptoms of angina. He gave a story of having had symptoms of a duodenal ulcer many years before. The symptoms consisted largely of epigastric distress that occurred some time after meals and was relieved by food. Repeated x-ray studies over a number of years failed to show any ulcer or any deformity which might indicate that an ulcer had existed. These symptoms had abruptly disappeared and had been replaced by substernal pain of a crushing nature which had continued for many years, but again with no evidences, by electrocardiogram or exercise tolerance, that the symptoms were related to his heart. The interesting feature of his history, however, was that the gastrointestinal symptoms had begun when his father had a duodenal ulcer, demonstrated on x-ray. The ulcer symptoms had disappeared and had been replaced by chest pain suggestive of angina when his father had angina related to arteriosclerotic heart disease. His father died as the result of a heart attack. The patient continued to have chest pains of the same nature thereafter. The mechanism would appear to have been identification with the father so that symptoms similar to his father's and coincident with them developed.

EFFECT ON EMOTIONS

Some of these mechanisms by which people handle their drives and emotions alter the intensity of the emotion. Some prevent any awareness of the emotion or drive whatever. Others may cause people to change their behavior to remove them from potentially stressful situations. Still others change the direction of the emotion or drive so that people may be unaware of what it is that has disturbed them. The emotion or drive itself may be altered in its expression, as when the desire for affection is expressed as hunger or sexual stimulation is expressed as anger. With all these alterations in form and intensity between the original feeling state and the expression of it, it is not surprising that the study of emotions is still in a state of confusion.

A problem which has troubled many investigators is the lack of precise correlation between the intensity of an emotion as reported by subjects and the degree of alteration in physiologic parameters studied. Though this lack of correspondence may in part be related to complex emotional states in which the overall physiologic changes are muted by conflicting emotions and antagonistic neurohumoral mechanisms, a part of it also lies in these mechanisms, which affect both the subjective evaluation of emotional intensity and the extent to which physiologic processes are altered.

MOTIVES FOR DEFENSE

These mechanisms of defense serve an important function in mental economy. They are utilized in order to avoid pain and anguish, whether imposed externally as physical punishment or internally through the arousal of anxiety or guilt. If through their use the person succeeds in avoiding pain, the defense may represent a source of such security to him that he clings to its use tenaciously even when it is not successful. A defense that has seemed to work well may be used repeatedly until it is established as a habitual defensive maneuver. Like behavior routines, habitual emotional reactions, or other habit patterns, the habitual use of a mental mechanism serves basically to reduce the energy necessary for daily living. If one had to make a conscious decision about each and every act during the day, life could become impossibly complex. However, in being reduced to a habit the act may continue to be carried out without thought or change. This conserves energy but may lead to continuation of the habit long after its usefulness has vanished.

SELECTION OF DEFENSE

Why should a person select one particular defense rather than another? The answer to this question is not yet known, but certain processes are known to contribute to the final outcome, and other factors may be presumed to play a part as well. The child with strong drives is apt to gratify these if allowed to do so. If he is raised in a family where discipline is rigid and severe, the drives may be displaced into an area where punishment does not occur. This may be in the form of sublimation into an acceptable activity or simply displacement of the response to a new object. If the drives are only moderate and the discipline is severe and rigid, they may be suppressed or repressed.

Often the selection of the mental mechanism seems to be quite fortuitous. Sullivan[2] has described the appearance of full-fledged sublimation during infancy. His example is the child who wished to suck on his thumb but sucked a toy instead. The new pattern of behavior seemed to be adopted "unwittingly" because it allowed gratification of a drive without the anxiety which more direct gratification would have occasioned. No conscious evaluation of alternative modes of behavior need be involved in this selection, the mechanism being utilized simply because it reduces anxiety.

That the mechanisms described are normal mechanisms used by everyone should be emphasized. The day-to-day behavior of everyone can be described in terms of them. The presence of a functional or psychosomatic complaint does not in itself imply a psychiatric disorder or a severe personality disturbance. Those mental mechanisms which intensify or prolong emotional responses also intensify or prolong physiologic changes and may thus produce symptoms. They may be used inappropriately, but they may equally well be appropriate to the circumstances and still put too great a strain on the organism. Thus a man who inhibits a display of anger may be acting quite appropriately in the circumstances in which he finds himself and yet, as a consequence, develop muscle tension with multiple aches and pains, a headache, or some other symptom.

Chapter 4

Emotions

EMOTIONS and feeling states are the focal point of psychosomatic medicine for they are an intimate welding of psychic and somatic processes. Definitions of emotions have often foundered on this welding of mind and body and there have been many arguments as to which aspect appears first and which represents the "true" experience. But only in thought can the two be separated and analyzed independently; as an experience they are inseparable. A thought process may have no peripheral manifestations by which to recognize it. As soon as it becomes associated with an emotion, it does. A pure thought disorder is a psychic problem; but emotional disorders are psychosomatic. Through the emotions aroused, events in the environment or ideas become associated with somatic manifestations.

Emotions are aroused under specific conditions.[41] The emotions pertinent to medical practice arise in a setting of frustration. When a drive is aroused, gratification is desired. If this is blocked, feelings of frustration are apt to develop. The block may be a physical, social, or psychologic barrier between the person and his goal. Such a barrier prevented Mrs. Bertrand (p. 26) from establishing friendships during her childhood. Gratification may not be achieved because the anticipated reward is not forthcoming, as with Mrs. Brown (p. 40) who got no praise for meticulous housekeeping. Gratification may be blocked by a competitive drive. In any of these circumstances, an emotion or feeling state may be aroused if the drive is of sufficient intensity. Whether it is anger, anxiety, depression, or some other emotion depends on the person's evaluation of the situation.

When frustration of a drive is associated with anger or anxiety, additional energy is made available and the effective force of the drive is increased. When frustration results from the antagonism of competitive drives, the energizing effect is usually concentrated in the stronger of the two, thus increasing any discrepancy between them. Since the intensity of frustration is greater the more nearly equal the competing drives, anger and fear tend to reduce the intensity of frustration and to lead to action resolving the conflict.

Emotions have other effects. Attention span and ability to concentrate are adversely affected by anger and anxiety. Perceptions are altered and the ability to recall what has been experienced is decreased. A selectivity in memory is introduced which may significantly distort reality. Because of these effects, emotions influence the evaluation of stimuli. An incident of little meaning under neutral circumstances may become a major stress if it occurs while the person is still reacting emotionally to a previous stress. The intensity of the emotion may determine whether the person succeeds or fails in his efforts and may thereby significantly alter subsequent evaluations of similar situations.

These facts are of immediate importance to physicians. A patient who is emotionally disturbed is apt to give an imcomplete or distorted history with no intent whatever of falsifying information. If he is already disturbed, minor irritations aroused by a physician may seem of major consequence and result in angry outbursts. The anxieties of office and hospital procedures may lead to panic. New symptoms may arise or previous ones be exacerbated as a result. It is well, therefore, to direct your attention to the emotional state of the patient at the very outset of your association with each other.

ANGER

Patients sometimes complain of tension, anxiety, or depression. They seldom complain of anger, yet anger is a common source of difficulty. So far anger has been discussed as though it were an entity that could be precisely defined. The term has been used in these pages in a broad sense to cover all aggressive and hostile feelings whose basic direction is riddance of the offending situation or circumstance. But within this broad category are many subtle variations which make more precise characterizations difficult.

Anger has been categorized in a number of ways: (1) according to the intent—whether bluster and sham or intent to do harm; (2) according to direction—whether turned inward against the self or outward against others; (3) according to control—whether well controlled or poorly controlled; (4) according to the manner in which it is expressed—for example, whether in antisocial behavior, psychophysiologic reaction, psychoneurosis, or "normal" goal-directed behavior. Anger usually arises when people wish to take aggressive action to change things. It arises when people feel frustrated, unduly restricted, or imposed upon. It is an outgoing emotion which can find adequate expression in physical activity. When discharged adequately it probably causes few if any symptoms. But when unexpressed or when expressed inadequately—for example, as a smoldering resentment or pouting—it may cause prolonged physiologic changes and be associated with symptoms.

Some people are repeatedly angered by little things, no one of which seems to justify an expression of anger. The trivial nature of each fresh insult may prevent adequate discharge of the irritations. The energy mobilized in anger then accumulates until it seems out of all proportion to the stimuli arousing it. At this point, any expression of anger is apt to be violent because of the amount of energy bound up in it.

Quite the opposite reaction may occur. Bettelheim,[42] studying behavior in a concentration camp, noted that some persons who expressed their irritations freely under ordinary circumstances showed no emotion whatever under nearly intolerable circumstances of extreme mistreatment. They seemed to accept these extreme situations as "right" or at least as beyond their control. Such a reaction is seen outside concentration camps, though on a less dramatic level. It is not uncommon to meet patients who admit that they are easily irritated by trivial events but feel no anger at all when things are seriously awry.

Anger may be aroused in a situation where expression of it would be entirely inappropriate or, indeed, where expression of it would prevent attainment of some goal. It then seems desirable to control or prevent expression of anger in order to preserve this goal. Free expression of anger is not the answer to the problem under such circumstances even though control of it is associated with illness. At such times, the physician plays the role of a neutral person to whom the patient can express his feelings openly and thus dissipate some of their violence so that he can consider his problem more objectively and logically.

Different kinds of anger have been found to be associated with somewhat different physiologic states, but they are by no means the extent of variation possible within the general category "anger." The problem is complicated by other feelings, especially anxiety. Feelings of anger may arouse anxiety lest the anger evoke expressions of disapproval from others. The act which one desires to commit in anger may arouse anxiety likewise. The reverse may also occur, as when someone tries to make a person feel shame or guilt (varieties of anxiety), and the person reacts with anger as well, knowing that it was intended he feel shame. There are, therefore, many guises in which anger may appear: guilt, humiliation, frustration, irritation, rage, ambitious striving, and resentment, to mention but a few.

The number of guises increases when the effects of the various mental mechanisms are added. Hostility may form a bristly façade, obvious to all who approach too closely but hidden from the person himself. It may be displaced from the actual stimulus which originally aroused it to some other part of the environment so that its aim becomes confused and its meaning lost though the anger remains. It may be projected onto others or introjected into oneself. It may be suppressed or repressed. And all of these transformations add to the complexity of the problem and the patient's difficulty in comprehending the nature of his conflict and dealing with it appropriately.

Because of these many guises the emotion "anger" cannot be equated with any specific physiologic pattern. If norepinephrine secretion accompanies angry outbursts directed at others, one might expect a fairly uniform response of generalized vasoconstriction. Yet the description quoted from Darwin (p. 50), a common observation to all of us, includes both flushing with anger and turning pale with anger—opposite vascular responses. And Darwin contrasted the confident, aggressive behavior of one person in anger with the tremulousness of another under similar circumstances.

Gellhorn,[24] discussing the reactions of vasoconstriction and vasodilatation in different people under the same external circumstances, suggested that the different vascular responses might reflect sympathetic or parasympathetic dominance. The "same" emotional response might then be associated with vasoconstriction in one person and vasodilatation in another. Lacey[43] demonstrated that the reaction is not specific for any one person but may vary from time to time in the same person with repetition of stress. This could well reflect differences in reaction and differences in physiologic state at the time the stress was applied.

The relation of these alterations to disease processes has been recognized for many years. John Hunter is said to have lamented that his life was in the hands of any fool who chose to annoy him. Many before and since his time have been aware of the importance of anger in precipitating angina. Peptic ulcer has commonly been related to anger, frequently under the label "oral aggression."[44] Vascular engorgement, increased secretion, and hypermotility of the stomach are associated with such feelings and are pertinent to exacerbations of duodenal ulceration.[27] Urticaria, a reaction of peripheral vasodilatation, has been linked with anger aroused when people felt mistreated,[5] but Raynaud's phenomenon, involving peripheral vasoconstriction, has also been linked with angry and hostile feelings.[45] Vascular headaches seem often to follow episodes arousing anger. Here the response is one of vasoconstriction followed by vasodilatation.[46] There is no easy answer at hand for this array of diverse vascular responses appearing rather selectively—at least insofar as signs or symptoms are concerned —in association with situations arousing anger.

ANXIETY

As with anger, anxiety may develop in frustrating situations in which gratification is blocked because of a barrier to or delay of gratification, a lack of adequate reward, or the presence of a competitive drive. Anxiety arises when frustration arouses uncertainty. Such uncertainty may be present when the threatening stimulus is perceived too vaguely to allow classification of it. At such times, the person cannot evaluate exactly what the threat is and therefore does not know what it will require of him. Even when perception is fairly clear, anxiety will be aroused if he cannot be sure which standard of conduct or which system of values should apply in determining his response. Anxiety will also be aroused, even with perception clear and values unequivocal, when he is not sure that he has the resources to meet the threat.

The stressful situations to which Fred (p. 56) was subjected were of all three types. When a rumor went through his Army unit that they would soon be sent to Korea, he was uncertain that they would leave and uncertain whether the outfit would see front line duty even if they did go. He may also have been concerned about his resources to meet front line duty, though this was not expressed. When he became engaged a few months later, he was torn between his love for the model and his ties of friendship with the boy who had been going with her before. He felt guilty and was not sure he was handling the situation properly. And when he contemplated the future of the marriage, he doubted that he would be able to hold her interest. Since treatment will differ according to the source of the anxiety, when a patient is anxious it is important to discover where the uncertainty lies—the nature of the threat, the principles of action, his endowment, or some combination of these.

In addition to the amount of uncertainty present, the intensity of anxiety depends on the motivation of the patient to perform well and on the immediacy of the threat. The fear of death may be an extremely potent source of anxiety, but if death seems relatively remote the fear of a needle puncture may have greater immediate force.

When anxiety arises from competitive drives within the patient, it may have no obvious precipitating cause. At such times, it often appears first as a "free-floating" anxiety, attached to no specific stimulus but pervading the patient with a dark foreboding of unpleasant things ahead. He feels anxious and fearful without knowing why. This is an extremely distressing feeling and acts as a powerful motivation for treatment.

The way in which the basic conflict of drives is handled is important. If gratification of one of the drives is quite unacceptable to the person, he may try to defend himself against this drive. When the drive is extremely threatening, the defense must be a potent counterforce to block expression of this drive completely. One of the strongest and most potent defense mechanisms available is repression, for here the emotion or drive is not permitted to enter consciousness at all. If the emotion that is being blocked is anger, for example, the person may be quiet and give no indication to himself or to others of the intense feelings which are being repressed. Free-floating anxiety often results when repression has proved inadequate to handle the energy present in an unacceptable drive. When the energy builds up sufficiently, it may break through the dam of repression in a sudden violent act which horrifies everyone who knows the person. This act, however, may bring so much relief and release of tension to the person himself that he looks upon it calmly.

Much commoner than such an occurrence, however, is for the drive to be expressed in some other form. If it can be expressed in some form that is acceptable socially, no symptoms at all may develop. But if the drive is deflected in another unacceptable direction, it may again arouse anxiety because the person has been made aware that there is something within himself which is stronger than his defenses against it. This is the reason for the common fear of loss of control.

There are impulses within himself which he does not fully understand and fears that he will be unable to cope with successfully.

Basic impulses are repressed because they are not acceptable to the person repressing them. That part of the energy which does find release is ordinarily expressed in a form which is more acceptable than the original impulse. The man who has hostile impulses and wishes to injure another may develop a fear of his own death. No matter how much anxiety the thought of dying engenders in him, it is more acceptable than the fear of killing someone else. In anxiety the fear of which the patient is conscious may not be the cause of his anxiety; therefore, no matter how much he discusses these specific fears, such as the fear of his own death, he does not relieve himself of the anxiety. For treatment to be of value it must be directed at the core of the problem, not at the secondary manifestations of which the patient is conscious.

Free-floating anxiety is a very distressing sensation which the patient cannot understand. Anything that will allay it is desirable so far as the patient is concerned. It is much easier for people to tolerate fears they can understand. If they know or think they know what is causing a fear, they have something concrete to evaluate and they can hope to find measures to cope with it. Consequently, it is not at all unusual for patients to seize upon anything which can be used as a rational explanation of their anxiety. If this is an external stimulus or a symbol of such a stimulus, the patient develops phobias or obsessive ruminations. If it is a symptom, hypochondriasis or an organ neurosis may result. In either case, the patient's attention is fixed on the phobia or symptom rather than on the anxiety itself. Under such circumstances, discussion and reassurance about the symptom will not allay the anxiety since it is not primarily aroused by the symptom in the first place. The person who feels that his anxiety is caused by a symptom "knows" that if he can get relief from that symptom he will be relieved of his anxiety. The symptom gives the patient a feeling that he understands. It removes some of the quality of the unknown from his experience and therefore relieves some of his anxiety. For this reason, symptoms can become very important to a patient with anxiety. The patient is still disturbed by anxiety but it is much less intense than if he did not have the symptom. The longer the symptoms persist, the more fixed they become, the more certain a patient is that these are the cause of his anxiety. If he has had such symptoms for 20 years or so, it may be extremely difficult to cure him. Relieving one symptom leaves the patient with free anxiety, and another symptom is quickly found to take its place. It is important that physicians recognize anxiety as early as possible and institute proper treatment for it, since treatment is much easier before firm fixation onto symptoms has occurred.

PAIN AND ANXIETY

Pain is so commonplace that we are apt to accept its existence without considering all its complexities. There is a marked difference, for instance, in superficial and deep pain. The end-organs, nerve-fibers and central pathways for superficial and deep pain are quite distinct. The reactions elicited by these types of pain are also quite distinct. Superficial pain, when intense, excites a number of reactions which seem to be mediated largely through the sympathetic nervous system. At such times blood is withdrawn from the skin and forced into the muscles. There is skin pallor, raised blood pressure, increased pulse rate, and, perhaps, dilated pupils. With superficial pain a person may be excited to increased activity. On the other hand, with deep aching pain these reactions are not apt to be seen. Instead there is weakness, prostration, lowered blood pressure, nausea, vomiting, sweating and pallor. Activity is usually markedly restricted during severe aching pain, particularly when visceral in origin. There are striking exceptions to this generalization, for the meaning of the pain to the patient seems to affect his reaction markedly.[47, 48] These physical reactions to pain may, if long continued, result in tissue damage and deleterious effects on vital organs. Recognition of this fact makes the physician use every agent at his command to stop the pain of a myocardial infarction, for instance, as quickly as possible.

One of the fascinating aspects of pain is the discrepancy between perception of pain and reaction to it. Though we are all familiar with this phenomenon we ordinarily give it little thought and seldom stop to realize its significance in medical practice. Harold Wolff and his associates at Cornell[34] determined the threshold stimulus producing just perceptible pain. They found little variation in the threshold to pain from one subject to another or in the same subject under a variety of situations. However, a subject's reaction to pain varied strikingly and his evaluation of the intensity of the pain varied accordingly. Thus the threshold stimulus which produced barely perceptible pain one day might produce pain of considerable severity on another day, though the threshold itself remained unchanged. This variation in reaction to pain was markedly affected by the emotional state of the subject. Feelings of anxiety and resentment were particularly apt to increase the intensity of pain reaction in the laboratory setting.

One clinical application of this discrepancy has been demonstrated experimentally. The cold pressor test is commonly used in medicine. In this test the patient plunges his forearm into a basin of ice water and holds it there for two or three minutes; blood pressures are recorded in the opposite arm before, during, and after immersion. The patient who is anxious, knowing that this test may determine whether he is to be operated upon or not, may have a very marked change in blood pressure and find the experience intensely painful. On another day, when this decision no longer hangs in the balance, the same test in the same patient may elicit little elevation of blood pressure and no pain.

There are occasions when anxiety aroused by anticipating pain may evoke a response before any pain is felt. This is seen in the child who cries at an uplifted hand or in the adult who winces at the sight of the dentist's drill. People who are apprehensive about dental work are more apt to experience severe pain than those who are not. Some dentists provide their patients with buttons that will turn off the drill. These give patients a feeling that the painful stimuli about to be experienced are, to some extent, under their control. By allaying anxiety somewhat, intensity of the pain is decreased.

People sometimes actually seek pain. It may be sought for exhilaration, as by people who belong to polar bear clubs and swim in ice water in January. Sometimes pain is sought as punishment to allay feelings of guilt, as in certain psychiatric disorders. I remember one patient on a psychiatric ward who bit large chunks of tissue out of his arms and thighs. His comment was "pain and suffering are good for the soul."

The influence of attitudes upon the intensity of pain is evident in other areas as well. People can learn to tolerate pain. A woman may wear shoes that are tight and painful or have her ears pierced for earrings in order to be stylish. A person may accept pain as a small price to pay for some important gain. This was apparently true of the martyrs who suffered intense pain for the principles in which they believed. It is seen, too, in the misbehaving child who knows he is going to be punished but is willing to accept the pain of punishment in order to have his little vengeance. Childbirth is frequently painful and yet the mother accepts pain for the pleasures of having a child. It is interesting to note that here is another instance in which the effect of anxiety is commonly recognized. The book *Child Birth Without Fear* is based on this realization. The author believes that elimination of the fear and anxiety relieves much of the pain associated with child birth.

Attitudes toward pain in the group to which an individual belongs are quite important in the reaction which pain elicits. Group feelings about stoicism and high individual motivations within a group are extremely significant in decreasing reaction to pain. A man's arm may be shot off in combat and he may experience little pain, busying himself instead with taking care of other wounded. A similar though less dramatic phenomenon is seen in sports. A man quite seriously injured in a football game may be unaware of pain at the time of injury and become very much aware of it later. Here clearly is an example of the power of motivation and group attitudes in determining response to painful stimuli.

It is plain that emotions and attitudes can affect reaction to pain enormously. It is equally true that the sensation of pain can arouse anxieties in most people. These anxieties are frequently focused around such questions as: How long is the pain going to last and how intense will it be? Can I tolerate this pain? What is the origin of it? Is it evidence of some serious disease? Does it presage death? Anxieties about one's ability to tolerate pain and the fear of death are two of the major anxieties aroused by pain. Thus a vicious circle is initiated, a circle which includes pain as a source of anxiety and anxiety as a factor increasing the intensity of the pain and thus arousing fresh anxieties.

TENSION

Tension as a feeling state is difficult to define. It does not have the dramatic qualities possessed by either anger or anxiety. It may, and often does, exist without awareness of its presence until it disappears, when recognition that it has been present comes only by contrast with the feeling of relief or relaxation. It may persist for days or weeks with little variation. Proposed definitions of tension are diverse and confusing. The word has been used to describe a basic drive, an emotional state, an attitude of mind, a physical condition, and a psychic force exerting a controlling influence over drives and emotions. Tension and anxiety are commonly experienced simultaneously, thus adding to the ease with which they can be confused. Anxiety is an emotion often considered to indicate "mental weakness," "neurosis," or inability to handle the problems of life. Many people avoid using the words anxiety or apprehension to describe their emotional state because of this connotation. They refer, therefore, to both anxiety and tension with the one word "tense." The distinction between them needs to be made clearly.

Psychiatrists in speaking of tension refer most often to sexual tension. The word is used as though it meant a drive seeking expression. When this drive achieves its goal, relaxation occurs and tension disappears. Though this may be an accurate description of the sequence of events, the sequence does not necessarily imply that drive and tension are synonymous. With opportunity for free expression of drives, sexual or otherwise, the sensations of tension and relaxation need not accompany the drive and its satisfaction. The longer the drive must wait before gratification is achieved, the greater the tension is apt to be. The more frequently the drive is aroused without gratification, the greater the tension which is evoked. These observations do not necessarily establish tension and drive as separable entities, but they do suggest that the matter deserves further consideration.

Many people use the words tension and anxiety as though they meant the same thing. And, indeed, the two are present simultaneously more often than not. But the more acute the anxiety, the less the degree of tension is apt to be; whereas with states of chronic anxiety, levels of tension are apt to be high. In medical practice one often sees people who are extremely tense and suffering from symptoms as a result who experience no anxiety whatever. The two cannot be synonymous, therefore, even though they are commonly associated.

Tension has also been defined as a state in which a person is alert and ready for action. Here, again, there is some difficulty. The person who is aroused with any strong emotion is in "a ready state," whether this is anger or anxiety or even joy. These states are associated with increased alertness, whether of a directed or undirected nature. Tension does not differ from these in being a state of readiness for action; the differentiating feature must lie elsewhere. The description of tension as muscular or psychic preparedness is merely another way of stating that it is "the ready state." Muscular and psychic preparedness are two components of one state. Attempts to separate them are useful only in making accurate description of both possible. Diethelm, Fleetwood and Milhorat[49] combined the muscular and psychic elements in their definition of tension as characterized by a feeling of tautness accompanied by a definite effort at control. They distinguished this clearly from anxiety which they described as characterized by subjective feelings of uneasiness and apprehension.

In a recent study of renal excretion[30] the relation of excretory patterns to emotional state was studied in 5 healthy subjects. Judgments of emotional state were made from observation of the subjects, discussions with them of personal events, and their reports of predominant feeling states during each collection period, using terms such as tension, uneasiness, apprehension, anxiety, excitement, depression, anger, and the like. Patterns of renal excretion were similar during collection periods characterized by feelings of uneasiness, apprehension, or anxiety, as would be expected from the definition of these terms given by Diethelm and his associates. There were marked differences, however, between these and patterns observed during periods characterized by tension. During these periods, urinary volume and urinary sodium were lower than rates observed during neutral periods. During periods of anxiety, apprehension, or uneasiness excretion rates of urinary volume and sodium were increased over those observed during neutral periods. And in subjects who reported the presence of both tension and anxiety simultaneously mean excretion rates for urinary volume and urinary sodium did not deviate significantly from those observed during neutral periods.

These studies suggested that tension and anxiety were two distinct states which could often be differentiated subjectively and were equally distinct physiologically. The excellent correlation between subjective evaluation of these states and renal excretion rates could not have been obtained unless both were clear and distinct.

When situations arousing tension and those arousing anxiety were compared, certain things became evident. The situations which aroused feelings of tension were, in general, familiar situations occurring repeatedly in the person's daily life. Feelings of tension were aroused when these routines were constantly being interrupted or when some extra load was imposed and had to be accomplished within a small amount of time. Thus child care aroused tension in a housewife when extra children were involved or when some planned, organized activity was being attempted with them. Driving aroused tension in heavy traffic. Shopping aroused tension when there were many items to be bought and time in which to accomplish it was limited. Tension seemed to be aroused when the person had to be alert and "on his toes" in order to get the job done but with no uncertainty about his ability to do so if he was alert.

Situations which aroused feelings of anxiety, on the contrary, were relatively new and unfamiliar situations with some degree of unpredictability about them. One subject reported apprehension when he made his first drive in a new automobile. But there was more unfamiliarity to this situation than just the new automobile. This was the first time he had driven any car in 2 years; it was the first time he had ever driven a left-hand drive automobile; and it was the first time he had driven in heavy traffic. Another subject reported anxiety during an evening when she was meeting some of her husband's relatives for the first time and on another occasion when she was preparing dinner for important guests. Another subject reported being apprehensive when her boy friend disappeared without leaving any word as to where he was going or how long he would be gone. These situations were not routine for the subjects. The striking feature in common was the uncertainty which surrounded them.

Despite these differences certain things were common for these two states. In all of the situations, whether arousing tension or anxiety, the person was motivated to perform well. In all there was a potential threat to his doing well. In all there was increased alertness. Thus the two feeling states, tension and anxiety, could not be differentiated in terms of these characteristics.

Since tension is characterized by tautness accompanied by a definite effort at control, the situations arousing tension should be examined in terms of the degree and type of control being exercised. In many instances specific motor activities were required to accomplish the task in hand and the person had to control his behavior in order to accomplish the task in the allotted time—as when shopping required that a large number of items be bought in a limited period or when extra jobs were imposed without extra time being allotted for them.

But in addition to this, many of the situations might be expected to have aroused feelings of anger or anxiety, even though no such emotion was consciously experienced. Sudden outbursts of emotion in a state of tension did occur on occasion. They suggest that these feelings were indeed being controlled by the state of tension. Where the controlling mechanism was completely successful, the emotion as such was not experienced. Where the defense mechanism was only partially successful, however, the person was aware both of tension and of some other emotional reaction, such as anger or anxiety, concomitant with the tension. Where the defense failed completely, even though only momentarily, there was a sudden outburst of anger or anxiety. Fear of loss of control is associated with anger or anxiety surprisingly often. If tension controls these strong emotional states, to some extent at least, it is not surprising that people with chronic anxiety states also commonly have some degree of tension. This common association of tension with chronic anxiety is probably the reason some people consider the two to be synonymous and why the term "tense and anxious" has become a cliché.

It is often stated that an underlying or unconscious anxiety is present in all threatening situations, whatever the conscious and overt reaction is. Nothing in the preceding discussion contradicts this point of view. When the controlling mechanisms are completely successful this underlying anxiety may never reach consciousness or awareness. Another conclusion naturally follows at this point, however.

Most, if not all, of the reported psychophysiologic observations are consistent with the view that the bodily changes associated with various emotional states are closely correlated also with the defense mechanism utilized. The type of threat may determine the choice of defense mechanism; but even if the defense is inappropriate to the threat the physiologic changes will still be consistent with the defense mechanism rather than with the threatening stimulus. The same external stimulus may arouse many different types of reactions in people, depending upon their evaluation of the stimulus in relation to their concept of themselves and their goals. If the threat is met with anger and a response appropriate to fighting, the physiologic changes are consistent with this defensive reaction. If met with fear and flight, the physiologic changes are those associated with fear and flight. A man may choose to avoid the situation entirely so that he will not have to resort either to fight or flight, or he may enter the situation knowingly but with the attitude of holding on, preparing for future action, or being "on guard" to control himself or the situation so that it does not lead to fight or flight. This controlling attitude is the one in which tension develops, and the physiologic changes are those appropriate to control or tension.

Some comment should be made also about the relation between tension and relaxation. Earlier it was stated that tension might be present without awareness of it except by contrast with later relaxation. The insidious appearance of tension is not surprising when one reviews the situations in which it was aroused in the studies on renal excretion (p. 93). Because these were usually familiar, routine situations ordinarily considered neutral or tranquil but disturbed by addition of new factors, the transition between tranquility and tension was vague and ill defined, though marked tension was easily recognized by an introspective person. In most subjects, however, a moderate degree of tension could be present before it was recognized. If the period ended abruptly, either because the clock reached 5:00 P.M. and the work day was over, or because the threat was terminated suddenly, the control was no longer needed. The subject relaxed his controls, felt relieved and at ease, and by contrast became aware that he must have been tense before. Such active relaxation was accompanied by a diuresis of water without corresponding amounts of sodium. Thus the physiologic state was quite different from that seen during neutral and tranquil periods.

One of the characteristic features of tension is muscular preparedness accompanied by increased muscle tone. This increase in muscle tone, if sufficiently intense or of sufficient duration, may lead to aching pain in voluntary muscles. The physiologic expression of tension however includes more than increased muscle tone. Renal excretion patterns reflect the presence of tension, as mentioned. Vascular changes at the glomerular level are almost certainly present, as indicated by decreased excretion of creatinine associated with this feeling state.[30] The state of tension is pertinent to cardiac failure[50] by virtue of the retention of water and sodium which accompanies it. Tension affects the response of the cardiac patient to therapy. This has long been recognized, as evidenced by the customary insistence upon physical and mental relaxation in the treatment of patients in cardiac failure. In addition the current theories concerning migraine and other extracranial vascular headaches ascribe a major role to vasoconstriction accompanying states of tension in setting the stage for the headache which occurs subsequently during periods of relaxation.[40]

DEPRESSION

Feelings of depression ordinarily lack the violent and dramatic qualities of anger and anxiety. They have more in common with feelings of tension, for they are frequently insidious in onset and may be present without awareness of them. They are apt to be chronic, lasting days, weeks, or months. And they may be hidden from the physician behind a screen of physical complaints.

The usual description of depression contains many physical manifestations. In addition to the lack of confidence, slow speech and difficult thinking that accompanies depression, there may be loss of appetite, disturbed sleep, weakness, fatigability, headache, and constipation. Muscle tone is decreased, the body stooped, the head flexed, the face immobile. Metabolic processes are decreased. Sexual desire is decreased and impotence may be present. The feeling state is one of hopelessness, despair, or despondency. Overt behavior is less one of avoidance than one of apathy and disinterest. Irregular or sighing respirations may accompany depression so that the symptoms of hyperventilation may be associated with this feeling state as well as with anxiety. Of the depressed person, Darwin[6] said, "The circulation becomes languid; the face pale; the muscles flaccid; the eyelids droop; the head hangs on the contracted chest; the lips, cheeks, and lower jaw all sink downwards from their own weight. Hence all the features are lengthened; and the face of the person who hears bad news is said to fall."

Depressive feelings are frequent in situations of deprivation, such as that after the death of a close friend or relative. Events resulting in loss of prestige, loss of money, or loss of self-esteem may also arouse feelings of depression. They may also arise when one feels a successful outcome is impossible and struggle futile. Here the deprivation is the failure to achieve something desired.

In all of these instances the person feels that he has been deprived of something which was his. One might expect this to arouse anger; such situations often do. But the person who is depressed has no desire to fight back. He is sad, discouraged, or dejected and feels that the fight is hopeless. He withdraws from the world, losing interest in his usual activities. His thinking and speech are slowed, muscle tone is decreased, and metabolic processes are retarded. Thus his body expresses the fact that he has "given up the fight."

But this simple state of depression, which might be called sadness or grief, needs to be differentiated from another form of depression. Freud made this distinction in his paper *Mourning and Melancholia:*[51] "The distinguishing features of melancholia are a profoundly painful dejection, abrogation of interest in the outside world, loss of the capacity to love, inhibition of all activity, and a lowering of the self-regarding feelings to a degree that finds utterance in self-reproaches and self-revilings. . . . The fall in self-esteem is absent in grief; but otherwise the features are the same." Thus the distinction between the two lies in a self-reproach, the presence of anger directed against the self.

It is true that many of the depressive reactions seen in association with loss of money, loss of prestige, loss of a loved one, or failure to achieve a goal show some anger directed against the self. But this is anger, not sadness or grief. It should be plain that anger directed against oneself is not synonymous with depression; for the depression of sadness or grief is distinguished by its very absence. The two can exist independently. The person who is striving to attain a goal and temporarily fails may well react with anger at himself if he feels he was responsible for the failure. If he is confident of mastery in the future, however, there need be no feeling of hopelessness or dejection. The anger then serves to spur him on to increased effort rather than leading to an inhibition of activity as is common with depression.

The physiologic changes observed in association with a simple depression are very different from those seen accompanying anger directed against the self. With depression, muscle tone is decreased; with anger it tends to be increased. With depression, constipation is frequent; with anger, diarrhea may occur. With depression, urinary excretion of sodium is markedly decreased; with anger, sodium excretion increases. With depression, pulse rate and blood pressure decrease; with anger directed inwardly, these increase. The physiologic correlates of the two states are therefore very different. Their combined occurrence should not lead one to confuse them any more than combined tension and anxiety.

Depressive reactions are extremely important in medical practice. The loss of satisfactions in life, which leads to the reaction, is associated with a depression of physiologic processes as well as a retardation of mental faculties. With decreased satisfactions from life, the individual loses his desire for health and activity. The decrease in motivation to get well interferes materially with the physician's work, which is directed toward improving his health. The physiologic changes which are a part of depression may also retard recovery. It is important, therefore, for the physician to recognize a depression when it exists and to take measures to relieve it.

MIXED EMOTIONS

Situations are often complex and the meaning of a situation to a patient will likewise be complex at such times. When Fred (p. 56) became engaged to the model he loved, the situation involved more than one step toward achieving a satisfaction which he desired. The situation involved not only his relation with the model but also his attitudes toward himself and the friend whom he had bested, attitudes which included feelings about friendship and competition. He reacted at each of these levels. He felt pride in his accomplishment of winning her but doubts of his ability to hold her and self-reproaches that he was unworthy of her. He felt guilty that he had bested his friend and feared to tell him that he was engaged lest he lose the friendship. His reaction in this situation was complex, combining many attitudes and emotions.

The physician commonly sees people with mixed emotions. The emotions and attitudes represent conflicting tendencies for action. The patient may be unable to decide which tendency to follow or may follow one after another in succession. As long as the conflict remains, the emotional expression of it remains, including the physiologic manifestations. Conflict prolongs the physiologic changes and this contributes to symptom formation. Emotional states in which one reaction clearly predominates are not unusual, but the physician is more apt to see the person who has conflicting emotions.

When two emotions are present simultaneously one might expect the physiologic changes to reflect both of them. This is true. Sometimes the two emotional components are associated with alterations in physiology which are in the same direction. The result may be a heightened effect. For instance, both anger and tension are associated with increased muscle tone. When anger and tension are present simultaneously, muscle tone may be markedly increased. The two emotional components may be associated with alterations in physiology which are in opposite directions. Thus anger is associated with increased urinary volume, whereas tension is associated with decreased volume. When anger and tension are present simultaneously, urinary volume may not differ from that observed during neutral and tranquil periods. Thus the same two emotions when present simultaneously may be associated with a heightened physiologic change when one variable is studied and with no change when another variable is studied. The problem becomes more complex when more emotions are intermixed.

EFFECT OF PHYSIOLOGIC CHANGES

In this discussion of the relation between emotions and physiology, the effect of emotional reactions on physiologic and biochemical patterns has been emphasized. Conversely, do physiologic changes alter emotional states? The answer is Yes. There are numerous ways in which alterations in the physiology and biochemistry of the body may affect response to a stressful situation. If an emotion is a composite of psychic and physiologic manifestations, when physiology is altered, on whatever basis, the person should react differently and perhaps even experience a different emotion. That differences in autonomic reactivity exist even in the newborn has been noted,[26] though this altered reactivity may be evidenced in one parameter and not another. It might be expected that the person with pronounced tachycardia as a part of his reaction in anxiety would experience anxiety differently than the person with less cardiac acceleration.

In addition to autonomic lability there is the factor of arousal. It is a common observation that people react in a different manner when drowsy than when excited. The meaning of an experience is different under these circumstances, and the emotional reaction is different. Part of this may also be related to autonomic tone, since arousal does have repercussions in the autonomic nervous system. But much of it seems related to increased neuronal activity emanating from the reticular formation. Certainly, alerting can precede any emotional reaction, and the reaction may be altered as a result of the alerting.

The effects of drugs on mood and emotional reaction to stress are well known, particularly since the advent of tranquilizers. Most of these act directly on central mechanisms. But it has also been noted that experimental subjects given ipecac reported feelings of discouragement and apathy with the nausea which followed administration of the drug.[52]

Perhaps the most obvious clinical illustration of the influence of disturbed physiology on emotional state is to be found in thyroid disease. One of the first evidences of hyperthyroidism may be an increased irritability, which combines both increased alertness and increased autonomic lability. The opposite occurs with hypothyroidism. In these instances, it is evident that chemical changes within the body do affect emotional reactions to external stimulation.

Another example has recently been studied. Workers interested in the problem of hypoparathyroidism[53] have gathered evidence which suggests that reaction to the stress of an interview or of psychologic testing may be intensified when serum calcium levels are low and that this becomes evident even before the levels have fallen sufficiently to produce signs and symptoms. Levels of anxiety, hostility, and depression were consistently higher in these studies during periods of hypocalcemia than during periods with normal calcium levels. Though changes in basic personality structure were not noted at such times, personality characteristics were accentuated. Thus a shy person became quite withdrawn while a resentful one became openly hostile.

If the energy made available during an emotional reaction is linked, even in part, to sympathetic activity, then people with more reactive sympathetic nervous systems might be expected to respond more energetically to stressful situations. Many other factors complicate the picture, for more than sympathetic activity is involved— the force of drives, hormonal activity, and the capacity for arousal. Whatever the origin of differences in vigor of response, it is certainly true that such differences exist. And the increase in vigor is apt to meet with a difference in response of parents and others close to the person, resulting in more or fewer controls and punishments, depending upon their feelings about vigorous reactions and their role in curbing them. Through interactions such as these, the physiologic processes can affect interpersonal relations and personality formation.

Chapter 5

Social and Cultural Forces

SOCIAL and cultural factors have a very important bearing on health, yet relatively little has been done to study these relationships in any detail. Studies have demonstrated a statistically significant increase in mental illness associated with population migration,[54] and some attention has been given to the effects of family mobility on health.[55] There have been few studies of the mechanisms involved in this relationship.

The story of Cy Logan illustrates the disruption of life which can occur with migration.

Cy Logan was an Oklahoma farmer born at about the turn of the century. He worked on his father's farm until his marriage in 1924 and then bought his own farm. Despite the depression, the dust-bowl years, and 5 children to raise, he managed fairly well. He worked hard but never accumulated much in the way of savings so that a few dry years put him under financial strain. In the midst of this, one of his daughters suddenly lost vision in one eye and required surgery for a detached retina. Crops were poor the next year, and they had insufficient feed for their cattle. Their home was badly in need of repairs. The well from which they got their water was declared unsafe. In view of all these troubles, Cy sold his farm and rented another. But he found that he did not have the same interest and pride in rented property. Consequently he began listening a little more to his wife's comments about being lonely on the farm. She wanted to move into town where there were more people and more things to do. The family left the farm and moved to the city. At 48, Cy had never known anything but farm life.

He didn't know what to do when he got to the city. He didn't know what kind of work to look for nor where to look for it. He had no ideas about what he was qualified to do. After a period of confusion he found a job working in a laundry. It didn't take him long to decide that this was no job for him. He didn't like working so close to other people; he resented being told what to do and when to do it. In addition, he began making mistakes on the job. He had known that his vision was a little blurred but had not realized quite how bad it was. He was slow in his work and those around him began putting pressure on him. He disliked this too. He wanted to quit but feared he would not find employment anywhere else. He stayed, hoping to save enough to be able to establish a laundry of his own.

He never saved enough. His son wrecked the car when driving while drunk and depleted the family's reserve cash. Then another daughter had a detached retina and the family went into debt with medical expenses. Things were going badly at work, and Cy was dismissed because his work was unsatisfactory. His vision was worse, his ambition was destroyed, his savings were gone, and he didn't know where to turn for help. He felt helpless in the face of these many blows. He noted that his heart was irregular, occasionally skipping a beat. Shortness of breath associated with a feeling of faintness developed. He slept poorly at night and had frequent headaches during the day. His back became sore and painful. And he developed a fear of crowds. Because of these symptoms, he sought medical aid.

The student who first saw this patient in the clinic considered him "constitutionally inadequate." He saw only a frail, middle-aged man who was unable to support his family and was suffering from symptoms of anxiety. He ignored the long years of adequate performance on the farm, the fact that this man had succeeded in raising and supporting a family through depression years that had proved too much for many others. Neither did he see the social factors which had contributed to this patient's illness.

The stresses involved in such a change can be of major proportions. The reasons for moving certainly influence the response of the person to stressful situations which he meets, as does the possibility of returning to the old way of life. He is uprooted, removed from the security of a familiar environment and from the security of knowing his way around in that environment. The roots one has in his community, the security one feels in knowing in a general way what the next day will bring are important forces for stability. With these gone, anxieties multiply, and when one fails to adjust adequately to new ways, discouragement and depression are almost inevitable. Cy Logan faced these problems and failed to meet their demands, largely because his way of life for 48 years had not prepared him to meet such problems. His past experience, in fact, led him to persist in the face of adversity rather than to seek other work. His anxiety and his depression were both understandable in this situation, and his symptoms stemmed from them.

The impact of social and cultural forces upon personality has been studied. Ruth Benedict's accounts of the interactions between individuals and cultural patterns in selected Indian groups[56] are fascinating. Margaret Mead has continued this type of study among native groups in the South Seas.[57] Kardiner has used a psychoanalytic approach to study the impact of minority status upon personal development.[58] These and many other studies have added much to our understanding of the interplay between culture and personality, but they are concerned only secondarily with the influence of culture upon health.

The focus of attention in psychophysiologic medicine must be on the stresses posed for the individual by the social and cultural system in which he lives. These include adjustments of personal aims which are required by society as well as contradictions inherent in the system. A start toward defining social and cultural forces of importance to psychophysiologic phenomena has been made by Talcott Parsons in his analysis of sources of hostility in our social system.[59]

FAMILY

The family is a basic social unit which performs not only the biologic function of propagating the human race but many social and cultural functions as well. Cultural ideas and beliefs are transmitted first within the family. All of the early learning process occurs here as well—not just the learning of skills such as walking and talking but the learning of values and affective relationships. Since many psychosomatic ills are rooted in emotional interpersonal relations, the affective habits learned in childhood are important as a groundwork for later health or disease. The earliest experiences with discipline and with the need to conform are in the family. They form the basis for later relationships with authority. In addition, children learn from parents about their role in the family and about their future roles as husband, wife, father, or mother.

These various functions are performed differently in families of different structure. The patriarchal family, with its numerous members living together or in close association tends to differ in its affective ties from the conjugal family consisting only of father, mother, and their children. Many factors which may at first seem only remotely related have affected family life. Industrial development led to increasing urbanization. Technologic advances made it possible for many persons from rural areas to move to cities. A combination of these and other forces brought with it a tremendous increase in the number of homes in urban and suburban areas. These homes, however, were not the large, rambling structures of old but small compact units to fit the needs of a new type of family. With the disappearance of family collateral lines from the home or immediate neighborhood, the demands upon the two remaining adults were intensified. The father was the only male to provide for the needs of the family. The economic burden fell solely upon him at first. To supplement his income, which was not always adequate, the mother might work outside the home. This was neither necessary nor considered desirable in the patriarchal family. Not only were all the economic burdens placed on a single male but all household and child-rearing demands were centered in a single female. Other adults of both sexes were no longer present to absorb or share these duties. Therefore, if the mother worked outside the home serious problems in housekeeping and child care arose. Baby sitters, nurseries, day schools, and various social agencies sprang up to help meet the economic and social problems which these changes brought.

The increase in population mobility and the concentration of population in urban areas put more emphasis on material possessions, since these were needed to establish status, to document adequacy, and to meet needs which formerly were met by other members of the family but were now displaced to the objects owned. In rural life, children were needed economically for help on the farm; not so in the city, where the responsibilities of having children were apt to outweigh the advantages. The number of children per family decreased during this period of change.

Many adjustments were required. The decrease in family size and the establishment of retirement policies left the older generation temporarily with no clearly defined role. Raised to become the focus of activities of a large family and to be dependent on the younger and more productive members, they found themselves with no work available to them, yet expected to be independent and to live alone. This led to many problems in adjustment for the older generation. Having anticipated a place of honor in the family in their later years, they found the pressures to remain independent and to live alone doubly difficult to accept. Often they felt rejected, unwanted, and useless. In many instances, they were a burden to their family and knew it. Feelings of depression, therefore, have been extremely common in this age group, and functional symptoms related to feelings of depression are regularly met by practicing physicians.

These changes brought many uncertainties and anxieties with them. Young men and women were faced with the problem of raising a family with no other adults around to help with the task and with few other families living in close enough association to give them an understanding of the normal variations in development or the phases and stages of growth. The experiences of their own childhood, under different circumstances, did not carry over into the new situation. Books and magazine articles, syndicated newspaper columns, high school and college courses, and adult education groups sprang up in profusion. Much of their reason for being lay in the need to dispel anxieties aroused by changing patterns of living.

Social change is often fraught with anxieties for those caught in the change. New problems require solution. Some people find satisfying solutions of their own. Cultural solutions may allay the anxieties, but the anxieties are there and the ways of allaying them may not be immediately present. Simmons has discussed this problem as it relates to the Hopi Indians[60] and states, "Whenever within a primitive society disruptions occur in cultural patterns and functions, the anxiety-inducing factors tend to outdo the anxiety-reducing factors, thus loading excessive fears upon individuals which, in turn, intensify bodily stresses."

Our society defines the role of husband and wife in broad general terms. For the family as a unit, the father is expected to be the economic provider, the mother the homemaker. This is not universally true, of course. Among American Negroes, though major changes are occurring, in many families the woman still acts as economic provider, despite the presence of an able-bodied male in the household. In this subcultural setting, such a relationship is acceptable. In most American households it would give rise to endless difficulties of adjustment, within both the family and the community. In one young girl raised in such a household marked feelings of social inadequacy developed. She would not take her friends home with her because her father cooked meals and washed dishes while her mother read current events magazines and discussed political issues.

Though these roles of the male provider and female homemaker remain broadly the same in our society, in the patriarchal family and the conjugal family, the way in which these functions are performed are quite different. In the former many adults of both sexes were present to share the duties. The duties allotted to male and female members were discreetly separated by sex though shared by several persons. In the conjugal family, the only person to share duties is of the opposite sex. The sharp differentiation of duties tends to break down, both sexes being more apt to contribute both economically and in the performance of housework. This blurring of male and female roles has required adjustments which have been quite difficult for some persons to make, especially those with conflicts around their masculine or feminine adequacy. Mr. Miller, (p. 75) the man who had neurodermatitis, illustrates the difficulties this may arouse. With increasing feminine demands made upon him, his conflicts about masculinity became sharply emphasized and symptoms developed.

In our society it is commonly considered proper for the male to be the dominant member of the family. He should make the important decisions and care for practical problems. The man who accepts this as an ideal but cannot assume the dominant role in the family may find this stressful. The woman who, aware of the cultural pattern, cannot accept the subordinate role it implies may find the situation equally stressful. The woman who feels that her husband is inadequate because he does not make decisions and handle practical problems in their life may feel depressed and unhappy in her marriage and may make her husband equally unhappy. Because some women resent taking a subordinate role in these matters, a highly competitive relationship may develop between husband and wife. All of these situations derive a great deal of their stressful significance from role differentiations which are culturally determined and are reinforced by social pressures acting through daily interpersonal relations.

The relation between parents and their children is also defined broadly. Parents are expected to give adequate care to their off-spring. Most parents wish to give their children everything they need or everything that the neighbors are providing for their children. Inability to do so may arouse feelings of inadequacy or engender arguments between parents. When the children become sufficiently aware of parental concern in this area, they may learn to manipulate the situation to their own advantage. When a person develops manipulation as a pattern for handling interpersonal relations, difficulties may arise in the doctor-patient relationship.

In child rearing, our society ordinarily expects the father to be the ultimate disciplinarian. Since he is gone most of the day, the mother may take over all of the daily disciplinary problems, but when the father is at home he is expected to take this duty upon himself in most households. This relegation of disciplinary authority to the father makes the male, by generalization, the symbol of authority for most children and affects the pattern of their relationships with other figures in authority. This, however, is affected markedly by the philosophy of child rearing subscribed to by the parents. In a highly authoritarian family, discipline will be handled very differently than it is handled in a family in which child-rearing practices are more indulgent. Obvious frictions arise when one parent has an authoritarian attitude and the other an indulgent attitude. The trend at present seems to be in the direction which Gesell[1] suggested as ideal: disciplinary measures guided by developmental considerations, suiting both what is punished and the way it is punished to the developmental stage of the child. This puts a considerable burden upon the parents, who must learn more about child development and need judgment as well as knowledge to put it into effect.

The source of authority in the family and the manner in which authority is wielded may have very important consequences in reaction patterns developed in the children. Funkenstein reports that, in his experimental setting, students who reacted initially with anger directed outward more frequently identified the father as the chief source of authority in their families and reported a poor relationship with him. Those who reacted initially with anger directed at themselves also more frequently identified the father as the chief source of authority but commonly reported a close and affectionate relationship with him. Those who reacted to the test situation with severe anxiety more frequently identified the mother as the chief source of authority, the father either being absent or perceived as a Casper Milquetoast. It was also of interest that the differentiation of parental roles was reported to be much more pronounced by the group who reacted with anger directed outward than in the group who reacted with anger directed inward. Though these studies relate to two laboratory stress situations using male subjects from a single university campus, the presence of such correlations suggests the possibility that emotional and physiologic reactions may be conditioned by cultural patterns within the family.[20]

In the definition of parental roles, society assigns to the mother the principal role of giving affection. Affection does not derive solely from the mother, but she is expected to be a more constant source of love and understanding than the father. Again, this is affected by the type of family, the number of adults in the household, and by cultural concepts of how affectionate one ought to be and how this should be expressed. There is a difference in the way parents express their affection toward boys and girls, partly based on feelings about masculinity and the desirability of boys being more independent and more stoic than girls and partly on personal factors. Affection can be expressed in many ways, as indicated by such adjectives as warm-hearted, seductive, over-protective, and indulgent. Affection may be used only as part of a reward system to insure obedience. It may be constantly present when needed or may be expressed one day and not another. The ways in which affection is expressed and the things which elicit its expression are quite revealing and tell us a good deal not only about the patient but also about his parents.

The balance between affection and discipline is as important as is each individually. The basic premise in child rearing is that the gains received must equal or exceed the frustrations involved if acquiescence is to be attained without undue strain. The gains are in terms of affection and approval; the frustrations are the demands made in training and discipline.

The background of Marian, the girl with rage attacks (p. 62), illustrates this point well. She described her father, manager of an industrial plant, as both stern and affectionate. However, his sternness was largely reserved for others, since she early learned ways of getting around his attempts at discipline. Her mother was a very inconsistent disciplinarian, wavering between extremes of being very strict and very lax. As a child, Marian had been required to recite verses for family friends and great emphasis was placed on being "a proper little lady." When she did not do what her mother wished, she was locked in a closet or ridiculed in front of others. On one occasion she was struck by the delightful combination of a red jacket and a white mink stole, which she put on and proudly showed her mother. Her mother, however, was horrified that anyone would put mink next to a jersey jacket and exclaimed for months to all her friends, in front of her daughter, at the complete lack of judgment she had shown in clothes. This understandably, aroused considerable hostility in the daughter.

Marian's parents were not happily married, nor was the marriage improved as it became evident that the father cared more for his daughter than he did for his wife. As the relation between father and daughter became closer, the relation between mother and daughter became cold and hostile. Punishment for minor offenses became frequent. When Marian was 8, her mother had a stroke and became a semi-invalid. Her father, apparently feeling guilty, did everything he could to satisfy his wife, and Marian had a secondary position in the family. This increased her feelings of being rejected and unwanted. She came to hate her mother and resented any efforts at discipline from either parent. She became rebellious and reacted to the smallest slight with violent outbursts of temper. She doubted the sincerity of any expression of approval or affection and was constantly testing her parents and her friends. Any failure to reaffirm their devotion to her reawakened her feelings of rejection and anger. Since the affection received was inconstant and inadequate to make up for the disciplinary methods used, Marian rebelled against her parents and all that they valued.

For children to learn their adult roles easily, parents should be persons with whom their children can identify satisfactorily. Much learning is by imitation, often quite unconscious, and children learn their future roles as adults from observing the adults around them. The boy brought up entirely in a female setting has little opportunity to learn masculine ways. Since in adolescence he will be judged by his peers partly in terms of "masculinity," his lack of these patterns of behavior may lead to considerable difficulty during the period of maturing and later. Similarly the boy brought up in an entirely masculine environment may learn little about relating to women as companions and must learn this before he can have a satisfying marriage. Similar problems arise for the girl brought up in a household entirely of one sex or the other. It is important, therefore, to have both a father and a mother in the household, or some substitute figure if death or divorce has dissolved the marriage.

Other important reasons make it desirable to have two or more adults in the household, preferably of different sexes. Children need both affection and discipline. When there is but a single adult in the family, who is therefore the sole source of affection, it may become very difficult, if not actually impossible, for the child to refuse to meet disciplinary demands since this means complete loss of approval. With all things balanced well, the family with a single adult may work out for the child, but a frequent outcome is for the child to become unusually dependent on the parent. This makes severance of the ties in the process of maturing very difficult. In addition, the child is apt to develop a very rigid conscience with a tendency to be compulsive and with great difficulty in expressing hostility. If adequate channels for displacement of anger are not made available, he is forced to suppress, repress, or deny his feelings, and symptoms readily develop in the process of doing this.

For reasons such as these death of a parent, divorce, or prolonged separations are often the focal points of emotional trouble. Fred (p. 56) was raised in such a household; his father was gone years at a time. He overcompensated by developing a very independent nature at a very early age. He displaced his anger easily into neighborhood fights, but he still had difficulties in adjustment and his basic insecurities were quite evident. Charles, the boy with ulcerative colitis (p. 73) spent his first two years alone with his mother and remained her favorite for 5 more years. During this time he became excessively dependent upon her and was totally unable to express any hostility toward her. In fact, for the most part, he was unable to permit himself even to feel any negative emotions for her. Consequently, when she transferred her affections to another and he felt angry at being rejected, the anger could be expressed only in a disguised form. It was displaced to his stepfather.

Society does not confine itself to establishing in a broad way how parents should care for their children. It also defines how children should react to parental discipline and expression of approval. It expects children to be obedient and respectful under most circumstances. The expectation of obedience and respect from children is also strongly supported by religious teachings. When children are raised with an intense awareness of this expectation but are unable to feel the love which they consider to be appropriate, much guilt may be engendered. The deep anxiety which accompanies guilt may cause severe and persistent symptoms.

Parent-child relationships are not the only ones of importance within the family. The relationship of siblings must also be considered. Children, it is believed, should not only love and respect their parents, they should love each other. The insistence on mutual affection is very strong in some families. It is an expression of a religious and cultural force in our society. Trouble comes when it is combined with highly competitive attitudes, especially when parents express their affection and approval only for accomplishments. When this occurs within the family, it may arouse intense sibling rivalry because the fight for the place of honor must be carried on in a setting of mutual love and affection. This combination is hard for some children to achieve. Again, hostilities may develop which are not permitted direct gratification. In the process of inhibiting expression of anger or altering its form, the physiologic changes accompanying anger may be prolonged and symptoms and illness ensue.

An example of this was seen in a 9 year old boy who was one of 5 children. He had an older brother who had done very well in school. He was unable to match his brother's record but found no substitute area in which to excel. Excelling in something was essential to gain approval and affection in the home. He was the best-behaved child in the family and obtained some measure of approval for this show of excellence. But his desire to excel required considerable effort and being "best behaved" meant careful control of his actions, particularly avoidance of any display of temper or rebellion. In this situation he had headaches which were sufficiently frequent and severe to lead to his hospitalization. His desire to excel and his need to inhibit expression of anger were basic factors in his headaches.

Sibling rivalry can have devastating results, particularly when the person who comes out second best is in a position in the family where he would be expected to be first. It is usually expected that older children will be ahead of younger ones in acquiring skills. In one family with two boys 16 months apart in age, the older boy was surpassed in all respects by his younger brother. The two boys were in the same grade in school, and the younger one got better grades with less effort. Besides this, he made friends more easily and was more popular in school. He was active in many extracurricular projects. As a result, he was very much favored at home. In the older of the two asthma and severe personality disturbances developed. A year or so after the older boy had failed his first year in college, while the younger one was getting a scholarship to attend the Massachusetts Institute of Technology, the load became too much. The older one committed suicide.

Spacing of children, which is related in part to cultural ideas, also affects sibling rivalry. The nearer two children are in age the more likely is rivalry to be strong. Successive sex of children is also a determinant of rivalry. Two boys or two girls in succession are more apt to be compared and to compete than are a boy and a girl. The number of children in the neighborhood, the age of joining preschool groups, the size of the family, the age of starting school—all these affect the amount and intensity of rivalry and the form which it takes.[61]

To a certain extent the process works both ways. Parents develop expectations of their children and children develop expectations of their parents. Mrs. Bertrand's complaint in childhood was "my mother never does any of the things for me that other mothers do for their children." This was a source of great resentment. She was not allowed to express this resentment without arousing anger in her grandmother. Many children complain occasionally in this way, and such complaining need not represent any serious deficiency in either parent or child. It does illustrate, however, that children develop expectations of what parents should do, quite apart from what the parents have taught them by their actions.

In the process of growing up, children meet a number of cultural patterns which play a part in shaping personality. The authority which age confers, as expressed in the privileges permitted to older members of the group, imposes frustrations and irritations on all children, whether it is a matter of starting to school, learning to drive an automobile, having the first date without a chaperon, or joining a sorority or fraternity. All of these are governed in general by age patterns that are cultural, though many individual factors affect the way in which it is finally effected. The cultural emphasis on heterosexuality is very important in our society. The anxieties aroused in those who feel homosexual tendencies within themselves may be intense. There are also anxieties in those who can accept heterosexuality but find their individual maturation is not timed exactly with that prescribed by cultural pattern.

Culture also prescribes certain types of sublimations as more desirable than others. High on the list for the younger age groups are competitive sports. Club activities also meet with approval. These are part of another cultural emphasis on extroversion. Introversion is tolerated, but preferably in small amounts and with a rapid return to a more "desirable" attitude toward life. The conflicts which may arise from these cultural emphases have been discussed in such books as Riesman's *The Lonely Crowd*[62] and Whyte's *The Organization Man*.[63] All of these cultural patterns mold personality. Those who lag find many opportunities in daily experiences for the development of anxiety, anger, or depression.

Some of the severest strains, however, occur during the period of seeking a mate and establishing a new family with which to repeat the entire cycle. Many patterns have been established to regulate this process. These begin at approximately puberty and prescribe the age at which dating begins, the roles of the girl and the boy in this process, and the type of behavior sanctioned.[64] Petting is expected and permitted. Though it may arouse intense sexual desires, the immediate gratification of these is usually frowned upon. If pregnancy occurs, the cultural patterns impose heavy pressures toward marriage, whether the union seems desirable from other standpoints or not. Because of the strong sexual taboos and frequent arousal of sexual desires during dating and courtship, symptoms may easily develop. Thus one girl, who had asthma early in adolescence, began to have fainting attacks while on dates late in adolescence. From her account of the sequence of events, it appeared that whenever sexual desires were aroused she fainted. This effectively protected her from participation in sexual activities. It also frequently ended "dating" with that particular boy, thus "protecting" her from repetition of the incident.

Choice of marital partner is supposed to be free in our society. But most parents prefer that marriage be within the same racial and religious group. Many also exert pressures to see that the choice be within the same social class and to a person of similar educational background. Some of these pressures are so strong that they do not need specific strengthening at the time of dating. Marital choice, therefore, is "free" but with many limitations. If the marriage is out of one's own class, social pressures operate to make this upward, though every upward marriage for one person is a downward marriage for the partner. The difficulties which may arise have already been illustrated by Mrs. Winters (p. 19), who became "the janitor" to her husband and children as the result of a marriage into a higher social class where she was not accepted. Choice of partner is much more important for the girl than for the boy, since the status of the husband determines in large part the status of the family. The girl is therefore dependent on choosing the right man for her way of life thenceforth.

Establishing a home brings many new problems—new roles to play, new responsibilities, and a close relationship in which many adjustments and compromises may be required. The potential stresses in this process are numerous though not sufficiently severe to deter most people. Symptoms sometimes develop during the period of adjustment, whether the bride breaks out in hives on the wedding night or the groom has episodes of vomiting during or following the honeymoon. Additional problems accompany pregnancy and the advent of children. The pattern of living may change completely after a child is born. At times, these changes may be difficult to accept. Viewed as frustrations or deprivations, they may give rise to marked or prolonged emotional reactions.

This discussion of the family has emphasized some aspects of life in our American family system which may be viewed as stressful. The physician must know these, not in vague and general terms but quite specifically, so that he will be able to ask appropriate questions and interpret the answers with a full understanding of the expectations and pressures imposed by society. This is as important in trying to ferret out the origins of psychophysiologic disorders as is a knowledge of liver function to an understanding of the manifestations of cirrhosis. If the physician has only a hazy picture of the social organization and cultural milieu in which he and his patients live, he has no point of departure for gaining an understanding of personality problems or of physical complaints which arise in conjunction with stressful life situations.

A system with so many inherent conflicts needs safety valves to allow accumulating tensions to drain off. Such safety valves do exist. The person who finds that hostility is aroused by relationships within the family may allow direct expression (gratification) of his hostility by dominating the family in one way or another. Culturally, this is easier for the father, who has the role of family leader.

It can be achieved in some families by children. It can also be achieved by any member who is ill, since he is then in a position in which society permits demands to be made more freely. Direct gratification occurs but is not socially acceptable when it is recognized as such. Cultural and religious prohibitions on the expression of anger and hostility act as strong deterrents for this type of behavior.

Hostilities may also be expressed indirectly by displacement. Society affords a number of opportunities for displacement of aggressive feelings. Thus hostility aroused in interpersonal relations within the family may be displaced into aggressive competition in sports or in hobbies. During childhood and into early adult life, it may be expressed as well in aggressive competition in school. Displacement into business competition in adulthood is not uncommon. In fact it has been suggested that parental rejection may be a potent spur toward occupational drive.[65] At such times the occupational drive represents an attempt to prove one's worth to oneself and one's family. The hostility manifest in such a drive is plain enough. In some segments of society, displacement of hostility to prejudices and biases toward minority groups is an acceptable mechanism allowing expression of anger which might otherwise go unexpressed.

Anxieties and insecurities aroused at home may be resolved similarly. One may achieve some sense of security by association with other groups, whether clubs at school, the boy scouts, sororities or fraternities, religious organizations, scientific groups, or the Elks Club or Kiwanis Club. All these groups, in addition to their avowed group purposes, are social institutions in which an individual may gain a sense of security through bonds with others. This function is most important when insecurities have been aroused in other relationships. A striking example of this was seen in the comfort and security which Mrs. Bertrand derived from her religious associations during adolescence.

OCCUPATION

Work is another important aspect of life. The satisfactions and dissatisfactions of work may have a considerable influence upon health. The ultimate goal of a physician is to return his patients to productive employment insofar as this is possible. He can often do a great deal to minimize the length of illness and facilitate return to work if he is aware of the motivating forces favoring return to work as well as the forces which tend to prevent or delay it. By strengthening the former forces and weakening the latter, he can sometimes exert a powerful effect upon a patient's motivation as well as upon his ability to work. Much depends upon the patient's concept of his own capacities for work and upon the satisfactions derived from it. These often determine whether he makes the attempt or not. A skillful physician, in the position of family friend and advisor, as well as family physician, can increase or decrease both of these factors. On occasion he can end a productive career by his advice. Such advice should be given sparingly indeed, with every effort bent to maintain productivity whenever possible.

Preparation for adult employment begins early in life in a number of experiences which are not always considered important to one's subsequent work record. Giving the child tasks, graded according to age and capacity and with appropriate approval for satisfactory completion, is considered one way to inculcate a sense of responsibility and a base of experience for occupational pursuits later. In addition to such planned activities, however, many unplanned contacts may strengthen or weaken this pattern. Daily contacts with the father, brief though these may be, give the child some idea of his father's attitude toward work, energy required in doing it, satisfaction gained, and the frustrations encountered. Comparison with other fathers adds more data as a check on what one may expect in hours and pay and how others regard work. If these unplanned contacts give a totally negative picture of the work world, they form a poor basis on which to build a strong motivation to work. However, many other forces are at work.

Another influence active over most of the formative years is the question put by friends, relatives, teachers, and even strangers, "What do you plan to do when you grow up?" This simple, oft-repeated question reiterates society's demand that the person work. Phrased in a way which makes it seem to be a completely open and free choice for the child, it ordinarily arouses no overt rebellion. Yet, by its phraseology, it prevents consideration of not working. The question is never, "Do you plan to work when you grow up?" Society's demand that people work is a powerful motivating force toward working. It should be noted, however, that certain groups and individuals are exempted from the demand for productivity. Among these are the handicapped and the ill. Physicians have frequent occasions to remember this.

Another potent influence in the direction of work is the emphasis put by our culture on achievement and success. For men, especially, success is ordinarily measured in terms of occupation and income. Competition is an integral part of life, fostered in the home, at school, in extramural sports, and in most group activities. Even when group goals require working smoothly together, prestige is accorded the leader, and there is usually competition for this position. In addition, one group is frequently in competition with another. The place where the outcome of that competition is individually most important is on the job. This becomes a potent area of trouble if a person falls short of his goal for himself, even though he may satisfy others.

The economic necessities of life require generally that work be done. The emphasis many segments of our society put upon material possessions increases the pressure to earn more money. In a mobile population with many new suburban communities springing up, possessions confer status more readily than family name and background. Once owned, they also give people a sense of security in having things of their own. Though these forces would seem almost universal in their application, there are people in the upper economic groups who would need do no work to have the possessions they desire, people in the lower economic group who have no desire for possessions, and a few other people on whom these forces operate weakly or negatively.

All of these influences and many others affect the drive toward work in a general sense. The specific type of work chosen is determined by other factors, frequently of a more personal nature and often based on the person's idea of where he is most apt to excel. To this extent, therefore, it is related also to the competitive urge instilled earlier in life. It is conditioned by the goals and standards of one's social class.[66] In addition, it usually is a choice made to satisfy certain desires—to work with people, to be one's own boss, to find variety, and so on. It is also related to family identifications and how satisfying these have been and to standards and goals of the social class from which one stems. But these personal drives toward specific work may be much weaker than the social forces compelling one to do some type of work. Many adolescents and young adults feel they want to do something, but they don't know what. And it should not be forgotten that many people finally drift into work only because they had to do something that was productive, had no great interest in any one thing, and so did whatever was most available.[67]

In our occupational system, choice is based largely on capacity rather than on family background or a caste system. It is therefore competitive. Though competition, when overemphasized, can lead to problems in adjustment, the child who has not been permitted to compete at all during childhood is poorly prepared for the occupational system he meets as an adult. Conflicts engendered within the family may be accentuated or ameliorated by experiences in the occupational field. A striking success vocationally may do much to soften the adverse effects of sibling rivalry in childhood. A good work situation with a sympathetic boss may help to smooth out difficulties which arose in relationships with authority in the family. By the same token, these conflicts may be accentuated and intensified by work experiences. In most work situations there is a hierarchy with discipline and a need to conform to what one's superiors require. There is competition for approval of the superior between the person and his colleagues. When conflicts in these areas are quite intense, a person may seek to avoid them by looking for work in which he is his own boss. This imposes additional responsibilities upon him, however, which sometimes he cannot meet. The competition is removed from the close personal one with colleagues and displaced to a competition with business rivals. Aggression is implicit in the system. Consequently, conflicts around aggression are easily mobilized.

There are additional strains in the occupational system. Ordinarily there is a separation of the sexes so that husband and wife are not working together as they might on the farm or in a small shop of their own. Their goals may be similar but they must go independent ways in trying to achieve them. The wife may have no comprehension at all of what her husband is doing and vice versa. The complete severance of technical aspects from the rest of life puts an additional strain on the family and on the individual. And success at work is important to the entire family. Success at work implies additional income and additional prestige. These carry with them more social and economic opportunities for the family, but the added obligations may put an added burden on the wage earner.

To illustrate how some of these factors affect health consider the story given by Mr. Roberts. He began having acute episodes of tachycardia when he was 27 years old. The first attack occurred when he was at work. He was managing a sales office at the time, a job which he liked. The attack occurred in the middle of one morning and began with a sudden racing of his heart, accompanied by cold perspiration and difficulty in breathing. He "fainted," falling to the ground without actual loss of consciousness. He remained semiconscious, unable to move or speak, for about 15 minutes, though he was fairly well recovered by the time a physician arrived to see him. He had no further attacks for almost a year, but then they became frequent and were associated with a variety of symptoms. In addition to palpitations, tachycardia, and shortness of breath, he had weakness in his hands and knees, numbness and tingling in his hands and around his mouth, a constricting sensation in his chest, pain in the front of his chest and down his left arm, and dizziness. All the early attacks occurred at work, but he soon began having them at home as well. Physical examination and laboratory studies gave no indication of the heart disease from which he thought he suffered.

What had been happening at work? He had never settled into any one job but had gone from one type of work to another, always looking for advancement and success. A year before his first attack he had found a job as manager of a sales office. He worked hard and enjoyed his work, but he soon learned that the salesmen earned more than he did and seemed to have a more relaxed schedule. He asked to be changed to a sales job but his boss refused because he considered him "too valuable in the office." He reacted with considerable bitterness to the boss, who he felt was holding him back. He finally left the job but only after considerable inner turmoil and his first attack of tachycardia. On his next job he found a man who was extremely difficult to deal with. There were numerous personal frictions between them, and when the boss expected him to cover up some shady deals for him he began having attacks again and quit this job. On the third job he was in a position of considerable responsibility but worked under a man who sat at his desk all day doing very little work. His employer took credit for all of the successes of the job, most of them successes which the patient considered were due to his own efforts. He resented this position tremendously, quit this job too, but only after frequent severe attacks. In his last job he again found himself in a position of continual irritations and frustrations with his employer. The attacks became so severe that he feared he was going to die; so he stopped work entirely and did not seek further employment.

A number of things strike anyone hearing this work record. It is quite possible for a person to have four successive bosses, all of whom are frustrating and irritating. It seems unlikely, however, and one wonders if the description is realistic or reflects Mr. Roberts' feelings about authority in general. It would appear that Mr. Roberts had some difficulties in his relationships with people in authority. Why should this be?

To understand his relationships with figures in authority, one asks quite naturally about his father and important male figures in his past. His father drank excessively and was abusive to the family. His mother and father were divorced when he was but a few years old. From then onward his mother's brother was the dominating male in his life. For many years his mother worked for the uncle, who had several businesses and was very successful financially. He hired his sister during the depression, at 50 dollars a month, to work 12-hour days. He never increased her pay. Consequently the patient's mother was out of the home most of her waking time, working for an inadequate salary, and the family was economically hard pressed. The patient felt economically and socially inferior to his classmates at school. He felt that he had been subjected to an unnecessarily hard youth and put the blame for all of this on his uncle.

When he started college his grandfather had cancer of the prostate with metastases to many of the bones of his body and was in constant pain. He needed frequent narcotic injections. The uncle refused to give these, saying that he loved his father too much to stick a needle in him. He therefore called the patient home from college, telling him that he would have to stay with the grandfather to give him morphine injections every 3 hours. Consequently, Mr. Roberts found himself for 6 months in the home of his dying grandfather, giving injections every 3 hours night and day. He could not go out to see a movie or have a date on Saturday night because there was no one else to give the injections. He resented this tremendously. In addition, he never got back to college and he blamed his uncle for his lack of education. With these early experiences in life, it is easy to understand why he had difficulties with authority. He viewed people in authority as frustrating and reacted to the demands they made in the same way he reacted to those made by his uncle. There is no need to give all the details of his work record. He had had many jobs before the first one recorded here and had gone through a similar emotional pattern with each of them. His relationship with his mother began as a very close one, but it gradually deteriorated. Though she had wanted to be a good mother, she was away from home 12 hours a day and was always worn out in the evenings. Thus she had little time or energy to give him the affection or care he needed. This was far less significant to him, however, than another difficulty which arose early in his life. By adolescence he was aware that his mother was "going steady" with a married man. They lived in a small town and he knew his friends at school were aware of what his mother was doing and disapproved of it. He also became aware during these years that his relatives disapproved very much and tried often to force his mother to break off the relationship. However, she seemed unable to do this, and he continued to live in fear of his classmates' comments. He was never quite able to forgive his mother. In any event, his ties to her were weak; his ties to his father were weaker. He had one sister, and his relationship with her was the only one he considered close.

His wife, on the other hand, came from a large, closely knit family. As people in her family got married they were inclined to settle close to the parental home. Ties were strong and there was much visiting back and forth. Mr. Roberts knew this when he married but did not stop to think of himself in such a situation. He had expected his wife to live with him and share his way of life. He found it very hard to accept her family's free and easy way of visiting. If any of them came to the town where he lived, they felt that they had to stay overnight in his home and they did so, invited or not. When he told his wife he would prefer that they stay at a motel, she found it impossible to suggest it to them. They certainly never thought it proper to do so themselves. Relatives came in from all directions. If there were not enough beds and couches available, they slept on the floor. Consequently, Mr. Roberts would come home from work at night for a quiet evening with his wife and stumble over two or three bodies on the living room floor as he came in the front door. It was at such times that his attacks of pain at home began. In addition to this, he knew that his wife's family did not have a high opinion of him. He had high goals and ambitions, but he had gone from one job to another without achieving any of the goals. He was very sensitive on this subject. He allowed his wife to work because she wanted to work and enjoyed it. But her family felt that this was merely another evidence of his failure to support her adequately. The comments about this were subtle or jesting, but the implications behind them were never lost on the patient. Consequently he hated to see his wife's family.

Here we have a clash between two people raised in different family structures and trying to establish a family of their own. We also have a man who, largely because of unsatisfactory relationships with authority in early life, found it impossible to work with his employers and whose early initiation into work was unsatisfying and whose work experiences were without real gratification. But such problems have been faced by others. Why is this patient unable to cope with these problems? If he has difficulties with employers and bosses, why not find a job where he can be his own boss? If he cannot tolerate his wife's family, why not avoid seeing them, either by asking them not to come or by moving to some place where they will not?

The answers to these questions are complex, but most of the difficulties stemmed from the fact that this patient, despite a fine physique and superior intelligence, felt inadequate and dependent on other people. Perhaps the pattern for this was set by his mother's reactions to her brother, for whom she worked for an inadequate salary for 12 or 15 years because she was afraid to leave the security of the town she knew and look for a job elsewhere. In short, she was afraid to do what Cy Logan had done. She felt inadequate to stand on her own feet. She felt dependent on her family for help. Mr. Roberts had similar feelings. With all his resentment of his uncle, he yet felt dependent on him. He felt forced to get along with him at all costs, lest his mother lose her security. His feelings of inferiority to his colleagues at school must also have made him feel inadequate. In any event, he reached adulthood feeling that he could not stand completely on his own despite a tremendous desire to do so and a deep resentment at being dependent on anyone else. His concept of himself as inadequate and his resentment at being in a dependent relationship to others could not do otherwise than lead him into successive dependent positions attended by frustration and resentment.

His life story is a long succession of such events. Successive frustrations and repeated arousal of anger were so intense that he feared they might overpower him. As an expression of this, anxiety attacks developed with all of the symptoms described. Thus we can trace the successive links in the chain between family structure and the occupational system, through difficulties in adjusting to both, to the probable release of epinephrine in association with anxiety, the development of hyperventilation, and the appearance of symptoms. He was accustomed to a few intense relationships and wished to have one with his wife. She was accustomed to diffuse emotional ties and could neither understand nor give what he desired. She was absorbed in her family, seemed to gain a sense of her own identity from it, and could not understand how anyone could love her and not also love her relatives. He had a distaste for relatives in general and saw in them only a threat to the close ties he wished to have with his wife. Their arguments on this score were frequent and at times violent. They had very different ideas on child rearing and on the type of home they wished to have. Much hostility was aroused in this situation and his anxiety attacks were in part related to his fear of losing control of the anger he felt toward both his wife and her relatives.

GROUP ASSOCIATIONS

While family and work relationships occupy a sizeable portion of life, another large segment is spent in group associations with neighbors, in clubs and organizations, and with other people of similar background and interests. These group associations and the relation of the individual to them are determined to a great extent by the social stratum in which the individual is placed, that is, by social class. Major factors in determining class position are income and occupation, though these are not the sole determinants. A family which for generations has had high social position in the community as a member of the upper class may maintain that position despite limited financial reserves. A family which has never had high social status does not achieve it through wealth alone. Yet occupation and income are the route by which change in position can be effected.

SOCIAL CLASSES

The features which distinguish one class from another have been described by Warner[68] and others.[69] Though this classification has been criticized, it is a useful starting point. Criteria of class vary from one section of the country to another and from one type of living to another. Thus class distinctions in urban and rural communities and in mining districts and farming regions differ. In addition, standards change from generation to generation. Yet class distinctions exist, even though the specific features differ from place to place and from time to time. Warner divides society into three major classes, upper, middle and lower and each of these into two segments, upper and lower.

The lower segment of the upper class has been described[70] as a group who are wealthy and spend their wealth in a quietly ostentatious way on large houses and expensive hobbies. They tend to marry late and to have relatively small families. A high percentage of their members hold professional or administrative positions. They belong to prominent clubs and organizations; their children attend private schools; their interests are broad and inclined to be national rather than purely local. They plan ahead, are interested in intellectual activities, and have a relatively low crime rate.

The upper segment of the lower class, on the other hand, is described as just getting by financially and spending their money on food and warmth. In general they live in poor housing, marry early, and have large families. Occupationally, they tend to be unskilled laborers. Their group associations are largely union memberships; their education is whatever is possible within their income. They have a high crime rate, especially against property. Their major concern is with their immediate security, and their interests apart from this are with sports, especially spectator sports.

The middle class between these two is made up largely of clerical workers and skilled laborers. Their ideology focuses around two major mottos; one is to keep up with the Jones's and the other emphasizes virtue and goodness, with the world painted largely in black and white. The upper middle class is most concerned with keeping up with the neighbors, and the lower with virtue.

It is probable that people's attitudes toward social position are more important to health in terms of psychophysiologic disorders than is actual social class. An attitude toward social position is present whether a person is aware of social class as such or not. He is aware in a general way of where he stands in relation to others. He is subjected repeatedly to cultural pressures to improve himself, to get ahead in the world, acquire more possessions, live in better housing and better areas. These goals are accepted socially and are the basic drives for rising in the social scale, "social climbing."

They are approved by society, but they represent an attitude toward social class. Less approved but more comfortable is contentment with one's status in life without a drive to alter it. An attitude allowing decline in status, even in the face of adversity, is discouraged.

The drives of "climbers" subject them to stresses.[70] Their goals force them to take on added responsibilities and to strive to do a little more all the time. Within limits, this need result in no symptoms and no illness. But it sets the stage for trouble, particularly if a man fails to improve his lot despite all his efforts or succeeds in improving it only by tremendous effort. This attitude toward social position, though culturally accepted, intensifies feelings of frustration when striving to improve one's position fails. It therefore is one of the factors determining what will be stressful and how stressful it will be.

The attitude conducive to social decline is, in our society, an indication of personality difficulty. Even in the face of disaster one is expected to maintain or try to improve one's position. Those who decline socially without trying not to usually do so by virtue of despair or hopelessness or because of rebellion against the pressures society has imposed. Mrs. Bertrand's father was such a person (p. 26). He felt completely overwhelmed by the demands and expectations of his parents, particularly his father, and removed himself as far as possible from all competition.

The people with whom one associates are determined in large part by one's social level. This determines where one lives and how well one is accepted there. It influences the schools one attends and the clubs and organizations one joins. It affects the church one attends. It influences one's chance meetings with other people. Belonging to a group confers the security of the group as well as the status of the group. Being a member of groups exposes one to varied attitudes and gives a clearer perspective of his position in the community at large. Security thus gained helps minimize problems of insecurity aroused in other relationships. Contrariwise, when security cannot be gained in this way, insecurities previously present may be acutely exacerbated and illness result. One girl of 19 had her first episode of ulcerative colitis when she failed to be pledged by the sorority of her choice even though accepted by other groups. She had had emotional problems before without symptoms. The seriousness to her of rejection by the sorority was evident in the fact that she dropped out of college and never completed her education.

The relation between social class and mental health has been studied in a number of surveys. A study undertaken in New York[71] reported that manifestations of anxiety have a fairly uniform distribution through all classes, though certain psychiatric entities appear to be concentrated in the lower classes. Depressions, hypochondriasis, alcoholism, latent psychosis, hypertension, arthritis, and "sciatica" were commoner in the lower classes. The same investigators found the incidence of peptic ulcer to be uniform at all social levels. Colitis, urticaria, and hay fever were commoner among members of the upper classes. The incidence of asthma showed peaks at both ends of the social scale. In terms of direction of movement, these workers found that severe psychiatric disturbances were much more frequent among people declining in the social scale than among those rising.

A study of social factors in rheumatoid arthritis has been reported by King and Cobb.[72] They found the disorder commoner when there was a marked discrepancy between education and income; they considered that this discrepancy probably represented social mobility. They also reported rheumatoid arthritis to be more common among women who had 4 or more children and who said that they had had no free time during the third decade of life. Since the correlation required the combination of these factors they felt that the pertinent factor might be the strain imposed by maintaining household duties and outside social obligations, since these double duties may easily arouse role conflicts and be associated with excessive demands and the accumulation of many tensions and frustrations.

SCHOOL

In addition to family and informal group relationships, school activities occupy a sizable portion of the time of children, adolescents and young adults. In this setting many of the problems which have been mentioned in connection with family life are met again. Discipline is involved in the learning process, and differences in age between teachers and students parallel those between parents and children. Teachers therefore may be substitutes for parents psychologically. The problems of affection, discipline, and identification are met again, and rebellions aroused at home may be expressed at school. The way in which these problems are handled determines whether problems arising at home are accentuated or alleviated at school. The child who feels rejected at home may find acceptance at school and achieve some sense of adequacy and security. Competitive drives aroused at home may be expressed freely at school in striving to excel. This may drain off some of the hostility aroused in competition at home. Emphasis on the spirit of fair play in school sports continues the rivalry amid mutual affection that has been stressed at home. Adequacy in performance is an important feature of school life. School activities help to broaden a child's concept of himself. That unsatisfactory school experiences may cause considerable difficulty was illustrated by the boy who did less well than his younger brother (p. 112).

RELIGION

Church activities play a somewhat similar role in many ways, but with other functions peculiarly their own. Religious practices of the family are important in setting the stage for the child's reaction to religion; but, as with other things, a child's feeling for his family affects his acceptance of these family attitudes. A child who feels rejected at home but accepted in the church may have strong religious attachment regardless of home attitudes. The church can give a sense of belonging, a feeling of having roots in society, and a sense of security which can be obtained nowhere else except in the family. When these are present in the family, religion can serve to strengthen them. Religion also gives solace in the face of acts of fate and disaster which might otherwise arouse feelings of anger or despair. Religion, by virtue of the solace and security it has to offer, can prevent or ameliorate suffering and illness.

Religion may mean many things. It may serve as a parent substitute, and people can act out their difficulties in adjustment in religion. Religion is a source of discipline, teaching moral precepts by which people guide their lives. Rebellion against authority may be expressed here. Because of the great security and the love which religion can offer, rebellion against its authority is difficult for anyone who has once felt security through it. When rebellion occurs, it is ordinarily expressed verbally in the form of arguments and discussions concerning free will and the tenets of religion. Religious teachers can do much to ease conflicts around authority and submission to it. In fact, rebellion against one's father and substitutes for him may be resolved in working out one's relationship to God.

One potent source of trouble in religion is the sense of guilt it may arouse. Guilt is used as a weapon by the church to help people do what is "right." But guilt is a form of anxiety and depression, and it can be associated with all of the symptoms of these emotional states. Thus it may give rise to illness or prolong illness. Religious strictures against the expression of hostile and sexual impulses strengthen the tendencies to deny and repress these feelings and the ideas associated with them. Some people try to deny the hardships with which they are faced as a way of avoiding any appearance of complaining against God. Repression of hostility avoids the sense of guilt which feeling the emotion and inhibiting its expression might arouse. To the extent that denial and repression are emphasized by religious teachings, they contribute to hysterical manifestations. The tendency to such manifestations is particularly strong when these strictures are prominent. One would expect to see them more frequently, therefore, in members of the Catholic Church and in evangelical sects of the Protestant Church. The religious coloring of some hysterical symptoms is a representation of the forces striving to control the repressed idea or affect.

VALUES

Value systems are closely linked with religion in our culture, though they are shaped by family and community associations as well. One of these value systems surrounds interpersonal relations. Thus we have different sets of standards for relationships with relatives, friends, business associates, and business rivals. We expect a different degree and a different kind of loyalty and honesty from these different people. We conduct our contacts with them with different values in mind. These standards control behavior largely without awareness, except when one set of standards conflicts with another in the same situation. At such times the person may have considerable conflict over what his behavior ought to be.

Values in regard to achievement[73] set up a hierarchy in which a person places financial, intellectual, spiritual and social success in terms of their relative importance and their pertinence to his own way of living. He will then judge his success or failure in terms of this hierarchy.

There are other value systems—those which set certain goals as more desirable than others, those that set certain gratifications as acceptable while others are not, and those that define the types of sublimation which are permissible in our culture. Whether a person sets up his own personal set of standards as preferable for him to what he perceives as socially accepted is also determined by a value judgment on his part. Whether one patterns his life for present benefits or is oriented to future rewards is also a value judgment and, like the others, determines how one reacts to situations.

These value judgments are extremely important in establishing what a person will be like and how he will act. They are often formulated without examination or even verbalization to himself of the basis for them. They set the goals toward which one will strive, both in personal behavior and in relationships with others. By determining goals and aims in life, they affect what is stressful. They are derived in large part from social sources, including religion, but they are deeply affected by personal conflicts and emotional problems. When goals lead one into a situation which he cannot handle adequately, intense feelings of frustration, severe anxiety, or utter despair and hopelessness may result. He must either seek new pathways by which to achieve the goals or must reexamine them in an attempt to solve the dilemma. At such times the physician may be able to help a patient examine his value systems and their sources, thereby giving him the opportunity of deciding whether pursuit of the goals is sufficiently important to justify its continuance in the face of emotional strain and physical illness.

As with social class, in addition to the value system itself there is personal orientation to the system. This can be a source of added stress and strain. If a person has a rather passive orientation to cultural values and social customs he accepts them as transmitted without any strong convictions about them and with no desire to force other people to live in the same fashion. Such an orientation ordinarily is associated with little stress or strain, either within the person or in his relationships with others.

On the other hand, some people have a very active orientation to values and customs. They not only accept what has been transmitted but take it upon themselves to teach these values and customs to others and to insist on conformance. Such people may be very disturbed when others do not play their roles in the approved fashion and do not accept the same standards which they accept, and may be extremely demanding of those around them. An active orientation is often considered more desirable, since it serves to maintain customs and value standards. However, certain limitations are ordinarily imposed upon the way values and customs are taught to others and the degree of conformance insisted upon.

Another active orientation is that of the person who has no interest in forcing others to conform but concentrates on satisfying his own desires in the most expedient way. He manipulates values, customs, and people to get his own way, using whatever value standard serves him best at the moment. This may not be approved socially but it is not an uncommon way of handling situations. The unwary physician may easily find himself being used by such a patient to achieve ends with which he has no sympathy. He must be able to recognize what is happening before he can handle such a situation.

Finally there is the deviator who makes his own rules in some area of living and ignores the socially accepted patterns. The stresses arising as a result of this depend largely upon how others react to these new rules.

In relation to the effects these orientations have on health, it can be seen that a passive orientation produces the least strain and an active one the most. The distinction between passive and active, though easily made in their extreme forms, is not a black and white one but a continuous progression from apathy to combinations of passivity in one realm and activity in another. However, the person who is actively oriented to his culture may find life quite stressful and may develop strong emotional reactions in the course of his daily activities.

Gladys was a 24 year old patient with many problems related to her orientation to social class and values. Her orientation to her way of life was active, and she expected others to conform and taught them to do so. She was striving to improve her social position. Her strong competitive drives and rigid value systems brought her into sharp conflict with her husband and prevented her from achieving any personal happiness. She came to the hospital because of frequent, excruciating, disabling headaches which began when she was 4. She was not sure of their exact nature before the age of 12, though she recalled that before that time the trouble was blamed on her stomach, since vomiting always relieved the headache. After the age of 12, however, she had two types of headaches and felt that she had had more days with headache than without. One type was a dull ache of mild intensity and long duration, usually temporal in location. These might continue for weeks or months at a time or might last but a few hours or days. The other headaches were vascular in nature. They came suddenly after a brief prodromal period in which she felt as though something within her were about to fly out through her head. The headaches which followed were intense, throbbing, and frontal. She was always nauseated with these headaches and might vomit repeatedly. Noises disturbed her greatly. These headaches were infrequent before her marriage at 18.

She had a son 4 years old who could read his own story books to himself. She had put him on an allowance of 10 cents a week. She felt this was very important because it was one of the things which she had not been taught. It disturbed her greatly when his father bought him candy bars after he had spent all of his allowance on a comic book. She did not feel that her husband understood the seriousness of what she was trying to teach their son. She was also disturbed that her husband would not spank the boy when he had been naughty but said that he was the best behaved boy in the neighborhood, so why punish him. She answered that he was the best behaved boy in the neighborhood because she had trained him to be. Training required discipline and discipline required cooperation of the two of them. Their discussions about child rearing were monologues during which he gave his undivided attention and seemed to hang on her every word. He never gave active assent, however, and never took an active part in discipline. She felt frustrated by this. She liked everything to be neat and orderly. She did not think that she was extreme on this point but said that she sometimes literally had to follow her husband around with an ashtray in order to keep things neat. She had taught her son to be neat and orderly. She started him right by teaching him not to climb on the furniture so that the furniture would not be marked or scuffed.

There were many other sources of friction with her husband. She had always wanted to associate with the "elite." They lived in a very good neighborhood but their neighbors were not "the best people" so she held herself aloof from them and tried to limit her son's play with neighborhood children. She would have liked moving to a better part of town but her husband could not stand "ritzy" people. He had already moved as far up the social ladder as he cared to go. Because of her feelings about the neighbors, they had few neighborhood friends. Since she and her husband could not agree on clubs, they belonged to none. She felt the social isolation keenly.

They also had disagreements over money and how it should be spent. She felt that the more expensive items lasted longer and therefore were cheaper in the long run. He seriously doubted this. She wanted whatever she bought—clothing for herself or furnishings for the home—to be the best. He believed she bought many needless things and spent money with abandon, and they had many heated arguments over financial matters.

One headache followed an argument with her husband while they were making a rapid vacation trip to Colorado. She felt they should visit some acquaintances en route so as not to hurt their feelings, though neither she nor her husband really wanted to spend their time in this way. A long argument ensued. Her complaints later were that he should have been willing to observe the social amenities whether pleasant or not, he should not have raised his voice in arguing with his wife nor have implied that she did not know what was proper under the circumstances. He should, in short, have known his role as husband better than that. Besides, she would have felt she was not living up to her social obligations had she not called. The argument lasted so long that they had no time to make the call. He therefore "won" the argument and she had a severe vascular headache.

On another occasion, after prolonged disagreements with her husband, she began sleeping with her son. She expected this to arouse some comment from her husband and thus open the way for a discussion of some of their difficulties. Her husband, however, made no comment. This unsatisfactory state of affairs continued for 6 weeks, during which she suffered from a constant muscle tension headache.

Gladys's story illustrates many of the statements made earlier in this chapter. She came from a middle-class background, was striving to reach the top socially, and saw everything in black and white. One either adhered to established manners and customs perfectly or one was unacceptable. There were no alternative solutions. She was a social climber by desire and was in conflict with her husband who had risen as far as he could without being acutely uncomfortable. She wished to use the family as a vehicle to social betterment; he wished to use the family as a haven of refuge from the stress and strain of daily living. Their ideas of child rearing were quite different, and therefore in her opinion he was not playing the role of father properly. She found it difficult to play her own role to her satisfaction since her ideas conflicted with those of her husband and son, and this gave rise to frequent arguments, which were contrary to her ideal of the good wife and mother.

Gladys had accepted these values from her parents without ever being aware of their origin nor ever having given them any thought. This was the "right" way. That there might be more than one right way had never occurred to her. The value system by which she lived placed propriety and social position above marital happiness. Yet when confronted with this fact she felt that a happy marriage was much more meaningful ultimately than social position. Her actions seemed to place "good behavior" above all else for her son, yet intellectually, at least, she recognized that this should be tempered considerably to allow him to develop into a normally active, healthy boy. She had not stopped to consider where her actions would lead nor on what they were based.

In treatment many of these matters were discussed with her in terms both of the social and cultural forces which influenced her behavior and of the conflicts within herself which found expression in this medium. Her orientation to society, her drive to make others conform to her way of life, her competitive nature, and her feelings about masculine and feminine roles in life all needed discussion. The discussion focused on the origins of these forces, the validity of them, the direction they carried her, and alternative ways of handling her problems. In this way she was able eventually to find a more satisfying way of life, less stressful to the whole family, and relatively free of symptoms.

Chapter 6

Constitution and Conflict

THE NEWBORN INFANT

THE newborn infant is sometimes described as though he were a colorless, amorphous chunk of protoplasm whose only activity was suckling. Such a description is wrong. Hooker's studies[74] on the appearance of reflexes and the order of behavioral development (using abortions, miscarriages, and premature deliveries) revealed an extensive behavioral development before full term delivery. Movements of individual parts of the body and specific reflexes appear quite early in fetal development. By the time of birth, many reflexes besides the sucking reflex are present, and many activities aside from nursing are possible. The description of the newborn which treats him as though he were formless and without personality seems to imply that all newborn infants are alike. It suggests that everyone begins the same way, with the same native endowments, though they mature in different fashion. But, just as newborn infants have different parents, who see their roles as mother and father differently and therefore meet infants' needs differently, so each infant has different endowments which make him respond in an individual manner to what his parents do. The interactions between an individual and his environment determine his course of development. Some of the factors in the environment which affect these interactions have been mentioned; but one must also be aware of a person's innate endowment if he is to understand the diversity of interactions which may occur.

Much has been said about the helplessness of the newborn. It is certainly true that, viewed in isolation, infants are completely dependent on those around them for care. However, when viewed in the social context in which an infant lives, his helplessness is a relative matter. Some infants are in complete command of the situation. Mrs. Bertrand's daughter for instance, was not helpless during her first 2 years of life. Strong social forces, as well as personal ones, bring about this situation, but the presence of these social forces means that the infant is not utterly helpless in the ordinary home. He may master the situation through vocalization, despite his inability to perform any of the necessary functions of care for himself. He soon learns that crying brings help. In a favorable situation he also learns in a few months that smiling and cooing bring affectionate responses from those around him. Perhaps the importance of vocalizing in infancy contributes to the significance of nonverbal communication later in life. A considerable amount of communication occurs between the infant and his parents through tone of voice and manner of handling, quite apart from any specific words or specific actions. This is true later in life as well. The tone of voice in speaking means far more than the words used. "Yes, dear," may be a source of exasperation or of delight. The nonverbal part of the communication is the essential message.

PHYSIQUE AND TEMPERAMENT

Though studies of physique have concentrated on young adults, it is a common observation that children vary similarly in physical build. The infant who is long and thin is apt to develop into an adult who is tall and thin rather than into one who is short and fat. The most extensive single mass of information about differences in body build is that of Sheldon.[75] After a study of several thousand young men of college age, he classified body build on a scale with three extremes rather than the conventional two. These three types could be called the fat, the lean, and the muscular. The fat body type is endomorphy; the lean is ectomorphy, and the muscular is mesomorphy. People usually are not of one body type to the exclusion of the other two. Ordinarily in any one person there are components of all three, but one predominates.

The person who is predominantly endomorphic has soft, rounded body contours, short limbs, and little muscle relief. The ectomorphic person is characterized by a delicate, linear frame, long extremities, and little muscle around the shoulder and pelvic girdles. The mesomorphic person is characterized by squareness and hardness of the body contours and prominent muscles on the trunk and extremities.

In addition to general body build, a conspicuous feature of physique is the extent to which traits of the opposite sex are noted. This is gynandromorphy. Such intrusion of traits of the opposite sex is most common in males who are endomorphic and in females who are mesomorphic, but it may occur with any type of body build. When present in the male, the hips are wider, body contours appear softer, the bones are smaller, and the curve of the thigh forms a full, even sweep. There may be some simulation of breast development. Changes such as these may be a source of considerable difficulty to a male in his social adjustment, especially during adolescence.

Sheldon [76] also described three types of temperament. Viscerotonic people are relaxed and slow and love physical comfort. They are amiable and have a rather even emotional flow. When in trouble, they like to be with other people. Somatotonic people are assertive and energetic and love physical adventure. They enjoy exercise, are somewhat callous emotionally, and are apt to have unrestrained voices. They are oriented to the goals and activities of youth and, when disturbed, feel the need of action. Cerebrotonic people are characterized by restraint in posture and movement. They like privacy and dislike social gatherings. It is hard for them to establish habits and their attitudes are somewhat unpredictable. Their orientation is apt to be to the later period of life, and when troubled they wish to be alone.

Sheldon tells us that these different types of people differ physiologically and in the types of symptoms they are prone to develop. Somatotonic people are apt to have hypertension but infrequently get gastrointestinal upsets. Cerebrotonic people have an overreactive gastrointestinal tract and their pulse and respiratory rates are extremely responsive to external stimuli such as pain. They get nauseated quickly and faint easily.

CONSTITUTIONAL CONFLICT

The three types of body build and the three temperaments distinguished by Sheldon were rated so that numbers could be assigned to patterns of body build and temperament. In a study of 200 persons selected for evaluation, it was found that perfect agreement between the two was not common (14 of the 200). But those in whom agreement was perfect were well integrated and generally well adjusted. No one with radical disagreement between body build and temperament had achieved a normal adjustment without considerable effort. When the rating of temperament fell outside the known patterns for physique, adjustment seemed to be hopeless.

These findings suggest that some people have inherent constitutional conflicts within themselves regardless of what problems are posed by their environment. A person of somatotonic temperament (one who is aggressive, loves physical adventure and sports, and is basically competitive in his orientation to others) who is of ectomorphic physique (with poor posture, flat chest, slender arms, and little muscle) is faced with a dilemma in which he must adjust his aggressive and competitive urges or accept failure as the outcome of his efforts. Such a struggle may be associated with great tension as he tries to reach a *modus operandi* between his desires and his capacities. On the other hand, where physique and temperament correspond there need be no problem. A somatotonic, mesomorphic person has the physique to match his temperament and need only adjust them both to social demands.

BEHAVIORAL CHARACTERISTICS

Some behavioral characteristics are determined before birth and may be evident very early in life. Gesell and his co-workers[1] say that certain traits can be readily appraised in infancy before the sixteenth week: (1) energy output, both amount and intensity; (2) motor demeanor; (3) self-dependence; (4) emotional expressiveness, and (5) readiness of smiling. Frequently, social responsiveness, communicativeness, and adaptability can also be evaluated during the first 4 months. These are early expressions of the behavioral and temperamental characteristics which Sheldon was studying in an older group. That the differences can be identified within the first weeks of life gives stronger weight to their hereditary nature than to their origin as a response to social and cultural molding.

Sleep patterns vary. Ilg and Ames[77] report that the endomorphic or viscerotonic person has a deep, easy sleep. He goes to sleep quickly and awakens with difficulty. The somatotonic person, on the other hand, loves to be awake and active. He has a low sleep requirement and is by nature an early riser. He goes to sleep fairly easily, however, sleeps well and seldom dreams. The cerebrotonic individual hates to go to sleep but once asleep hates to wake up. It is hard for him to go to sleep, and he awakens easily. His sleep is light and unrelaxed. He is apt to dream a good deal and is apt to need more hours of sleep than somatotonic people.

Eating patterns vary from person to person as well, and these differences are evident early in life. There are differences in the vigor with which newborn infants nurse, in the quantity of food taken at one time, in the interval between feedings, in the ease with which an infant is weaned, and in the willingness to suck on nipples, bottles, thumbs, and other objects. The viscerotonic person is seldom, if ever, a feeding problem. He eats well and has a good digestion. The somatotonic person is a hearty eater and may readily overeat. The cerebrotonic eats little, eats rapidly, gains little, but somehow remains healthy.

Differences in emotional display and ability to socialize with others are evident early in life. Some infants are very responsive to people around them, while others are not. Viscerotonic people are apt to be warm in their relations to people, affectionate, communicative and loving. Cerebrotonic children, on the other hand, are secretive, unaffectionate, restrained, and apt to suffer in silence and to be emotionally inhibited. While the somatotonic child is noisy, vigorous and assertive, the cerebrotonic is apt to be very sensitive, to be overly aware of stimuli about him, and to have a relatively low threshold of attention, though once interested he can concentrate intently.

A difference in response to painful stimuli is also evident in infancy. Some infants will cry vigorously after a slight painful stimulus, whereas others will endure this easily. The difference in response to pain is clearly evident during childhood, though it is difficult from this time on to separate social conditioning from innate sensitivity to painful stimuli.

But how do these innate constitutional differences influence the occurrence of stress or contribute to the formation of conflicts? Because of the relative helplessness of infants, every child is raised by adults, whether his parents or others. If they subscribe to an authoritarian philosophy of child rearing, their way of fulfilling their role is apt to be quite different than it would be if they saw their role as one of allowing the child to develop on his own insofar as possible. If a parent believes that children should be seen but not heard, the noisy, assertive, destructive child of somatotonic temperament is apt to have a difficult time. Many stresses will arise; many punishments will be given. The cerebrotonic or viscerotonic child will have less difficulty over this particular injunction. If the parent feels that children should sleep a certain amount each day and the child is one who needs little sleep or naps with difficulty, there may be conflicts between the child and his environment. If feeding is on a rigid schedule and the infant's eating pattern does not fit this schedule, another stressful situation arises. If the parents feel that children should be affectionate and the child is restrained and emotionally inhibited, there may be further difficulties. All of these traits, therefore, can produce stresses when they do not coincide with the expectations or demands of the family in which the child is being reared.

Here, then, we have the individual in conflict with his environment rather than in conflict with himself as in the case of difficulties arising between temperament and physique. Mrs. Bertrand (p. 26) had had difficulty of this sort in childhood. She had been an active and assertive child, predominantly somatotonic in temperament. Her grandparents had imposed many restrictions upon her in an effort to curb these traits. They wished her to "act like an adult," for they found noise and youthful activity disturbing.

Even when no open conflict results from these behavior traits, they serve to establish the pattern of interpersonal relations and reactions to stressful situations. Fred (p. 56) seemed to be both cerebrotonic and ectomorphic, a tall, thin, small-boned youth who liked to be by himself. When his father left home, he responded by withdrawing into himself. By nature unaffectionate, the events of his early years led him to be even more so. His mother therefore gave her attention and affection to his younger brother. Consequently he matured without having had a close or warm relationship with either parent.

When pain is associated with expression of a drive, whether the pain of disapproval or physical punishment, the child tends to alter his behavior so as to avoid the pain. If he repeats similar behavior, he will usually feel anxiety in anticipation of punishment. In altering the behavior so as to avoid punishment in the future, any of the mental mechanisms may be called into play. The child may avoid the activity, even to the point of refusing to eat. He may try to suppress or inhibit his destructive tendencies or to fit his eating patterns to the demands of those rearing him. Or he may repress the undesirable impulse. Symptoms, therefore, may result from this initial conflict between the self and the environment.

A parent who is concentrating on teaching his child some behavioral pattern, such as sitting quietly, not being destructive, or meeting a particular eating schedule, is actually teaching his child much more than this. He is also teaching the type and severity of disciplinary measures which will be used, the degree of conformance which is required, the amount of understanding he has for the child, and the amount of affection. In the process of interaction, the child forms some idea of how "good" he is and how adequately he meets the expectations of his parents. Discipline is necessary. The undisciplined child is not socialized adequately to live in society easily. But the parent who is concentrating only on the behavioral pattern which he is trying to teach his child may lose sight of the fact that he is also teaching him that his parents are harsh and rigid with little affection or understanding. This was true for Marian (p. 62), who was forced to recite verses for her mother's friends and who was punished by ridicule or by being locked in a closet. The lack of understanding and affection was clearly evident in the type of punishment meted out.

DEVELOPMENTAL PATTERNS

In addition to certain features of body build and certain traits of temperament which may be constitutionally determined and influence one's reaction to his environment, there are also developmental patterns. The rapidity with which a person matures is largely innately determined and these patterns vary from one person to another. Puberty changes are perhaps the most dramatic of these maturation processes and illustrate the point well. Though the overwhelming majority of people experience puberty during their teens, there is nonetheless much variation in its exact time. Pubertal changes are of great importance and the variations from one person to another may on occasion have considerable emotional impact. Developmental patterns of physical, intellectual, emotional, and social growth are of great importance in determining a person's relationship with others and his evaluation of himself.

Early learning experiences seem to be of overwhelming importance in personality formation and in creating the philosophy by which the problems of life are met. Because of the importance of this philosophy and its permeation through all stages of development, the physician who traces a conflict in adult life back to its origins is apt to find these rooted in the earliest learning experiences. In addition, there is a difference in early and later learning processes. When one learns something new, having learned something in the same area previously, he must first unlearn the old and then learn the new. Thus two processes are involved, whereas in the earliest learning period there is only one. This should not lead us to ignore the importance of later learning experience, for the solution to early conflicts may lie in such experience. Were this not so there would be little value to psychotherapy.

The developmental patterns by which one matures may be a source of stress in themselves. The slow child is urged on to more rapid development. The child who is developing more rapidly than others of his age group is cheered on to further acceleration. This process of pushing to greater and greater effort, whether one is slow in development or rapid, may result in nervousness, irritability, and tension, accompanied by physical symptoms such as headache or behavioral difficulties such as stammering, enuresis, bullying, or vengeful behavior.

Physical maturation is perhaps the most obvious of the developmental processes. Everyone develops a general body build which seems relatively fixed for him, regardless of food intake. A very short person may feel inferior, being "the runt" of the group, and may overcompensate for this. A very large person may have an equal problem. He cannot fight with other children of his own age without being called a bully. Frequent, not always complimentary, remarks may be made about his size. He may become self-conscious and temper his general behavior considerably. Muscular coordination also matures during childhood. There is a tendency to push children to more and more highly coordinated activities, and frustration or tension frequently result. Sports also require considerable muscular coordination, and the child who develops slowly in this regard may be at a great disadvantage in something which has considerable social approval attached to it. This again may be a source of tension or frustration.

There are other far-reaching effects of this difference in physical maturation. People at the extremes of all three types of body build are apt to mature relatively late. The child who matures early is in a more favorable social position. If he appears older than his age he is apt to be treated as older by his colleagues and by adults. When this does not place undue strains, leading him to try to act older than he is, it has favorable effects in making him a leader of his group. A study of correlations between level of maturation and leadership has demonstrated that people who mature early physically are apt to be socially and emotionally mature and to have positions of leadership in the groups to which they belong.[78] The late maturers physically are somewhat immature in their behavior as well and are apt to be followers.

Sexual maturation is closely linked to physical maturation, though sexual behavior is determined to a great degree by social factors. A certain amount of curiosity about sexual matters in early childhood increases as the child recognizes the intense concern of society in general with the problem of sex. This can be markedly accentuated by the attitude of parents toward sexual problems. The more restrictions and taboos placed on sexual activities by the parents, the more important these activities seem to the child, whether he accepts the restrictions and taboos or not.

Orville was the son of a pious Englishwoman and an Irish laborer living near the Atlantic seaboard. He was their first child and had been a problem to them from the day of his birth. Perhaps the most serious difficulty, however, arose when he was 5 and his mother discovered him in the back yard sucking a neighbor boy's penis. She was horrified, spanked him as hard as she could, and then gave him a lecture on how evil he was and the eternal damnation toward which he was headed. He was deeply affected by this experience and could scarcely eat for the next 6 months. He gradually regained his appetite and the weight he had lost and seemed to forget the experience. He was shy, however, made friends with difficulty, and withdrew into himself whenever troubles arose. He formed one close and lasting friendship, however.

At puberty, this friend introduced him to mutual masturbation, in which he engaged with intense feelings of guilt. One day the friend was making some idle boast to a group of schoolmates and Orville scoffingly remarked that what he said was not true. The friend laughed and turned to the group saying, "You can't believe anything he says. He masturbates." Orville turned pale and fled as everyone joined in general laughter. He could scarcely return to class after this episode. When called upon to recite, he found his mouth pursing in a strange fashion which made speech almost impossible while his left hand turned awkwardly back with fingers spread wide apart. His left leg became rigid so that he had to walk stiff-legged to the blackboard. His classmates howled with laughter when this first happened, and he begged his parents to let him drop out of school. But he could not explain to them why he wished to leave school and they saw no reason why he should not continue to attend. After several repetitions of this experience at school, however, he ran away from home. His flight was short lived. He felt quite unable to cope with the world alone and was relieved when picked up by police and returned to his parents.

Orville's early expression of sexual drives in childhood resulted in conflict with his environment and the clear statement that such activities were taboo. The outcome of this initial conflict was the development of a symptom, anorexia. In puberty, when again introduced to sexual activity, the conflict aroused was expressed in guilt feelings. Again stress was aroused between himself and his environment when the fact of his sexual activity was used against him punitively. Symptoms arose, this time of a hysterical nature, with behavior which combined re-enactment of the original act, sucking, with involuntary behavior of his left arm and leg which seemed to express both sexual excitement and denial of any part in it himself. This led to further trouble and panic.

The development of secondary sexual characteristics at puberty is a period of very complex changes and reaction patterns. There are problems to be met both by the girl who is flat chested and masculine in appearance and by the girl who feels self-conscious because she is too well developed. Among boys there is much comparison of development, and feelings of inferiority or worries about sexual inadequacies may be quite intense. In this period there may be a good deal of social value to be gained from having sexual information. In some groups, the one who can dispense information to others may achieve status in this way. In other groups, sexual experience is considered evidence of maturity and sought for its social value. With girls, sexual activity may be a means of getting affection and attention which is not obtainable otherwise. Sexual activity may also be used as a means of expressing rebellion against parental authority.

In addition to sexual and physical maturation, there is also intellectual maturation. During the early years, individual differences in intellectual development cause little trouble to children so long as they are not disappointing to their parents. However, the problem may become quite acute at 6 or 7 when the child is sent to school. Social patterns are again important as potential sources of trouble. The age of starting school, which in some areas is rigidly fixed regardless of intellectual level, is one of these. The policy in some school systems of advancing children automatically regardless of whether they have learned the material is another. Automatic advancements avoid the necessity of facing failure openly but lead to other problems in the process of doing so. The child who has a low IQ may react to the school situation with acute rebellion because of disappointment aroused in his family and the need to keep up with his classmates when his capacity does not permit him to do so. The child whose IQ is only slightly low is less apt to rebel and more apt to develop severe degrees of tension while trying to keep up the pace of those who have a somewhat higher intellectual endowment. Disorders of eating, sleeping, and speech, as well as gastrointestinal and muscular symptoms are prone to develop at this time.

But it is not only the person of low IQ who may have trouble. The child with a high IQ who is put into this standard situation may be disinterested in school if it represents no challenge to him. And, on the other hand, even the child with a high IQ may have nervousness and physical symptoms if his attention span is not sufficiently long to meet the demands of the classroom.

ADEQUACY

All of these aspects are closely bound together in the problem of adequacy, a personal evaluation with which the physician must deal repeatedly. Adequacy is more than endowment—whether one is fat or thin, intelligent or dull, sociable or reclusive, happy-go-lucky or easily upset—but endowment is the background on which an idea of adequacy is to be formed. The concept of adequacy does not depend on how slowly or rapidly one matures, though this certainly affects it. Nor is it a matter only of experiences—whether these have been met easily, have been challenging but surmountable, or have proved too much for the person to cope with successfully. The concept of adequacy is all these things—endowment, maturation, and experiences. It is also the timing of experiences in relation to the level of development. But this is not all. Adequacy also involves the attitude of the parents toward the child.

The problem of adequacy usually begins at about the age of 2 or 3, but the stage has been set even before birth. The reason for the pregnancy may influence later feelings of adequacy. If the child was conceived in order to cement a marriage and is unable to do this, he is apt to feel the disappointment of his parents and therefore feel that he is inadequate. Marian had this problem, for she was supposed to cement an unhappy marriage. Actually her coming had the opposite effect, since her father gave her the love which should have been her mother's. This aroused anger and jealousy in the mother that resulted in rejection and feelings of inadequacy and insecurity in the patient. If a child is conceived in order to make up for an inadequate spouse, a heavy load is placed upon him before he is born and is apt to result in feelings of inadequacy. If the birth is to justify marriage or fulfill family traditions, again a burden is placed on the child. And if the child is totally unwanted, as was true of Mrs. Bertrand, he is bound to be affected.

Rivalry with siblings and neighborhood children also affects adequacy, particularly as it influences the way parents handle the child. This was clearly demonstrated by the boy whose younger brother did better than he in all spheres—at school, in extracurricular activities, and socially. This was so disturbing to the older boy that eventually he committed suicide. All of the things which affect sibling rivalry and competition, therefore, have some effect upon feelings of adequacy. This competition is not limited to personal competition of the child but includes, as well, the position of the family and the family's competition with its neighborhood group. The material possessions of a family in relation to those of others in the immediate area affect the child's evaluation of his family's adequacy and secondarily of his own.

The problem of adequacy, therefore, has many facets. If the physician wishes to understand the patient who feels inadequate, he may have to examine all of these facets, including constitutional endowment, patterns of maturation, experiences which the patient has had, the time at which these experiences came, the attitude of parents toward the child (including the reason for having the child), sibling rivalry, competition in the neighborhood and at school, and the position of the family in the community.

Gladys (p. 131) was faced with a major problem in her feelings of inadequacy. Many of the demands she made upon herself, her husband, and her son were related to her efforts to prove herself adequate in every sphere. Her basic endowments were good. Though not beautiful, she had a trim figure and a pleasant face. She was intelligent and honest. She had her share of friends. She was married, had a son, and lived in a very substantial neighborhood. Despite this, she felt inadequate. The background for this feeling had been laid early in her life.

She was an adopted child. She had been told that her mother was from an upper-class family and was a very beautiful girl who was unmarried. She learned of her adoption at the age of 4, which was the time her headaches began. She said, however, that she was told in a "beautiful fashion." Her mother explained to her that she had been selected from a number of children and had been named Gladys because they were so glad to have her. Her parents were never harsh or demanding. They made few specific demands upon her and yet she was given the feeling that she must make up to them for the fact that they had no children of their own. Because she was not their own child, she was expected to be much better than other children and her behavior and general development were compared frequently with children of relatives and friends.

Her father ran a successful grocery store when she was a young child. She was always given everything that she wanted materially. During high school she was very active. She was a good student, took an active part in athletics, and was well liked socially. She went with the "better" group of girls and belonged to the "best" clubs. She was always poised and well controlled, yet she had nightmares, many of which suggested fear of loss of control. Her demands on herself were great but caused relatively little trouble during her high school days.

She went to college but stayed there for only a few months. She gave two reasons for dropping out—she was doing B instead of A work and did not feel that this level of work justified the money her parents were spending on her, and she did not get into the sorority she wished to join.

Gladys was adopted to make up for the lack of children. To do this, she had to be a little bit better than any of the neighborhood children. She learned to set her standards in life in terms of her associates, but always "a little bit better" than they were. Though perfectly mannered, active socially and in athletics, and a good student, she still never felt that she had quite succeeded in making up to her foster parents for the fact that she was not really their child.

Soon after leaving college because of her scholastic and social "failure," she met her husband. She quite frankly stated to her physician that she had not been in love with him at the time of their marriage. She felt insecure and inadequate and found in him a source of emotional strength. She felt at ease with him because he made no demands on her but accepted her as she was. Unfortunately she could not accept him just as he was. He came from a lower-class family. His father had lived openly with many women. Gladys held him in contempt and could not abide any traits in her husband which resembled his father. She tried to make him over. He made no demands on her but neither did he make sufficient demands on himself. He was content with moderate success. He did not have to be the best. He was not a strict disciplinarian for their son. He was not perfectionistic about the house. He had no use for social climbing and could not understand the drives which motivated her. Her need to have the best husband, the best-behaved son, and to live in the best part of town was bound to arouse friction between them.

Her feelings of inadequacy were expressed in all these ways—unflinching poise for herself, neatness and order in her home, her material possessions, and her family. But her conflicts with her husband over these things aroused another set of feelings of inadequacy. Though she wanted him to be authoritarian toward the child, she could not tolerate such an attitude toward herself. "I won't take that from any man," was her statement; and she would then decry the inferior status of women in our society. However, these feelings were tempered by her picture of the ideal marital relationship. When she took the dominant role, she felt guilty for being more aggressive than a "nice" woman should be and inadequate as a wife for not letting her husband assume the dominant role. A lady should always be poised; she frequently was not when she got into an argument. Every wife should love her husband; she wasn't always sure she did. So she felt inadequate to play her feminine roles in life.

It is plain that stresses such as these can lead to a variety of emotional reactions and be associated with many types of physiologic changes and symptoms dependent on the mixture of feeling states and their relative intensity. She felt that her desire to be loved could only be met by proving her adequacy. In childhood this had been true in order to receive love from her mother. In adulthood, her respect for herself still was dependent on proving her adequacy. Many of her arguments with her husband were over matters whose importance to her was largely related to adequacy—fine clothes, a well furnished home, an upstanding husband, and a well-behaved son. Many of her headaches followed an argument in which she had lost her dignity and poise and had spoken in a manner ill befitting a well-bred "lady." Adequacy to her meant being just a little bit better than others in actions as well as possessions.

Most children identify with their parents or with parent substitutes, imitating their ways and trying to be like them, though the child is not aware of most of this. Identification is the unconscious counterpart of imitation. By identifying with the parents, the child assumes some of their attributes. One of these attributes is the critical, punishing, disciplinary one. With the first step of identification, this critical attitude is not turned upon oneself but upon others, as was the parents' criticism. At this point there may be great intolerance for the same traits in others which have been the object of criticism in oneself. From these beginnings conscience appears. Then the parents' attitudes toward their child have become, by identification, the child's attitude toward himself. The conflict which formerly was between the child and his parents has become an internal conflict with himself. Henceforth, no reinforcement is necessary from the environment; he reinforces the prohibitions himself with each new awakening of the impulse. An intrapersonal conflict has appeared, which, if not adequately resolved, perpetuates the original stress. This process was evident in Orville. The original conflict between himself and his mother became internalized. When the situation recurred at puberty, he punished himself with feelings of guilt.

In addition to introducing new conflicts into the personality, the process of identification obviously affects a person's feelings of adequacy. He forms an evaluation of his moral adequacy, to be added to his feelings of adequacy in the intellectual, physical, emotional, and social realms. This is not dependent solely on the attitudes of the actual parents but is affected as well by parent substitutes, such as teachers, and by religious instruction. Any one of these may work to soften the judgment of another or to intensify it.

Feelings about personal adequacy form a major part of one's concept of himself and are of great significance to psychosomatic medicine. The person who has doubts about his adequacy in any sphere is likely to find experiences in this area stressful. If feelings of inadequacy are mild and the person expects to be able to deal with the situation, the result of inadequacy will be feelings of tension and striving, with the attendant physical manifestations of tension. If the feelings of inadequacy are intense, anger at being placed in such a situation or depression at the thought of the failure to come will have the physiologic responses associated with these emotional states.

Intense striving to overcome feelings of inadequacy is expressed behaviorally as overcompensation. Thus a person with a mild speech impediment may strive to become a great orator, as did Demosthenes; one who is considered weak physically may concentrate on physical activities to disprove this weakness, as did Theodore Roosevelt. Perhaps a more common reaction, however, is to avoid activities in which one feels inadequate and to concentrate instead on activities in which one feels adequate and the chance of success is correspondingly better. Thus, most people who feel physically weak or poorly coordinated will avoid sports and compensate in some other sphere, such as intellectual endeavors. The individual who does not feel that he is intellectually brilliant is apt to concentrate on sports or on occupational pursuits which do not require high levels of intelligence.

SECURITY

Another very important aspect of personality and of one's concept of himself is the feeling of security. Security and adequacy are frequently confused. Certainly feelings of inadequacy and insecurity are commonly associated. However, a person may feel inadequate for some specific task and yet be firm in the assurance that he is accepted despite this inadequacy. He is secure though feeling inadequate. One dictionary defines the word secure as "so strong, stable, or firm as to ensure safety" and another definition is "freedom from anxiety." This feeling of security seems to come primarily from the parents and to a very small extent from other sources. It is fostered by a parental attitude of acceptance and love of the child for what he is and not solely for what he does. They love him for being their child. They do not express approval and affection only for excelling in some activity or successfully competing with siblings or other children. When the expression of love is reserved for success, feelings of insecurity and inadequacy are likely to become closely associated.

Other factors affect security, though probably to a lesser extent. For example, when the position of eldest son carries with it certain privileges and prestige, the eldest son may feel quite secure regardless of what he does, since his position cannot be wrested from him. Contrariwise, intense sibling rivalry may, if handled improperly by the parents, lead to feelings of insecurity.

In addition to the attitude of the parents, the stability of the family seems to have a great deal to do with feelings of security. Thus even a child who is loved for himself may feel insecure if the home is insecure. Constant parental discord may give all of the feelings of rejection present in actual desertion. Desertion seems to have much more serious repercussions for the child than actual death, though the parent is absent from the family in either case. The insecurity aroused by separation from a parent seems to depend largely on the reasons for that separation and the attitudes of the parents toward it. Desertion implies rejection and says quite openly that the person who has deserted does not love his family. This has an entirely different meaning from a separation which is necessary for economic reasons but does not represent rejection by the parent.

Patients frequently recount childhood experiences which document these statements. A young woman closely attached to her father told of frequent violent arguments between her parents that culminated in her father stalking out of the house and not returning until the small hours of the morning. She lived in fear that he might never return or that her parents would be divorced and she would not see him afterwards. For years during childhood she would weep and scream whenever her parents tried to leave her in the evenings to visit their friends. A young man whose father had deserted the family when he was 2 said he knew where he could find his father but had never looked him up because "if he didn't care any more than that for me, I don't want to meet him."

DEPENDENCE

Several areas of conflict cannot be avoided and seem to have almost universal applicability. These conflicts are based on constitutional endowment and maturing processes and are markedly accentuated by social forces. They cannot be solved in the sense of one side of the conflict triumphing over the other. Each person must find a way of living with these conflicts in a manner satisfactory to himself. A satisfactory adjustment in one set of circumstances may not be a satisfactory adjustment in another. Consequently, there are apt to be changes in the way a person adjusts from time to time. A certain amount of plasticity is necessary to maintain a satisfactory adjustment with these conflicts. One of the most important of these conflicts concerns dependence and independence.

The biologic basis for this conflict begins with the physical dependence of the infant on those around him for care. At the same time he has certain drives toward independence. He has energy which will find expression, in part, in trying to master his environment, whether by vocal commands or by doing things for himself. It will be remembered that the degree of independence was one of the characteristics which Gesell[1] said could be evaluated in an infant during the first 4 months of life. Reaching for objects, learning to walk and talk, and dressing oneself are part of mastering one's environment. They lead to independence. Thus there are biologic bases for both dependence and independence.

The social basis for this conflict lies in the dependence of each individual on others in his social group. The division of labor and of responsibilities in any community group means that each individual is dependent on those around him to carry out their activities. At the same time, he must do his part so that others can depend on him for his part. This requires that a balance be struck between independence and dependence, neither of them being absolute.

The similarity of the infantile state of dependency to severe illness or handicap in the adult should be noted. In the adult who is ill there may again be physical dependence upon others. Yet, as with the infant, the adult may be completely in command of the situation, despite his physical helplessness, through verbal communication. Such a person may be demanding of those around him and childish in his emotional reactions. Whether this similarity in reaction of the patient means that he has regressed to an infantile level or whether it is simply a similar reaction in similar circumstances depends on one's point of view. In the infant, this situation soon leads to emotional dependence on others. This state of emotional dependency has been defined by one author[70] as an inner desire to monopolize the flow of love and affection from one or more other human beings.

It should be noted that dependency at this level imposes no discomforts and no failures except when the situation or the environment requires independent action. If the environment, specifically the parents, meet all of the needs and demands of the infant willingly, there is no incentive for the child to develop independence except for his own inner energy and drives, and these may not be very insistent if the satisfactions from the state of dependency are great. This is one way of attaining mastery over the environment, though this mastery is somewhat tenuous. It should be noted that from the start there is a confusion between dependency and love. This can be a major stumbling block in developing independence later in life. All too often the adolescent who is struggling to develop independence is met by the plaintive plea of his mother or father, "You don't love me any more or you wouldn't do that."

Obviously many things affect the conflict of dependency. One of these is the child-rearing philosophy of the parents. It is not any single act which is important but rather the emotional atmosphere permeating the relation between parent and child. Parent substitutes are likewise important. In the extended family, parent substitutes are already present within the family; in the small nuclear family, this is not true. If teachers and neighbors can be parent substitutes for the child, they may ease the problem considerably. Teachers are inconstant parts of the environment. If dependency conflicts can be displaced to teachers they may be easier to resolve, since it is easier to break this relationship. Maturing demands that a person develop a certain amount of independence of his own. A problem which faces physicians repeatedly is handling the patient who has not developed a normal amount of independence but is still tied to his family and dependent on them for approval.

Since everyone starts out in a dependent position and must develop a certain amount of independence before he can function in society as an adult, many social and cultural pressures are brought to bear to foster independence. These play upon innate energy which needs discharge in some sort of activity and upon the desire for gratifying one's needs and for mastering one's environment. These social pressures are so great that people sometimes feel that their goal should be complete independence.

The person who feels a strong need to be independent will commonly take certain measures to prove that he is independent. The physician should be aware of these behavior patterns and their significance, since they may be an early clue to a major conflict. The presence of many of these signs or of some of them repeatedly throughout a case history should suggest that the patient has been sufficiently disturbed by his dependent needs to try to deny them. They therefore indicate a fairly intense conflict around dependency. The behavior patterns used to emphasize independence include repeated assumption of unnecessary responsibilities or of responsibilities which put a heavy strain on the patient; breaking of ties, such as frequent change in jobs; broken friendships; divorces and separations in marriage; frequent change of residence; avoidance of close ties insofar as possible; negativism; antisocial behavior; and social climbing.

These behavior patterns were evident in Fred (p. 56) at the age of 4. When his father disappeared the first time, he suddenly became very independent. By the age of 6, he was preparing his own breakfast and taking care of himself throughout the day. He would not let his mother express affection for him or make decisions for him as she did for his younger brother. He roamed the town by day, justifying his goings and comings to no one. He had many companions but no close friends.

As he grew into adulthood, he had a succession of jobs, one of which he left, interestingly enough, because he was developing too close a friendship with his boss (a woman). He became engaged but broke the engagement because he felt unworthy of the girl. His pattern of living, therefore, had been one of trying to be independent, since no one could be depended on. Exacerbations of diabetes were closely related to stressful situations which he interpreted as a threat to his independence.

The other side of the conflict may be equally troublesome. Some people fear the responsibilities imposed by independence or fear that striving to become independent will destroy an important relationship. Such a person tries to emphasize his dependence by assuming a dependent role within the family or at work, by marrying a domineering and controlling spouse or by compulsive failures at work. He may develop strong feelings of guilt. The very dependent person may also indulge in antisocial behavior, particularly in alcoholism and promiscuity. The behavior patterns which emphasize dependence should also be recognized, since they, too, indicate the presence of a problem and tell the physician that the patient needs help in achieving a more satisfying adjustment between his dependent needs and his independent strivings. That these two patterns of behavior may sometimes alternate in the same person is not surprising, since both sides of the conflict are always present.

When the conflict is intense it can lead to considerable turmoil. The person who is anxious to prove his independence may be led to assume increasing responsibilities requiring considerable expenditure of energy and accompanied by tension and anxiety. If he has succeeded in shouldering one responsibility satisfactorily, there is little time for pleasure in success for he must continue proving his independence. Therefore satisfaction is short lived and he must seek other areas in which to prove again that he has not lapsed back into a dependent state. The person who picks this road has a long and arduous journey. Similarly with the breaking of ties and friendships. There are considerable satisfactions in having friends and being close to other people. Yet this closeness, despite its satisfactions, is threatening because it means a growing dependence emotionally on someone else. Consequently, the person feels forced to dissolve his marriage or break up his friendship. This may be accompanied by marked emotional disturbances, with uncertainty about why he has broken the tie.

There are also troubles for the person who is stressing his dependency. He cannot avoid being aware of the strong social pressures toward independence. This may arouse shame, guilt, and depression as he compares the social ideal with his own actions. Intense dependency almost invariably is associated with great hostility toward the person on whom one is dependent. This is true despite the satisfactions achieved through dependency. Being dependent requires that one subordinate his own desires in order to maintain the flow of affection from the other person. His activities are therefore restricted. Though he may do nothing to destroy the dependent relationship, he yet feels frustrated in his own personal goals and hostile toward the person who demands that he conform in order to receive his attentions. The dependent role is considered a submissive and inferior one in our culture. This increases the hostility in the situation. In addition the one who cares for the dependent person usually feels that he deserves to be loved. The feeling that one is obliged to love a person who has put one in an inferior and frustrating situation leads to further feelings of hostility. It is for reasons such as these that a dependent relationship is almost invariably associated with considerable hostility if it has existed for any length of time.

SELF-LOVE

Another conflict which appears early in life is that between love of oneself and love of others, the conflict around narcissism. The infant, it is said, considers the whole world continuous with himself and does not distinguish what is "I" from what is "not I." At this stage, he uses others to master his environment without any true awareness of their existence apart from himself. Though physically dependent on others from the start, the infant cannot develop emotional dependence until aware that other people and other things exist. Emotional dependence is the first step away from love of oneself toward love of someone else.

In the infant narcissism is simply a lack of awareness that anything exists except himself. Later in life the narcissist is aware that others exist but has, in a sense, fallen in love with himself. He regards himself with the same devotion and admiration that is ordinarily reserved for someone else. In this stage, which is common during adolescence, he is preoccupied first with his physical development and appearance, then with his own ideas, and, finally with mystical concepts and ideas of finding himself through losing himself in something greater. The egocentricity of this period resembles paranoia in many ways, and paranoid ideas are not rare during the adolescent period.

Ordinarily this is worked out satisfactorily and a person falls in love with someone of the opposite sex. The psychoanalysts tell us that there are two common types of object-choice.[36] One of these is a narcissistic choice in which the person falls in love with someone who is very like himself or what he would like to be. The other object-choice is related to the dependency conflict, and the person falls in love with someone who will take care of him and do things for him. It is obvious that narcissistic preoccupation with one's own ideas and desires can introduce considerable stress into a marital situation, particularly if both partners have this trouble. The physician should recognize this problem so that he can deal with it appropriately.

To be loved by another increases one's self-esteem and self-love. Therefore the narcissistic person will do all he can to obtain love from other people. This may be expressed by letting others know that he feels rejected and abused in the hope that expressions of affection and love will be elicited to counteract these feelings. Narcissism may also be expressed in gratifying one's desires. On the other hand, the person who is trying to deny his self-love will go to an extreme in those activities which seem to emphasize altruism and love of others. Such people are overprotective of others, identify with them and their problems easily, engage in many charitable activities, relinquish their own personal goals easily, and extol the spiritual side of life. No one of these manifestations alone is diagnostic of conflict in this area; but the person who carries this mode of life to an extreme may have narcissistic conflicts which he is trying to solve. As with dependency, there is no solution by one triumphing over the other. The person must seek a satisfactory balance between his own desires and self-love and the requirements of others and love for them.

Gladys (p. 131) had not found a satisfactory equilibrium for herself in this problem of narcissism. Her self-love was intimately interwoven with her feelings of inadequacy. It was expressed in her manner of dress and concern about her personal appearance, in her aggressive drive to achieve her own goals with no willingness to compromise with her husband, in her emphasis on material possessions, and in her concern for the symbols of love and success. She had great difficulty in loving anyone else, even her husband, and felt this as a lack within herself. She needed his love to bolster her own self-respect but her rigid demands decreased his expressions of love. When she felt uncertain of his love, as was commonly true after an argument, she would indulge herself by buying a new hat or some new household article. Thereby she would try to give herself the love which she did not get from her husband. This often led to further troubles and a resurgence of the conflict around self-love and object-love.

MASCULINITY

Another area of conflict concerns masculinity and femininity. It is generally conceded that feminine and masculine traits combine in the physique and in the temperament of most people. Male and female hormones are found in both sexes. The conflict is expressed almost entirely in terms of adequacy for the masculine and feminine roles in life. These are prescribed by the culture in which one lives. Masculine and feminine ideals exist; certain deviations are permitted; but gross deviations are frowned upon. One of the gross deviations in our culture is homosexuality. This is much more serious for men than for women. In addition, more evidences of masculinity are accepted in a woman than evidences of femininity in a man. However, the conflict may be intense in either sex and is greatly affected by social and cultural forces.

Men who are threatened by the feminine tendencies in themselves may develop behavior patterns to emphasize masculinity in an attempt to allay this anxiety. Their behavior is aggressive, and they tend to be especially punitive toward feminine men or homosexuals. They are unable to admit their weaknesses and engage almost exclusively in activities which are considered to be male pursuits. They often refuse to let their wives work, since this is a reflection on their adequacy as a male and provider.

On the other hand, men who are afraid to compete in the masculine world or who, for any reason, wish to minimize their masculinity may express this wish in a number of ways. Marriage to a masculine or domineering woman is one of these. Avoidance of competitive activity or engaging in ritualistic or repetitive work is another. Incapacitating disease, impotence, excessive fears also minimize masculinity.

Mrs. Bertrand's father (p. 26) exemplified this. In childhood he was completely overwhelmed by his father and his father's aggressive approach to life. He felt unable to compete with him or to meet any of his standards. In general, he avoided competitive or masculine activities. He was a complete failure in the businesses which his father gave him. He could not supervise other men working under him nor take competitive action in business. His first wife was a girl who could not have been attractive to anyone in his social group. When he found another man in bed with her after their marriage, he made no protest but left, leaving the other man in command of the situation. His second wife was a woman who was perfectly willing to work and support them while he stayed at home and did the housework. This reversal of roles did not disturb the two of them but did arouse comment among their friends. This made them socially uncomfortable and cut them off from other people. The only job he held for any length of time as an adult was a job as a secretary.

Conflicts play an important part in determining what will be stressful. The dependent person who is striving to appear independent will find any situation in which he must take a dependent role, or in which he feels that he does so, a stressful one. To such a person, marriage may be stressful for the emotional dependence it entails. The narcissistic person who is striving to prove his ability to love others will find a situation stressful in which he must aggressively hold on to his own goals and not relinquish them in favor of someone else. The man who is trying to appear very masculine will find any situation in which he cannot maintain masculine activities to be stressful. Impotence, even transitory, will be a severe stress to such a man. Incapacitating disease prevents a person from being aggressive and from competing. Consequently, the man who is striving to appear masculine will be threatened by such a disease while the man who fears aggressive competition may welcome it.

Similar conflicts, with a biologic and social basis, of course exist also for women. The woman who is troubled with a conflict about masculine drives may try to emphasize her femininity by emphasizing childbearing and feminine activities, by confining herself largely to masculine companionship, by being flirtatious, coy, submissive, and perhaps by promiscuity or by a denial of intellectual interests. No one of these alone indicates a conflict over masculinity, but the person who carries them to an extreme is apt to have such a conflict and these are signs which the physician should keep in mind in interviewing patients.

MASOCHISM

Among other conflicts of which the physician should be aware is that of masochism and sadism. Mrs. Bertrand's grandmother (p. 26) had a good many masochistic traits. She felt she had sinned gravely and deserved lifelong punishment. She lived with a husband who was violent and demanding and who often beat her and the children. She accepted this as her proper lot in life and exerted herself to please him in any way she could. The masochistic person who feels a need for suffering and punishment may find illness an appropriate vehicle to achieve his ends. Such people are especially difficult to treat and may demand one surgical procedure after another. They willingly submit to suffering and even seek it out. The physician should be aware that such problems exist and avoid playing directly into the conflict.

Such a patient was Mrs. Cowan, a 63 year old widow. She had lived 22 years with an abusive husband for whom she had contempt and by whom she had had nine children. She said she had stayed with him because it was her duty. However, when he was sent to a tuberculosis sanatorium where he could no longer abuse her, she divorced him. She promptly married another man who was almost as bad. He died a few years later. She married a third time to a husband who was "good" but chronically ill. He died soon after the marriage. When first seen she had lived alone 13 years in a large house. She never had anyone join her because she "liked to be alone," though she had been a nurse for many years because she "liked to be with people and listen to their troubles." During the years after her second husband's death, her "good" years, she had suffered almost continuous poor health. She had had five major operations and six or eight (she couldn't be quite sure of the number) minor operations. In addition she had had severe insomnia, being unable to sleep for a week at a time and then dropping with exhaustion to sleep for 7 hours or so. During the episodes of insomnia she beat the pillow or paced the floor, her "only thought" being, "Why should I be punished so!"

She came to her physician complaining of insomnia and of painful hemorrhoids—which were not the cause of her insomnia, she insisted. She thought surgery would probably relieve her. The surgeon should make his decision for or against surgery entirely on the physical findings in such a case. A desire for surgery should not enter into the decision, since it is based on a desire to be punished, even though such patients cannot decide why. The results of surgery are apt to be poor, as the results of previous operations had been for Mrs. Cowan.

All of these conflicts impair the ability to make logical, clear decisions. The person who has a conflict over dependency and is striving to appear independent will be impelled when faced with a situation involving this conflict to make the decision which emphasizes independence, whether this is a logical decision or not. The man who has conflicts about his masculinity may find it impossible to let his wife work even though the logic almost demands that she be economically productive. The masochistic person will choose the alternative which punishes him.

All of these conflicts affect one's feelings of adequacy and his concept of himself. They are potent forces in determining what will be stressful and what will not. All of them, then, may affect health. In addition, by virtue of the force which they give goals in a person's life and the value systems which they set for him, they in large part determine what his life will be. Though everyone has elements of the same conflicts within himself and must find a working relationship with these conflicts, the physician should not feel that they are unimportant to health. When he finds that a patient is obviously struggling with such a conflict, he should do whatever he can to help him find an appropriate equilibrium. In doing so he is giving good medical care and may be helping to prevent subsequent illness.

Chapter 7

Reaction to Illness

ILLNESS is often stressful and the reaction to it is conditioned by all the factors which affect reaction to any other stress. The patient's endowment, his concept of himself, his feelings of adequacy and security, and his conflicts about dependency, masculinity, narcissism, or masochism affect the meaning of illness to him. The mental mechanisms which he is accustomed to use in dealing with other stresses—denial, avoidance, displacement, and the like—are apt to be used in the response to illness as well. And throughout it all are social and cultural forces which affect his ideas about health and disease as well as shape his personality to determine what sort of stress the particular illness will be. The physiologic changes associated with this reaction are similar to those which accompany reactions to other stresses, use the same pathways, and may result in similar symptoms. Thus reaction to illness may intensify and prolong the symptoms of the illness or ameliorate them, depending on the type of reaction elicited.

THE MEANING OF ILLNESS

To understand the reaction of a patient to illness, one must understand the meaning of illness. To know this, one must understand the social and cultural forces related to health and illness as well as the patient's past experience as it affects his reaction to illness. Any generalization about reaction to illness that may be true for the group is not necessarily true for any single individual within it.

Our society believes that health is the right of everyone. It places considerable responsibility upon parents to maintain the health of children. Through magazines and newspapers pressures are exerted upon people to maintain their own health. Articles dealing with matters of health, proper nutrition for children, the appropriate amount of exercise and sleep, and ways to stay healthy are common. Magazines are filled with advertisements about vitamins, health remedies, the advisability of using cathartics, and the wisdom of "staying regular." Many of these advertisements are far from accurate in what they say, and their recommendations have more pertinence to the sale of the product than to the health of the individual. However, implied in each is the desirability of staying healthy and the person's responsibility to maintain his own health. The recent emphasis on routine physical examinations and periodic checkups is another community force acting upon people to impress them with their responsibility for their own health.

This emphasis on health is generally beneficial, for it encourages people to develop sound habits of personal hygiene and to seek medical aid early in the course of illness. Minor variations from a state of well-being become more significant for people with this philosophy of health and disease than the same variations do for people who believe that a certain number of aches and pains are the normal lot of mankind and should be accepted without complaint. Most people combine the two philosophies, leaving the division between a "normal" ache or pain and an "illness" somewhat vague at best.

The popular definition of illness thus becomes of major importance. And this dividing line between health and disease is particularly vague for mental and emotional illness. People commonly believe that an ambulatory person with no obvious disability is not sick. A person with an emotional illness, such as a psychoneurosis, is therefore not considered ill. He is not relieved from his responsibilities and he frequently experiences considerable conflict over this. He does not feel able to work and yet cannot point to anything which seems to justify stopping. Such a person may lament his robust appearance and castigate himself for his symptoms. Mr. Roberts (p. 119) did exactly this. It was a point of great concern to him that he looked so healthy when he felt so ill. But his distress was sufficiently great to force him to seek help despite his robust appearance and the comments of family and friends that they could not believe him ill when he looked so well.

Despite the popular emphasis on health, patients not infrequently delay their first visit to a physician for weeks or months after the appearance of a symptom. Part of this delay may be related to the difficulty in defining illness; but when the delay means that a malignant growth has become inoperable or that a patient suffering from angina for months appears in the doctor's office only after a myocardial infarction, the factors contributing to the delay become of vital importance to physicians and all others interested in the health of the community. What are these factors?

One group of factors is found in social and cultural attitudes. It is not uncommon to find people looking upon an unbroken record of robust health as a sign of masculinity.[79] Why should this be true? If in some way illness is equated with loss of masculinity then any person concerned with his masculinity might be expected to deny illness as long as possible. One cultural attitude operating to equate illness with loss of masculinity is the value placed on stoicism. Though we may consider our society weak in comparison with others, a certain amount of stoicism is imparted to children. When a mother tells her son who has just hurt himself that he is a big boy and must not cry, she is teaching him stoicism. This is carried into adult life in the feeling that one should not give in too easily to infirmities and should limit requests for help from other people. Such an attitude obviously affects the time at which a patient decides to consult his physician. The more stoic a person has learned to be, the longer he will tolerate a symptom before seeking aid. He is reluctant to seek help until his symptoms have become sufficiently severe for him to feel that no one could criticize him for complaining. Since all of us have minor symptoms that come and go and which can be ignored without harm, this attitude has many beneficial effects. But when it delays the first visit of a man to his physician until it is too late to effect a cure, it is harmful.

Another attitude which may accentuate this problem is the cultural goal of independence. Responsibility for economic independence devolves principally upon the men of our society. Closely allied to this are social concepts concerning work, career, and vocational choice. It is considered proper for every adult to engage in some productive activity. Women now take a more active part in vocations; even those who are not helping to secure economic independence for a family are expected to be occupied and busy during the day. If they do not have a family to care for, it is considered proper for them to engage in activites of social meaning. This includes social gatherings, church activities, school activities, and community projects. Independence and productive activity are closely allied and have many repercussions. They may keep a man at work long after he should have stopped. Even after accepting the fact of illness they may make it impossible for him to relax and gain the full benefits of a therapeutic regimen. The physician who understands this may be able to deal with the situation by making immediate rest and loss of income acceptable in order to achieve long-term independence.

In addition to these social pressures toward stoicism and independence and their psychologic counterparts, there are other psychologic reasons for delaying a visit to the physician. In a study of the reasons for delay in seeking surgical care,[80] it was found that the conflict around independence influenced a significant number of patients to delay seeing a physician. An even larger number delayed surgery because of fear of the surgical procedure or of death. These patients frequently viewed surgery as a punishment, a retribution for hostility toward significant people in their lives. The fear of death was present even when it was unrealistic in terms of the type of surgery needed. Shame and the fear of disclosing behavior about which guilt existed delayed a number of patients, especially those with symptoms referable to the genital area. And, unfortunately, an unsatisfactory relationship with the physician deterred other patients from visiting him even when the need existed. This list is not comprehensive but it indicates the many factors which must be assayed in any consideration of the reasons people fail to avail themselves of medical care when it is needed.

Once a person and those about him have accepted the fact that he is ill, new standards surround his conduct.[81] Generally, illness is a deviation from health which decreases one's energy level and his ability to cope with his environment and interferes with his ability to be productive and independent. Society recognizes this and relaxes its demands. It is permissible for the sick person to be dependent on those about him and to make demands on their time and energy. He is relieved of his social responsibility for independence and productivity. Illness, therefore, permits him to give up the struggle with the harsh realities of life if this is desired. The person who is ambitious and successful in his strivings may find illness a major frustration, a barrier between himself and a goal almost within reach. He may be impatient and demand immediate and lasting relief. When the nature of the illness requires bed rest and dependence on others, as after a heart attack, the physician may need to spend considerable time helping the patient relinquish his goals of independence and productivity. On the other hand, a patient who finds that it takes more energy to reach his goal than the goal seems worth may accept illness as a refuge from a life of constant striving. At such times the physician may need to strengthen the drives toward independence and productivity, minimize social attitudes which relieve the patient of responsibility, and help him adjust his goal so that he can achieve them without exhausting his energies.

It should be remembered, too, that there are times when illness or disability may offer a patient and his family more independence and security than would health and work. In our clinic a young man was seen who was receiving relief payments because of a number of rather vague complaints. He had, in addition, a hernia which could easily have been repaired. He complained little about his symptoms himself, but his wife emphasized them repeatedly and insisted that it would be impossible for him to work until they were relieved. He had never worked at any steady occupation and had had no job satisfactions. Though his father had been a steady worker and provided well for his family, he seemed unable to do this himself. His wife insisted that he was too ill to work and opposed surgical correction of the hernia. Her attitude was, at least in part, an expression of her feeling that "A regular relief check is better than irregular wages." His "illness" was an adequate reason for them to be on relief.

Illness may also be used to cover feelings of inadequacy. One of our patients, approaching 60, had put much emphasis on accomplishment through his early adult life. As he grew older he found it difficult to accept the decline in his capabilities which came with age. He felt inadequate and could not face his inability to maintain his previous hours and standards of work. He became ill. His illness need not have been disabling but it was, since illness allowed him to avoid feelings of inadequacy by making it unnecessary to meet his former standards. It gave him an acceptable reason for demanding support from state funds. And demand it he did, stating vociferously that it was his just due. Actually, this man was not inadequate except as many men nearing 60 are inadequate to maintain the standards and accomplishments of which they were capable at 30.

Illness may also be used to express rebellion. Patients who have been in conflict with figures in authority may continue this conflict in their relationship with their physician. Such a patient may make endless demands for treatment and relief of symptoms yet never cooperate by carrying out the treatments suggested. Or the rebellion may be against society in general, as by the patient who uses a relatively minor illness as justification for demanding that society support him.

The sick person is allowed to increase demands on those about him. It is usually expected that he will limit these demands to what is made necessary by the severity of his illness, but this is an ill defined area in which the patient himself is allowed considerable freedom of decision. The sick or disabled person who does more than the group expects is approved and admired for doing so, but there is usually no disapproval for taking advantage of the lack of responsibilities which go along with illness. In fact, it may be approved if it is seen as one way to reattain the state of health.

A 77 year old woman was seen in our clinic for multiple complaints, a year after she had married a retired minister. For years she had had hypertension. Three cerebrovascular accidents had left her with a partial left hemiplegia. She came complaining of shortness of breath and swelling of her ankles and was found to be in congestive failure. Adequate digitalization made it physically possible for her to be on her feet doing light housework. However, she made no move in this direction. She got out of bed only to move to a rocking chair near the fire. Her husband did all of the housework, prepared all of the meals, washed all of the dishes, and took care of her every need or desire. Whatever her capabilities, they both considered her to be an invalid. She played her part as an invalid who needed care and attention. He played his part equally well, giving her the attention she wanted and felt she needed.

In this patient, the effect of her attitude and her husband's attitude toward her illness on treatment and convalescence is quite obvious. She had been in poor health a long while and felt a need for dependence on someone else. She was not going to jeopardize this relationship by exerting herself when she might be needing care again at any moment. She knew she could do more than she did; but she also knew that, as an invalid, she would not be required to do more. Her husband had spent many years tending his previous wife through a long, terminal illness. He got certain satisfactions from caring for others. He would have appreciated more assistance from his wife but was certainly not going to force her into activity. She was ill, after all, and no one should expect her to do more than she was doing. To him it was remarkable that anyone so ill could remain so cheerful. Could one ask more than this?

Illness may represent a release from the need to assume responsibilities and therefore be accepted with pleasure. An example of this was a middle-aged man who was admitted to the hospital because of a myocardial infarction. When told that he had had a heart attack and would have to stay in bed for several weeks, he beamed with pleasure. He relaxed in bed and seemed to enjoy his illness to the full. His family was quite distressed by this reaction. They doubted that he had had a heart attack but thought instead that he had put on such a good act he had fooled all of his doctors. Instead of being sympathetic, they did all they could to arouse feelings of guilt and inadequacy in him. They felt it was unseemly of him to be so happy at having had a heart attack.

The background for this rather strange reaction to illness included several years of trying to run a business jointly with his uncle, without much success. He felt that the uncle was giving him all the unpleasant jobs to do. The uncle shirked his own responsibilities and, in addition, took the greater share of the profits on the grounds that he was the senior member of the firm. The patient had come to detest his uncle and to hate the work that he was doing. Yet he was unable to break up the business association. To do so would have made a rift in family relations, and the ties in his family were very strong. To do so would be to gamble with his future and to expose his family to the possibility of financial insecurity. To do so would also mean admitting failure to adjust to an unpleasant situation. He was happy at having a heart attack because this relieved him of the responsibility of making the decision to break up the partnership. Here is a man who would rather be a cardiac invalid than to take the responsibilities of opposing social pressures in his life. His case gives abundant evidence of the strength of social pressures.

The family had also been in a situation which affected their reaction to his illness. The patient had for years been complaining of symptoms which were not sufficient to incapacitate him but sufficient to arouse complaint. He had been fearful of a heart attack for some time before the actual illness and had had chest pain. He feared that he might have coronary difficulty. They had not taken these symptoms seriously since he had had them for some time and coronary disease had never been proved. They felt that he was a chronic complainer and that his illness was "neurotic." Consequently when he had a myocardial infarction they were suspicious of it. They considered it to be another neurotic manifestation and his attitude toward his illness merely confirmed this opinion. They thought his enjoyment of illness reflected his pleasure in having fooled the doctors into thinking that he had actually had the heart attack he had predicted to his family.

In such a situation, the physician must do many things besides treat the heart disease. He must see that the patient does not become a chronic invalid unnecessarily, even though he may not be able to return to the pressures of his former job. He must see that the family understands that the heart attack has been a real one and that some of the prior chest pains may very well have been anginal. A discussion with the family of the meaning of the illness to the patient and the reasons for his reaction to it may or may not be appropriate. The physician must decide this from his knowledge of the family. Both the patient and his family need help before an adequate adjustment can be made.

We have spoken thus far of illness as though it were an entity which could be defined. Certain attitudes do apply to illnesses generally. However, within this broad category are many variations which depend on the type of illness. This can be seen in the different attitudes commonly taken toward an illness that follows an abortion and the same illness following a normal delivery. Cancer commonly arouses fear; venereal disease, shame. Epilepsy is a disease to be hidden from others, if possible, while a broken leg is not. A mother may be ashamed of her diabetic child because diabetes marks him as different from other children. Many people consider illnesses which develop in a setting of emotional stress to be evidence of weakness on the part of the person having them. He should be able to cope with his environment without developing symptoms. If he cannot, there is something wrong with him. Physicians frequently share this view.

Closely allied to this is the feeling that loss of a part of the body means loss of one's ability to cope with his environment.[82] Though this is true at times, the feeling is frequently much more intense than is justified by the actual loss. This is again a matter of self-concept. A person who has lost a leg, whether surgically or as a result of disease, may be perfectly able to cope with his environment but feel unable to do so. A woman who has had a hysterectomy may become quite depressed afterwards in the fear that she has lost her sexual desirability. She may feel unable to attract men or to hold her husband's interest. And, indeed, this may at times be true. Mrs. Guarneri had a hysterectomy when she was 38. After surgery her husband refused to have intercourse with her. He said that to him she was "just the shell of a woman" and physically repulsive. He felt so strongly about it that they never had intercourse thereafter. Much of this is related to cultural ideas about parts of the body, their necessity, and their use. The reactions are related, of course, to personal evaluation as well. The personal evaluation here, as elsewhere, however, is strongly conditioned by the social attitudes toward these matters.

The need to consider a patient's reaction to illness and what it means to him is well illustrated by a young farmer of 24 who had one child. During adolescence he had had epiphysitis, and a fairly marked kyphosis resulted. This put his back at a slight mechanical disadvantage so that hard physical work resulted in muscle soreness, which, however, was not sufficient to keep him from continuing work. One day a farm accident resulted in a back injury. He received medical treatment and recovered from the immediate disability, but when he tried to return to heavy farm labor, he found that he had considerable back pain. When seen in the clinic his family was receiving emergency relief and he was trying to get classified as permanently disabled. He wanted to work but had never done anything but farm labor. The fact that many kinds of jobs within his capacity were available had not occurred to him. Besides, his physician had told him that he could never work again, probably meaning only that he would be unable to do farm labor. In his concept of himself, therefore, he was a farmer who could never farm. He was markedly depressed, even at times to the point of suicidal thoughts. The future looked hopeless to him. He saw no chance of being independent or productive; he could not fulfill his obligations as husband or father. Though little could be done for the back pain, much could be done for the patient. Because of his depression, his drive toward work and his capacity for it were decreased. A major part of his treatment was dealing with his reaction to illness so that he could make the initial steps toward return to productive employment.

MEDICAL CARE

Another large area affecting the patient's reaction to illness is the problem of medical care. Physicians increasingly tend to see patients only in their offices and only during office hours. They make fewer house calls and do less night work. This is of obvious benefit to the physician and, at times, is greatly to the advantage of the patient as well. Necessary instruments or drugs and the help of an office nurse are available in the office; their absence in the home may handicap care and an office visit be necessary as well as the house call. However, when this trend is enforced as a general policy, it decreases the availability of medical care and increases apprehension when medical emergencies arise.

The distance a person lives from a place where he can receive adequate medical care has considerable effect on his reaction to illness. This is particularly true in an illness in which emergencies may arise. A person who lives in the country with miles of rough road between him and the doctor and with inadequate means of transportation has a very different problem than the one who lives in a city with many public modes of transportation or his own personal car available to take him to the doctor. A person who lives on a farm with no telephone has an added barrier between him and medical care for himself or his family. At such times the problem of caring for an invalid who may have a sudden turn for the worse becomes a matter of major concern. When this is combined with a physician who makes no house calls, the problem is even more acute.

The ramifications of these problems may be quite extensive. A 62 year old woman appeared in the clinic with symptoms of fatigue, anorexia, and constipation of five years' duration. Though pleasant and cooperative, she seemed somewhat depressed, an emotional state which might well be pertinent to her complaints. Questioning disclosed that her husband had been ill for 7 years. Up to that time they had lived on a farm 15 miles from town. They had enjoyed country living, had raised 5 children, and had been well and widely known in their area. As his illness dragged on, it became evident that he would never return to farm work. The children were married and gone. The farm lay idle. Their savings gradually dwindled. In addition, frequent trips to the doctor were necessary and the 30 miles to and from the office were a drain on his energies. Though he was eligible for state relief and could remain in his home while receiving it, everyone agreed that it would be wise for them to move to town where they would be nearer the doctor. So they had sold their house and moved to town 5 years before. At this time her symptoms began.

This move of 15 miles disrupted their entire mode of living. While in the country, their nearest neighbors were a quarter of a mile away, but these neighbors were close friends. In town they were surrounded by neighbors on all sides, but they were strangers. The patient had been very active in church work in her small country church. In their new church she felt strange and had no position of importance. She simply attended the church. On the farm there had always been plenty of work to keep her occupied. In town there was nothing but housework and sewing, activities which soon lost their interest for her. Through her husband's illness she had lost her home, her friends, her work, her position in her community. She still had her husband and knew she was better off than many others. She did not complain at what had come to pass. But it is small wonder that she felt depressed, had no enthusiasm for living, tired easily, and had symptoms of depression.

The economic problems of medical care complicate the matter further. Illness ordinarily means economic loss and increased responsibility for other members of the family. The problem is considerably different for acute and chronic illnesses, and the effect on economic status and responsibility may be different as well. A family of moderate means may well stand the medical expenses of an acute illness even though it costs several hundred dollars. This expenditure can be spread out over many months and, since it is not cumulative, the hardship is not great. However, an illness which costs much less for any one month but which lasts for months or years, puts a constant strain upon finances which even people in moderate circumstances may not be able to meet. The attempt to meet such costs may result in a lowered standard of living and loss of social status. Prolonged physiotherapy, orthopedic appliances, and long-term nursing care may be desirable in treatment but difficult to obtain because of cost. And in the cost of illness one must include the loss of income from inability to work. The patient and his family are bound to approach the prospect of a chronic illness or chronic disability very differently than they do an acute illness.

The significance of financial problems goes beyond cost and social status. Worries about financial problems and their effect on the life of the family may have deleterious effects on the health of the patient. In a recent study of cardiac patients who had had episodes of congestive failure,[50] it was found that financial problems were a frequent source of worry. Whether these were discussed with others or not, their contemplation was associated with fluid and sodium retention, sometimes with significant weight gain, changes at least potentially detrimental to the status and welfare of the patients.

In addition, the quality of care and the patient's confidence in the physician make considerable difference in his reaction to illness. The patient who thinks his physician is competent and will do the best possible for him regardless of what happens reacts differently to illness than one who is unsure of his physician and constantly wondering if he might not get better care if he went elsewhere.

Illness frequently arouses fear of pain or death, of the unknown, of an uncertain future. Such fears are often readily understandable when they are recognized. When they appear out of proportion to the threat present, the physician should recall that one effect of internal conflicts is to intensify or prolong reactions to stress. He should seek the source of the trouble, for only in this way can he deal with the problem intelligently.

When Mrs. Bertrand (p. 26) visited the neurosurgical clinic for evaluation for sympathectomy, she had been told she had but 2 years to live, whether she had surgery or not. This aroused intense anxiety, almost precipitating a panic. She had no operation, choosing to diet instead. She lost 50 pounds and maintained her weight at its new level. Anginal attacks became less frequent, and she even tried to go back to work for a time. Her blood pressure fell to a more moderate level though not back to normal. In every way she seemed to be responding very well to weight loss and a favorable doctor-patient relationship. Improvement with minor fluctuations continued for many months. Blood pressure then began rising. Angina became more frequent and more severe. She began to fatigue easily and limited her activities drastically. She seemed depressed at times and more easily upset. Because of this, her doctor began seeing her more frequently, wondering what caused her increasing troubles. On one visit, he thought her disc margins were becoming blurred. She told him on that visit that she had a strange feeling that she was about to die. And with that remark he suddenly understood what was the matter. The second anniversary of her visit to the neurosurgical clinic was only 2 weeks away. Her death had been predicted within 2 years, and her angina was a constant reminder of that possibility. She had not consciously brooded over the prediction, but as the time approached the original anxiety surged back. A frank discussion of this prediction, the fear it had aroused, and its recurrence as the time drew near, coupled with reassurance about her physical status on the basis of objective changes rather than symptomatology reassured her. Symptomatically, she gradually returned to her previous baseline and again felt cheerful and able to cope with the world.

ILLNESS AND SOCIAL ROLES

The reaction of a patient and his family is conditioned by the role which the ill member has played in the family. It makes considerable difference whether a child, the mother, the father, or some elderly person in the family is ill. When there is only one adult female in the household, it is most important that she be able to perform her duties as homemaker. When there is only one adult male in the family, it becomes important that he remain on the job and bring home his wages. Illness of the mother may require that some other person take care of the house and children; illness of the wage-earner may require that some other source of funds be found while he is ill.

There is little place in the modern family for the elderly person—the grandparent, aunt, or uncle. He has few duties and responsibilities to perform; he is an outsider who is tolerated in time of necessity but seldom desired as an important member of the household.[83] When he is ill, he increases the burdens imposed upon other members of the family. The mother, already harried by her many duties of housekeeping and child care, suddenly finds herself forced to care for a sick relative as well. The father, already feeling the pressures of providing adequately for his wife and children, suddenly finds medical expenses in addition. Thus, when an elderly person in the household becomes sick, the other members are apt to react with irritation and a feeling of being imposed upon. This is often communicated to the patient who feels rejected, unwanted, and depressed. Feelings of depression are a frequent and difficult problem in treating elderly patients.

People therefore react to illness in terms of attitudes toward health and illness in general, goals in terms of work and independence, feelings about the acceptability of a particular type of illness, the role within the family, feelings about that role, and what the outcome of illness means in terms of the future. Illness may seem to represent a weakness or inferiority, an inadequacy for meeting the needs of living. A patient may react with anger or guilt, with anxiety or depression. His reaction depends on his concept of how this illness affects his goals and standards.

Illness brings with it many new experiences and the patients' concept of his ability to meet such experiences is an important part of his reaction to them. Diagnostic procedures such as venipunctures, lumbar punctures, thoracenteses, paracenteses, bone marrow aspirations, liver biopsies, or splenic punctures all involving introduction of needles into the body—may arouse tension, apprehension, or frank anxiety. Cardiac catheterizations and various visualization procedures may arouse similar feelings even more dramatically. The factors involved in these reactions have been studied by Kaplan,[84] who reports that unfamiliarity with procedures or with the environment in which these procedures are carried out accounts for some of the anxiety but that psychologic problems of the patient and poor doctor-patient relationship add to the intensity of the reaction.

HOSPITALIZATION

Hospitalization is a special problem which partakes of these features. But, in addition, hospitalization entails a way of life which is quite foreign to most people. Some adapt more readily than others to this way of living. Hospitalized patients depend on others for food, companionship, and care. The way in which these needs are met partly determine how secure or how anxious they feel. Some patients find it hard to accept dependency or to allow others to make their decisions for them. Even those who accept the dependent state will become anxious or angry if the care given them seems inadequate or lacking in attention to individual needs. The independent person may rebel against the subordinate and submissive role. Allowing him some power of decision, if only over what he will eat at mealtime, may alleviate this situation. A feeling that his desires are important to the physician, even if acquiescence to his requests is not always possible, also alleviates a part of his distress in this regard.

In addition to the dependent role which hospitalization necessitates, there is a great deal of routine and regimentation. The person who habitually arises at 8 o'clock and hurries through breakfast in order to arrive at work on time may find the hospital routine of being awakened at 5:30 with no breakfast until 8:30 irritating. The person who has directed his schedule by the whim of the moment may also find the regular routine of hospital existence disturbing. Dependency and regimentation are aspects of hospital living which require adjustment.

Hospitalization also entails separation from family and friends. This may necessitate a greater adjustment for children than dependency and routine. It is also difficult, however, for some adult patients. This difficulty is accentuated if visiting hours are severely restricted or the hospital is far from the patient's home. It is accentuated when patients depend to a great extent on their friends and family for stimulation of interest in living and for companionship. If hospitalization represents rejection by the family, it may elicit a depressive reaction or marked irritability which makes relationships on the ward difficult. This is more apt to be the case with patients in state institutions or nursing homes, but it is sometimes met in general hospitals as well.

In a hospital there is also the stress of what happens to other patients. It is easy for patients to identify with each other since they are undergoing a new and strange experience together. Consequently, the reaction to what happens to the patient in the next bed or in the next room may be quite intense. Sometimes the reaction is beneficial. A patient who becomes absorbed in someone else's problems may see his own illness in broader perspective and accept it more philosophically. But the reaction is often not beneficial and one must be alert to these circumstances.

The family also reacts to having one of its members hospitalized, and its reaction may be every bit as complex. Separation is difficult; but when it is combined with uncertainty about what is happening to the patient, worries about the adequacy of care, fears about diagnostic or therapeutic procedures, or distress at the patient's reaction to his illness, hospitalization can become a major emotional upheaval.

REHABILITATION

When the acute phase of illness is over and the person must return to work, with or without residual disability, the process of adjustment must begin all over again. After a prolonged illness there is apt to be loss of work skills. These must be regained if the person is to return to his previous employment. If new type of skilled work is indicated because of disability, these skills must be acquired. The skills of work, therefore, may pose a real problem in rehabilitation. If the illness began at work, the patient may fear return to it; if the work is new, he may question his adequacy for it. The sudden jump from convalescence and little activity to working an 8-hour day in competition with others is a big one, and it is not surprising that some patients view it with apprehension. Overcoming these barriers requires a fairly strong motivation for return to work.

Motivation is sometimes discussed as though it were a fixed and unchanging entity which could be evaluated quantitatively. Thus a patient may be called "well motivated" with the statement that he will do well in rehabilitation or "poorly motivated" with the statement that nothing can therefore be done for him. This is a considerable oversimplification. Motivation is a composite of many forces, sometimes working at cross purposes, and one can strengthen or weaken it. The motivation to work depends on the balance between the personal gains deriving from work and the losses incurred because of it. On the positive side we have the obvious factor of economic gain. There is also the satisfaction in doing something productive and the social prestige and approval which may come from this. In many instances long-term goals can only be satisfied by employment. There are personal gains that depend on the type of work done and the pleasure in exercising authority and assuming responsibility or demonstrating skill at a particular kind of work.

Work also has its negative side. It is frequently routine and a certain amount of freedom is lost by working. A great deal of uncertainty is involved in some types of work, and the person is not sure from one week to the next that he will be employed. The constant supervision of one's activities may be felt as a restriction and a frustration. In general the gains in terms of personal satisfaction, pay, and social approval far outweigh the losses, but this is not always true.

A study of motivation among factory workers[67] showed that 30 per cent of them were in their jobs largely because they had no particular interest in doing anything else. They became factory workers by default. In this situation job satisfactions are apt to be minimal. Nor is the economic gain always a major one. As illustrated in a case mentioned earlier, relief payments may offer more security than work payments. At such a time dependency obviously offers far more security than does work. Where no social opprobrium is connected with dependency there is far less need for working, since the forces acting to get a person back to productive activity are weak. And if life is viewed in terms of living from one day to the next rather than of achieving long-term goals, another motivation for work is lacking.

If a person has never had satisfaction on the job, if he has lost his previous skills or must learn a new trade, if his relief payments are higher than the income he would make by working, if he has no long-term goals, and if there is little social approval for working, then the routine, the loss of freedom, and the uncertainty involved in working outweigh the gains potentially present, and the motivation for work is low. Such a person requires considerable efforts before rehabilitation can be effective. But if you analyze the forces which are acting for and against getting him back to work, many avenues of approach to the problem become evident. If you can find work which will give him satisfaction his motivation may increase. If he can be helped to relearn old skills before return to full-time employment, as is done in sheltered workshops, one of the fears which block return to work may be allayed. If you can give him approval for working to make up for the lack of approval in his own social group, another factor which influences his motivation to work is affected. If you can find something he would like from life which he has not attained but could by working, a long-term goal may act again as incentive for work. Minimizing his loss of freedom in work also will affect his motivation. Avoidance of the routine types of work or the uncertainty of seasonal labor also may affect motivation. All of these factors do not apply to any one patient. You must evaluate what has accounted for "poor motivation" and try to correct this deficiency.

The effect of social pressures varies among people for personal reasons. Fred (p. 56) had an intense need to appear independent. Diabetes threatened his independence, particularly when it seemed to be interfering with his chances of getting a job as fireman or policeman. Though somewhat depressed at not getting the kind of work he wanted, he also felt insecure and uncertain of the future. Anxiety resulted in an exacerbation of his diabetes. As the day neared for the Veterans Administration to decide on his disability and pension, the same conflict was activated and his insulin requirements reached their peak. With a decision in his favor and arrival of the first check, his anxiety decreased. He felt secure and able to take care of himself, assured that a check would arrive regularly from the government. With Fred, social pressures to work reinforced his own needs to be independent. Motivating him to work was no problem for the physician. Despite his regular Veterans Administration check and frequent changes of job, he was never without work for more than a few days at a time.

Quite the contrary was true for Mr. Benson. He had been a very successful traveling salesman who enjoyed meeting people and prided himself on his ability to influence others. He had a fine physique, enjoyed athletics, and was proud of his physical capacities. In the prime of life he suffered a stroke which left one side of his body weak. Physically he could have continued his work, for his disability was very slight. However, he never returned to work of any sort. He said he had lost his confidence, wanted to avoid people, and had no interest in any type of work. This reaction, strange at first thought, becomes understandable viewed in terms of the basis for his previous "excellent" adjustment. He was very narcissistic and had been proud of his physique and prowess. Much of his confidence lay in his feeling that others admired him for his appearance before ever speaking to him. This made it easy for him to approach others with a warm, friendly, confident manner. The slight physical disability was therefore a major stress to him and one which he could not fight or change. His conflicts about masculinity and his narcissism were both severely strained by his illness and he wanted to hide so that others would not see him. Social pressures toward work and independence were not of sufficient strength to overcome the inner forces which prevented his return to work. He therefore remained a chronic invalid despite almost complete physical recovery.

Another factor which needs attention is the patient's environment during convalescence and after recovery from illness. The social milieu in which he lives can strikingly affect health and the adequacy of adjustment following illness. This has been studied particularly for patients who have had mental illness. The effect of family expectations on the success or failure of return to community living was well demonstrated in the study of Freeman and Simmons,[85] who found that even patients with a low performance level were more apt to adjust adequately upon return to a parental family than to a conjugal one. Sutherland, studying a group of patients with colostomies,[86] found that family relationships had a very marked effect upon the patient's adjustment to a colostomy. Such data is needed for other conditions as well.

We tend to think of social factors in life in rather abstract terms forgetting their dynamic quality. We look upon personal attitudes as rather indifferent matters which we can change tomorrow if we so desire. This is far from the truth, except in the most minor of matters. Our aims, ambitions, and ideals affect our behavior from day to day and become the guiding principles and goals of our life. We consider attitudes to be indifferent matters largely because they are so well molded by the social pressures in which we live that their major direction is seldom directly opposed. Their strength is most evident when they are frustrated, and it is at such times that the physician sees his patient. It is most important that the physician recognize the dynamic quality and the potency of a patient's attitudes and goals.

The effects of attitudes and emotional reactions on a patient's response to treatment may spell the difference between success and failure. Emotional disturbance of any sort can prevent a patient from being able to rest mentally or physically. With patients suffering from cardiac decompensation, thyrotoxicosis, or other disease requiring rest, this may become a matter of major importance. When an illness is related to suppressed anger, as is duodenal ulcer, or when symtoms may be precipitated by anger, as in coronary atherosclerosis with angina, the irritations and frustrations of hospital regimens may seriously interfere with recovery. If such a person sees his illness as a frustration and reacts to it with anger, the illness may be prolonged whether he is hospitalized or not. The patient who is anxious or depressed and has symptoms related to these emotions may get significantly worse on admission to the hospital because of apprehension about what is to come. The symptoms of a patient with arthritis or with muscular aches and pains may be exaggerated by muscular tensions engendered by the stresses of being ill. These are matters, therefore, which deserve the serious consideration of every physician. The physiologic concomitants of attitudes and emotions are complicating features of illness whether the illness is primarily emotional or not. One cannot separate the patient from his reactions to being ill. When a reaction interferes with therapy and rehabilitation, it behooves the physician to be aware of it and to treat the reaction to illness as vigorously as he treats the illness itself.

Chapter 8

Interviewing

I N the practice of medicine the physician relies heavily upon information obtained from the patient in interviews. To arrive at a correct diagnosis you must be able to get the pertinent information and to interpret its meaning. You cannot expect to do this if you do not know what information is pertinent, nor can you succeed if communication between you and the patient is hampered. The process by which information is gathered is of great importance and deserves more emphasis than it is usually accorded in medical education. Though interviewing is a part of therapy as well as of diagnosis, it will be discussed here primarily as a source of information about the patient.

During interviews, you wish to gain all information which will contribute to a full understanding of the patient and his illness. You want to know about the symptoms from which he seeks relief, the circumstances in which these arose or became aggravated, his response to these situations, and features of his personality and past experience which affect this response. With such information at hand, you will be able to evaluate the problem and institute appropriate therapy.

RELATIONSHIP

The act of history taking and the type of doctor-patient relationship are inseparable. Relationship develops through communication, both verbal and nonverbal. In the course of questioning a patient about his symptoms, you convey your feeling of respect for him as a person or your lack of it and your interest in his problems or your preoccupation with other matters. In doing so, you establish a relationship with him which affects the history you obtain. The patient who feels at ease with his doctor and knows that he is respected will give a more complete and meaningful history than the one who is only answering yes or no to what is asked. Thus a circle of reinforcement is established between history taking and relationship. Though you may intuitively do the right thing, intuition cannot be relied upon to meet every situation perfectly. An awareness of the effects of questioning on the patient and of factors affecting the relation between physician and patient can greatly assist you in achieving your goal of relieving him of his symptoms and helping him realize the full extent of his potentialities—physical, emotional, intellectual and social. The two basic tools which you constantly use to achieve this goal are the process of history taking and the doctor-patient relationship.

In any interview, a keen ear, a sharp eye, an alert mind, and a sympathetic interest in others are the keystones to success. The last is by far the most important. The person who is interested and understanding will be courteous and considerate and will preserve the dignity of the patient. He will have a warm, friendly approach and will be responsive to the emotions he finds in the patient. Sympathetic interest in others implies some awareness of basic motivations and some warmth of feeling for human frailties. It implies, as well, a deep respect for others.

Not all communication between doctor and patient is contained in the words which are spoken. Your warmth and interest are expressed in your tone of voice, facial expressions, and gestures. These express better than any words how you feel toward your patient. It is not necessary to tell him that you respect him and will honor his confidences. In fact it will probably arouse suspicion if you do. Respect ordinarily is best expressed nonverbally.

The interviewer should maintain an accepting attitude. This does not mean that you must always agree with the patient. It does mean that you should avoid criticism insofar as possible. An accepting attitude means more than merely refraining from verbal criticism. Criticism can be expressed in many ways—by demeanor, by facial expression, by a lifted eyebrow, or by a chance inflection on some key word. All of these may express a critical attitude without your awareness that you have expressed it.

THE SETTING

Your setting is familiar to you, and it is easy to forget that the surroundings are strange to the patient or that they may arouse tension or anxiety. A tense patient is also controlled and inhibited in expressing himself. Anxiety tends to impair memory and to lead to faulty recollection of symptoms and past experiences. It therefore is important to put the patient at ease. A prime requisite for interviewing is a friendly atmosphere. A warm approach by the first person the patient meets in this new setting can do much to relieve tension or anxiety. And a friendly attitude on the part of the interviewer is the best assurance of a productive interview.

Privacy is important. When a private room is not available, conversation should be carried on in quiet tones which do not attract the attention of others in the room. A person may give his name easily in a group, but a woman may prefer not even to state her age if her neighbor will overhear it. More intimate information than this may be withheld if the conversation can be heard by others.

STARTING

Once introductions have been completed and the patient and you are both seated comfortably, attention is directed to the problem which has brought the patient to you. If he has come because of an accident, the details of the accident are discussed. If he has come because of a symptom, the symptom is discussed. If he has come in upon the order of his superior or the insistence of his wife, their reasons are discussed. Ordinarily this is the smoothest and most productive way of proceeding. If a patient is tremendously upset emotionally, it may be better to let him express some of this emotion first. Then he can attend to the practical questions. In such a case it is perfectly acceptable to start with a comment such as "You look depressed. What is the matter?" or "You seem to resent coming here. Why?" Questions of this sort, sympathetically posed, can often be of considerable benefit.

The physician must appraise the emotional state of the patient and adapt himself to it if the interview is to be successful. To treat all situations alike can only lead to difficulty. The person who actively seeks help will give information freely, and the interviewer needs only to indicate what information is desired. It is quite a different matter to interview a basically belligerent person, even though on the surface he may be calm and friendly. The person who has come at the insistence of someone else needs a brief period of adjustment. You need not point out to him that he is being uncooperative or belligerent. It is only necessary to be aware that the anger is justified and is not directed at you though it is interfering with your functions. The patient did not want to come; he was forced to come. If you view his hostility as understandable under the circumstances, his acceptance of your understanding will be communicated in his manner even though no comment is made about it. Similarly, the timid person needs to have a few minutes to get acquainted with the surroundings and with the interviewer before questions are put to him. Launching immediately into a long list of routine questions—your name, your age, your job, your symptoms—without preliminaries is not conducive to obtaining pertinent information later in the interview.

MAKING QUESTIONS MEANINGFUL

Questions, especially those concerning social and emotional data, should be meaningful to the patient. If the patient sees no connection between his physical complaints and the circumstances in which he works and lives, he is apt to treat questions about these matters as unimportant and give perfunctory answers to them. It is not necessary, however, to discuss psychophysiologic concepts to make these relationships meaningful. If you start with the presenting complaint and identify the situation in which this arose, questions about this situation are at once pertinent to the illness. If you use the ordinary outline of history taking and complete your questioning about the Present Illness, Past History, and System Review before asking about the patient's family and his relationships with others, the questions no longer seem pertinent to the symptom which brought him to you. He is apt to give less complete and less informative answers, since these questions seem to be unnecessary, asked more as a routine than for any value the information may have for understanding his illness. The same questions become significant to him if they are incorporated as part of gathering information about his symptoms. Questions must have significance to the patient to assure a complete answer in which he does not gloss over stresses he is struggling unsuccessfully to meet.

The same considerations hold throughout the interview. It is necessary to understand the patient well. You must evaluate his intellectual and emotional resources and must understand his attitudes toward life, his values and goals, his concept of himself, his conflicts and defenses, and the social forces which have impinged upon him. To maintain his interest and cooperation during this process, you must constantly make questions seem pertinent. This can be done by maintaining a logical sequence of questioning in which the illness of the patient is constantly kept in focus. Thus, having learned the symptoms which trouble him and the circumstances in which they arose you then inquire why this has been stressful. This question leads to a discussion of attitudes, values, and goals; conflicts and defenses; and past experiences, including childhood events and relationships. Answering this question fully may require extensive exploration of the patient's background. Nevertheless, identification of the stress and the reasons for its being stressful are part of your job. For almost any stressful situation it can be said that others have met similar situations without illness. You should therefore seek to understand why the patient has been unable to cope with this situation without symptoms. This entails an evaluation of constitutional endowment and of the defense mechanisms he uses. It also requires consideration of the blocks and resistances which prevent him from using other defenses or taking direct action in the situation. What is stressful? Why is it stressful? Why do symptoms develop in association with this stress? Only when these 3 questions have been explored in detail are you ready for the fourth question—What can be done to help the patient avoid a recurrence of symptoms when next he meets this stressful situation?

Each new point should ordinarily be approached with an open question which permits a wide range of answers. Specific questions can then be asked in order to clarify any point which seems vague. Starting with a specific question may prevent the patient from discussing related issues of importance and thus prevent you from getting needed information. When first asking the patient about his symptoms, do not begin with, "Do you have pain in your stomach?" but rather "What is the trouble?" or "What are your symptoms?" If pain is mentioned, then specific questions are asked to characterize it more clearly. Emotional and social data should be approached in the same way— general questions first, specific and direct questions only when necessary.

NONVERBAL COMMUNICATION

You can direct conversation by what you do not say as well as by the questions you ask. Ordinarily a physician directs the patient's conversation by questions which lead to avenues which must be explored before the illness can be understood. When a patient dwells on apparently irrelevant details the conversation is directed into other channels, but usually not by telling him you are not interested in those details. To do so would break the free flow of communication and might arouse considerable resentment as well. Instead, listen quietly to what is said but direct all questions away from the irrelevant. Save your interest, which is in a sense your approval, for things you consider important. The patient will note, even if not consciously, the lack of response and will soon adjust his conversation accordingly.

An interesting study with considerable pertinence to this point has been reported.[87] The investigator instructed subjects to say as many different words as they could. Whenever they gave a plural noun, he would murmur "mmm-hmm" in an approving manner. He found that the frequency of plural nouns correlated directly with his murmurs though none of the subjects seemed to be aware of the "mmm-hmm's" to which they responded. In extending these observations,[88] it was found that expressing approval of an opinion, or paraphrasing the opinion back to the subject without direct expression of approval or disapproval, resulted in a marked increase in the number of opinions and attitudes expressed during ordinary conversations. Omitting approval or repetition led to extinction of this response and a decrease in the number of attitudes expressed. This is an experimental confirmation of the importance of nonverbal communication and its effect in determining the type of information obtained during interviews and discussions. By such nonverbal cues you can encourage or discourage the expression of feelings or attitudes from your patients and thus alter the sort of data elicited and thereby aid evaluation of the patient.

CLUES TO HEED

Physicians must be acute observers and good listeners to get maximal information from an interview. They must listen closely to patients' answers and comments, never lapsing into the role of passive recipients of information. Clues to important facts are often contained in subtle changes of inflection. Unusual words, an unusual succession of ideas, hesitation in speech, recurrent references to a topic, inconsistencies in facts, inconsistencies between what is said and what is done may all be signposts pointing to emotional meanings never clearly verbalized. The skillful interviewer must be alert to these clues and investigate them with further questions.

A young girl with vague gastrointestinal complaints when asked to describe her stepfather replied, "Oh, he's all right. He's a little jealous but we get along very well together. We've never had an argument." Despite the tenor of amicability in this reply, the word "jealous" seemed unusual applied to a father or stepfather. Inquiry revealed the pertinent fact that she was her mother's favorite, her stepfather clearly holding a second place. It also became evident that she used her symptoms as a means of reassuring herself that she retained this position. In this instance a single unusual word led to uncovering an important and abnormal relationship.

As I was starting a physical examination of a young man with acne, he asked me what my special interest was in medicine. I told him I was an internist particularly interested in psychosomatic phenomena. He then said, "I'm not sure I believe in psychosomatic medicine." After a brief pause, he continued, "I went to a psychiatrist once and he told me my acne was an expression of a desire for self-punishment. I don't go along with that. My dermatologist has been treating me with salves and diet." He paused again and a peculiar grin spread over his face, "I asked him, if diet was the cause of acne, why it only appeared on my face!" Here, in a short succession of sentences, no one of which is particularly revealing, the patient may have indicated a major area of conflict, his relationship with authority. The succession of rejections of "authoritative" statements is a clue to this possibility. Further questioning is indicated in such circumstances.

When various statements of the patient are inconsistent it is not uncommon to be somewhat irritated. Yet inconsistencies may indicate emotional ambivalence toward the matter being discussed. Questions to clarify the inconsistency should be asked in a manner of friendly inquiry and not to determine which is "true" and which is "false." Similarly, inconsistency between what is said and what is done may be the clue which reveals conflicts or blocks and resistances to action that might otherwise go unremarked. They should be noted and explored.

Perhaps the most difficult clues to capture are those to be found in things unsaid. As the patient talks, you should try to recreate for yourself the situations and emotions being described. Is the reaction one which might be anticipated from the person who is talking? Are there discrepancies? What elements have been omitted from the description to account for these discrepancies? From questions such as these, you may discover new areas which deserve investigation.

In addition to listening, you should observe the physical reactions

of the patient. Nervous movements of the face or hands, gesticula-
tions, musclar tension, blushing or blanching may all be evidences of
emotional meanings to material being discussed. A young man with
anxiety attacks broke into goose flesh repeatedly during a discussion
with his physician. He had no idea what precipitated his attacks of
anxiety and his tone of voice remained well controlled and carefully
modulated no matter what subject was being discussed. But his physician noted that goose flesh, evidence of an autonomic reaction, appeared each time he mentioned his father. Investigation of this clue
led quickly to the discovery that his father was the center of a number
of conflicts of intense emotional significance. These would doubtless
have been uncovered in time without recognizing the autonomic response, but they were revealed during the initial interview because
the physician noted it and recognized it as a significant clue worthy of
investigation.

OBSTACLES

One obstacle which may hamper communication between physician
and patient is haste. Though the busy physician would like to get
information as quickly as possible he must not do it in a brusque
manner or with questions which prevent the patient from giving pertinent information. Direct questions with a yes-or-no answer, a rapid
succession of questions which cut off the patient in the middle of
his answer, too much talking from the interviewer, all those things
which we do to save time usually have quite the opposite result. In
the long run these steps prove to be wasteful and inefficient because
they prevent you from obtaining needed information and you then
must retrace your steps in order to get it. The old adage, "make haste
slowly," is a good one.

Some people have a great deal of difficulty putting their feelings or
ideas into words. If you understand what the patient wants to say, you
may verbalize it for him. However, in doing so you must remember
that these are your words, not the patient's. Always check with the
patient to be certain that this is really what he means. If he uses any
new or unusual phrase in his assent, it is wise to question him about
this to be sure that you and he mean the same thing. In any verbalization, it is most important to avoid offense and to avoid expressing biases and prejudices. These verbalizations are used to clarify the
matter and not to express your own opinions on it.

You should also avoid phrasing questions in terms of everyday conversation or making them sound like casual, social questions. Questions such as "Are there any tensions at home?" or "How do you like your work?" are ones which arise in social conversations in one form or another every day. When we pass a person on the street and say, "Hi Joe, how are things at home?" we do not expect a full and detailed answer. More often that not the patient will interpret such questions in the light of previous everyday experience. He will give some bland, uninformative reply, such as "Oh, we get along fine. We have no more troubles than any other married couple." Such an answer really tells you nothing and you must recognize that it does not. What the patient considers to be the normal number of tensions in a married couple's life can only be judged by his own experience and it is, of course, no greater than what has been customary for him. If you ask such a question and get an essentially meaningless answer, you can proceed with "What sort of troubles do you have?" or drop the matter temporarily and wait for another opportunity to pose the same question in a different form. You must always be watchful for the bland, sociable answer and recognize that it does not give the information wanted.

It is important to realize that talking can be used as a defense against divulging personal information. The garrulous person may prevent pertinent questions being put to him by deflecting the conversation to a more neutral area. When this happens, it is most important to be aware of it; for it is just at these times that you have hit upon an important area of difficulty. To be sidetracked without being aware of being sidetracked is to miss important material. To confront a patient with the fact that he is sidestepping the question or talking around the issue is to create a hostile and belligerent frame of mind. This again will cut off the information that is desired. It is better to direct the conversation back to the subject being avoided until the reason for avoiding it has been determined.

Jesting can be used very shrewdly by some people as a defense. When a person finds himself confronted with an awkward situation or a topic of conversation which embarrasses him, he often turns to a jesting reply. In our amusement at the wit, we may fail to see that he has avoided what is potentially embarrassing. In jesting, he has made use of an acceptable social amenity. We do not ask him to explain why he has answered jokingly, so a jest usually ends the conversation on that subject. This, of course, is why jesting is an excellent defense.

An illustration of jesting as a defense against discussing an emotionally painful subject was afforded by a patient with progressive degeneration of the retina. Blindness was increasing as the months and years passed. When a medical student obtained his history, he was impressed by how well this man had adjusted to his handicap. He was impressed because this patient, when asked about his inevitable blindness, had retorted in jest. He had said with a laugh that he had been looking around for a good seeing-eye dog. He thought that a good dog would be able to find his way in and out of beer taverns and so his life would not be greatly different when he was blind than it was now. Actually this patient was so overwhelmed by the thought of being blind that he was completely unable to face the practical problems before him. He used the jest as a defense and had made no preparation for the blindness that was to come. Extensive treatment was necessary before he was able to consider essential arrangements. He needed to learn braille. He needed to find some occupation for the sightless years ahead. He needed to make living arrangements. All of these things could be planned in advance and some preparations made, since he knew that blindness was to come. When confronted with the same question put in a way that required a serious answer, he said that when he became blind he could see no alternative but suicide.

IDENTIFYING THE STRESS

Psychophysiologic phenomena are often referred to as "disorders of stress" because they are commonly related to circumstances viewed as stressful. Patients, however, usually complain about a symptom rather than about the situation with which it was associated. Yet, to deal intelligently with the symptom, you must understand the situation and the response of the patient to that situation. It is not always an easy matter to identify the stressful factor, but the temporal association of symptom and stress usually gives a convenient starting point. It should be emphasized, however, that you have not achieved understanding simply by identifying "the stress." You must go well beyond this to gain sufficient understanding to help the patient.

Ordinarily you will start by asking a question which gives the patient a chance to talk about what bothers him and then listening carefully to his answer. You ask not only when the complaint first appeared but also what was going on at that time. You may ask whether the symptom occurred more commonly while he was at work or while he was at home. If while at work, what are the stresses on the job, how does he get along with his boss, who are his colleagues? If while at home, what are the problems he and his wife disagree on, how are the children, and so on.

The simplest circumstance is that in which the patient's complaint is clearly associated with some stressful circumstance in his life. The connection, however, may not be so obvious. Mrs. Curtis, a middle-aged woman, came to the clinic complaining of intermittent difficulty in swallowing since a hysterectomy 3 years before. Though it was soon apparent that she was suffering from globus hystericus, the connection of such a symptom with uterine surgery was not immediately evident. How does one proceed in finding out what this connection may be? The first question put to this patient concerned the symptoms which had led to the operation. Questions were then directed toward the operation and how disturbing this had been to her. It was not difficult to proceed directly from this point to her sexual desires before and after the operation. Her answers to these questions did not indicate that the hysterectomy itself had been particularly stressful to her.

However, to the next question, which concerned her husband's feelings about the operation, she answered that he had not appeared to care one way or the other. Her tone of voice emphasized the extent of her husband's indifference. Following this clue led to the disclosure that her husband was indeed completely disinterested in her. He had not visited her in the hospital at the time of her operation. They had had no sexual intercourse since the surgery. He had no interest in her except as someone to keep the house clean and prepare his meals. Her attempts to break through the barrier between them had been met by avoidance and withdrawal, and it seemed to her that she would never be able to achieve happiness with him. Thus the physician had uncovered a stress which was an adequate reason for the symptom of globus. The stress was an unsatisfactory marital relationship based in part, but only in part, on the fact that her husband found her sexually repulsive after her uterus had been removed. Identification of the stressful circumstances pertinent to her complaint was the starting point for further discussions aimed at understanding all the factors which had led to this state of affairs. It was a starting point which added meaning to those discussions.

At times, you may not be able to learn the circumstances surrounding the first appearance of a symptom but will be able to identify the stressful circumstances under which it recurs. An example of this was a man in his early thirties who went to see his physician because of shortness of breath on exertion. There are many possible causes for this symptom, but the description given by the patient made it unlikely that the symptoms arose from any cardiac or pulmonary disease. Associated with his shortness of breath were numbness and tingling of his fingers, a generalized feeling of weakness most severe in his legs, some blurring of vision, and dizziness. These symptoms suggested hyperventilation. Patients who chronically overventilate slightly may have an exaggerated response to exercise. Symptoms are then precipitated by exertion. Hyperventilation, however, is usually related basically to emotional factors, such as anxiety and depression.

This patient was obviously "nervous." A discussion of emotional factors was started by asking him if he thought that he was a nervous person. He readily admitted this and added that his nervousness was most apt to be aggravated by his children. He had six children and found their noise and confusion almost more than he could tolerate. Yet he could not discipline them at all, leaving all punishment for his wife to administer. He said that spanking them was harder on him than it was on them. When he got angry, he broke into a cold sweat and had all of the symptoms which he had just described in association with exercise. In this patient the stress was internal. Feelings of anger aroused anxiety which blocked any adequate expression of the anger and was associated with hyperventilation.

More difficult is the symptom which recurs but has no relationship to stressful situations so far as the patient can recognize. A very common example is the patient with vascular headaches. These may occur in the evening, during the night, or early in the morning. They are common when the patient is relaxed on weekends or is anticipating a pleasant evening with friends. Their lack of correlation with stress is an obvious feature to the patient and makes it difficult for him to recognize that there are emotional backgrounds to this symptom. Vascular headaches are more apt to occur after a stressful period has ended, when the patient is relaxing; so one must go back several hours, or even a few days, to find the episode which laid the groundwork for the headache. If headaches are frequent these stresses are often found to be the daily circumstances of living. They therefore do not appear as stresses to the patient even when his attention is directed to them. At such times it may be helpful to ask him to describe his daily routine. The case of Mrs. Brown (p. 40) was an example of this.

Another situation is presented by the complaint which is insidious in onset and constant and thus has no temporal relationship to use as a starting point. Such a situation was presented by a 53 year old man who complained of chronic fatigability for 3 years without associated symptoms. Fatigability of this duration without other signs or symptoms is most apt to be related to stressful life situations. Consequently, questions pertaining to emotional stresses must take their place alongside questions evaluating the possibilities of chronic disease. Home and work are the two major areas of most people's lives; therefore, you may start by asking questions about these.

What about his home? He lived with his wife and teen-age daughter in a pleasant bungalow which had been paid for. How did he get along with his wife? They had occasional frictions but no major arguments and he thought they got along quite well together. He stated that sexual relations were satisfactory to both of them. His daughter was a fine girl who had done extremely well in school and had lots of friends. What about his work? He had been a carpenter for 5 years or so. He said he was quite satisfied with his job and had a fine boss. His pay was adequate and he was in no financial distress.

The question which unlocked the floodgates of information in this patient and demonstrated how careful one must be in evaluating bland responses of the sort just noted was "what had you planned to do as a young man starting out in life?" He began to talk more freely at this point and told the following story.

He was the oldest of 4 brothers living on a farm. His parents were poor but industrious and had high goals for their children. However, when he was 14 his father died. As the oldest of the children he took the responsibility of running the farm. He put his 3 younger brothers through college. One of them became an engineer and all 3 achieved financial and social success. He himself had no education beyond the eighth grade. By the time the youngest brother was through college the patient was married and continuation of his education did not seem feasible. He disliked farm work. He didn't want to do outdoor work of any sort. He had wanted to have a small business of his own where he could be his own boss. He needed money to get started in such an enterprise. If he had had his way, he would have gone to college and majored in business administration. But none of these things were possible for him. So he started out trying to make money—quick money—any way he could. He worked on the farm. He took extra jobs. When he had saved a little money he looked around for some way to double that money. He tried anything which he thought would make money. Consequently, he worked hard and saved all of the money that he could for investment in various projects, but since none of them were particularly successful he never had money for the things which make life more comfortable and pleasant. His relatives, however, did well, and his wife, in looking around at their circumstances and comparing her own, considered her husband a ne'er-do-well and a failure. His daughter had contempt for him as a provider. His efforts to improve himself, therefore, became increasingly desperate. Life went on in this totally unsatisfactory manner for years without his ever managing to accumulate the funds he felt he needed to start a business of his own, which had been his goal in life.

When his fiftieth birthday came along, he suddenly began to feel old. The years in which he could do hard labor were numbered. He had passed the prime of life and the chances of his attaining any success in achieving his goals had become slight indeed. He realized that not only had each individual venture failed to get him what he had wanted but that the sum of his activities in life had failed. He had not achieved the security and financial position for which he had aimed; and in his efforts to get there he had alienated his family so that his wife and daughter were contemptuous of him. It was in this setting that he became depressed and fatigued, finding it hard to continue at his work as carpenter.

Nothing was really right in this man's life. Why did he give such bland information in response to the initial questions? He had said that he and his wife got along fairly well together. They had occasional frictions but no fights. This was perfectly true. His wife had trouble containing her anger and contempt at his lack of success in the world; but she expressed this in a general irritability. He felt he was a failure and that her irritation was perfectly justified. He accepted it without complaint; consequently, they had no arguments. His daughter had done well in school and had friends. No one asked if she was contemptuous of him, and he didn't volunteer the information. His job was the best he had ever had. It offered security and he did have a good boss. There was no logical reason to complain about this job. It just didn't fit his goals and aims in life. He wanted to be his own boss. He wanted to work inside, not outside. He wanted to have an executive position with prestige, not to be a common laborer. But if he had to work for someone else, this was as good a job as any he could hope to get. His statement that sexual relations were satisfactory to his wife and himself was likewise a statement which he could justify, though it gave a very false impression. They had had no sexual relations for at least a year. Before that time, relations had been infrequent. His wife did not want to have relations with him. This was part of her rejection of everything he was. He felt depressed and discouraged. Part of being depressed is a decrease in sexual desire, if not actual impotence. Consequently, he also was satisfied with the state of affairs. He felt reticent in discussing these matters and the question had been asked in such a way that he could avoid the facts without actually stating something which was not true.

In attempting to identify the pertinent stress, you must be careful not to interpret events through your own eyes. The nature of stress is subjective and personal. You must understand the patient's reaction fully, making no assumptions, or you may find that you are treating yourself rather than the patient. At the same time it should be emphasized that the "stressful situation" may not seem unpleasant to the patient even though it has led to a symptom or an illness. This may cause considerable difficulty in identifying the pertinent circumstances. An illustration will help to clarify this point.

A hospital ward clerk sought medical aid because of muscle tension headaches which she had had for 5 months. She had not had headaches before; in fact, she had always enjoyed excellent health. Interestingly enough, she had started her work as ward clerk exactly 5 months before. When the time relationship was pointed out to her and she was asked if she thought the two might be related, she was quick to respond that, though the headaches had never been present before she started her job and had appeared within a week after starting it, there could not possibly be any association between the two since she enjoyed her work so much. She said in rapid succession that it was the best job she had ever had, paid better, had more security, and gave her more responsibility. She had never thought that she would have as good a job. She wasn't sure that she was capable of holding it. She had worked extremely hard to be sure that her work was always perfect and in the 5 months no one had ever criticized anything she had done. She was trying to do the best possible work because she wanted to be assured of keeping the job.

This patient enjoyed her work to be sure. But even in saying this she revealed much of her trouble. She had never had as good a job; she had some doubt about her ability to hold it. She was extremely careful, trying always to turn in a perfect performance. What better attitude to engender tension than this one of always being alert and on guard so that no error is ever made? And what attitude is more likely to be associated with muscle tension than this? Here we have a person putting herself under stress. The rewards are such that the total effect is pleasant for her, but the stress is there nonetheless.

These few sentences contain information which answers two questions: What is stressful and why is it stressful? The first of these—what —is usually answered in terms of current happenings, the history of the present illness. The second—why—is answered in terms of past experiences of the patient and his basic endowment. Investigation of pertinent past experiences may take you into the patient's childhood and his relationships with his parents. At times this sort of intensive delving into a patient's past may require the assistance of a psychiatrist, but in many instances it can be obtained quickly and easily, as in the case just described. One must always keep in mind the intensely personal quality of stress. Few physicians would find the job of ward clerk one to arouse enthusiasm or one they would perceive as a challenge. This patient did. All of us, when we meet an experience which we consider to be challenging and in which we want particularly to do well, react with a certain amount of tension, as this patient did. An understanding of her attitude toward her job makes her response to it understandable, and an understanding of these matters is extremely important to therapy.

The third question is yet to be answered. Why does the patient have symptoms with the stress? The answer to this usually lies in the intensity of the response or in its duration. Sometimes both factors are important. In the ward clerk, the duration of the response was particularly important. Her headaches occurred in the middle of the afternoon. She was able to carry the tension developed at her work for several hours before symptoms resulted. In her case, decreasing the intensity of her response slightly or finding ways to decrease its duration would alleviate the symptom. This was relatively easy to do because her evaluation of her capacity to handle the situation was based on an underestimation of her own abilities. Pointing out to her that she may have needed to be this careful during the first few days on the job, when everything was new and unfamiliar to her, but now that it was routinized she should be able to relax somewhat without making errors, helped diminish her tension. Reminding her that for 5 months she had turned in a performance near enough perfection so that no one had complained about it and indicating that this was evidence of her ability to handle the job also helped. It was not necessary for her to change her job to get relief from her headaches.

A SAMPLE INTERVIEW

The comments and suggestions which have been made about interviewing are not rules to be observed rigidly. Interviewing requires flexibility and ease in human relations. No two patients are exactly alike; no two interviews will be the same. Nor will two physicians proceed in the same manner even when interviewing the same patient. The interview is an expression of the physician as well as of the patient. The example which follows illustrates one way an interview might proceed.

Dr. Bailey extended his hand in greeting as he said in a quiet but warm and friendly voice, "How do you do, Mr. Laird. Have a seat." Dr. Bailey's quick eye noted that Mr. Laird seemed ill at ease, that he was probably in his early fifties, and that he was neatly dressed in conservative, well tailored clothes. He noted, too, that his handshake was returned in a rather perfunctory fashion and that his greeting had not been returned at all. Mr. Laird had moved to town 2 years before and this was the first time he had come to see the doctor. But Dr. Bailey knew that he lived in one of the more fashionable new developments just out of town and worked for a large corporation. The lack of cordiality was strange under the circumstances, but Mr. Laird was obviously troubled and preoccupied. He sat uncomfortably in the chair offered him, waiting for Dr. Bailey to open the conversation.

"Well, what seems to be the trouble?" Dr. Bailey asked, his tone of voice indicating interest and concern as to what should trouble Mr. Laird so deeply.

"Oh, I just seem to be nervous all the time." Mr. Laird sighed as he spoke and his fingers clutched nervously at the arms of his chair. It was reassuring, though, to meet a doctor who could see that he was disturbed and was ready to take it seriously. "Can't do my work the way I should. I don't know what's the matter but I've got to do something about it." His left cheek twitched involuntarily as he spoke.

"How long have you been nervous?"

"Well, I've always been a little nervous, I guess. But it's been much worse during the past 6 months." Mr. Laird sighed again.

"What happened then?"

"I don't know. My work was going fine then. I just got nervous and couldn't keep up the pace." The nervousness was plain enough as Mr. Laird shifted uneasily in his chair, his face continuing to twitch at intervals. But he was obviously depressed as well. His tone of voice sounded almost despairing.

"What sort of nervousness is it?" asked Dr. Bailey sympathetically.

Mr. Laird hesitated, "Well, it's mostly my hands. They tremble. Sometimes they tremble so badly I feel like hiding from people." He was watching the doctor as he spoke, gauging the effect of what he said. Could he speak freely about the nervousness that embarrassed him so much or was he going to be told to get control of himself and forget it? He wished he could. Dr. Bailey seemed to be taking it as a serious complaint, however.

"What makes you nervous?"

"I don't know." He paused. "Well, whenever I'm under pressure my hands start to tremble a bit."

"What sort of pressure?"

"Oh, well, when someone doesn't like what I tell them to do. If they begin to argue, I start trembling and have to leave. But, really, that shouldn't be the cause of it. It always has made me a little nervous to have someone argue with me but it's happened often enough that I should be used to it. And it never made me *this* nervous before."

"Are you only nervous at work?"

"No. It's just as bad at home. I seem to be nervous all the time." Mr. Laird seemed more comfortable, though his fingers continued to move restlessly along the arm of his chair. The tic seemed a little less frequent, too.

"What makes it worse at home?" Dr. Bailey's voice was quiet and friendly but his whole manner indicated his interest in getting to the bottom of the trouble.

"Oh, I'm not sure I know. I guess its the bills." He hesitated, obviously about to say more, so Dr. Bailey waited quietly. "You know, there are an awful lot of things to pay for when you get married and start a new home at my age."

"You got married recently?"

"About two and a half years ago."

"Really." Dr. Bailey's tone indicated his interest and desire to know more.

"Yes, we went together as youngsters but we each got married to someone else. My first wife died after 7 years. That was more than 20 years ago. Her husband died several years ago. When I heard about it, I wrote to her. We started going together and then we got married about two and a half years ago. We've been married two and a half years and we're still adjusting—but I guess that's to be expected."

"What kind of adjustments?"

"Well," he hesitated, as though deciding where he ought to start and how much to say. "Well, for one thing we built a house a year ago. It's a nice home, worth about 30 thousand dollars. I had a little savings and put all I had into it. She had more and put a part of hers in. We have a pretty big mortgage and our monthly payments are more than a third of my income." He sighed as he continued, "It doesn't leave much for the rest of the bills."

"What about using her savings to help out?"

"No, those are hers. She only has a few thousand dollars, though she does get a monthly income from some property she owns. That goes into her savings too. She says it's hers and so she keeps it. Her attorney told her the man should pay the bills."

"Attorney?" Dr. Bailey's voice expressed surprise and interest as he directed the conversation toward apparent marital difficulties.

"Yes, she went to one 6 months ago to get a divorce. He said she was right—the man should pay the bills. If he couldn't meet his financial obligations she had a good basis for a divorce. I guess he was right. A man should pay the bills."

Dr. Bailey noted the three-fold repetition of "a man should pay the bills" and also that Mrs. Laird had gone to her lawyer 6 months before seeking a divorce. That was the length of time his nervousness had been severe. The two could well be related. But he did not break the flow of conversation with these ruminations. "Those bills are pretty big for your salary, aren't they?"

"Yes, it seems a bit unreasonable to me. But she doesn't think much of my job. It can't ever pay much. Her first husband did much better financially. She came from a poor farm family just like I did but he left her with money and property. I can't do that."

"And she wanted a divorce because of your financial troubles?"

"I guess so." His words expressed agreement but his tone of voice left some doubt as to whether he really believed this. He seemed to dismiss it as unimportant and hurried on. "But we've got things straightened out now. She's decided we can sell the house and get something I can afford payments on. We'll live more simply. But she says she is willing to try it."

Because of the doubtful tone in which Mr. Laird had agreed that the reason for seeking divorce was finances the physician thought it well to ask questions about other problems in their adjustment.

"What about your sexual adjustment?"

"Not too good. I don't have much pep. We haven't had any at all in 6 months. But she's understanding." There was a short pause and then, as though clarifying what he had said, "She says I don't seem to have any pep—not like her first husband."

"She compares you with him frequently?"

The question, meant to be bland and merely a request for factual information, nevertheless carried an implication of criticism of his wife for making invidious comparisons. Mr. Laird was quick to recognize this and the tone of his answer was more a response to the criticism than to the question.

"Oh, not every day. I couldn't stand that. No, but she mentions it occasionally. She doesn't overdo it, just mentions it."

"Do you think the trouble at home could affect your work?"

"I suppose so. I do think about it an awful lot. I think the medicine caused most of the trouble, though."

"Medicine?"

"Yes, I got pretty nervous about 5 or 6 months ago. The company doctor put me on equanil. I didn't go back, just kept getting a refill at the drug store. He put me on 3 a day but I kept feeling more and more depressed and would take more pills hoping they would relieve it." A pause followed in which he seemed to be considering his next words. When he spoke again it was hesitantly with an eye kept watchfully on Dr. Bailey for his reaction. "I was having crying spells. I don't know what started them but they embarrassed me and when I felt one coming on I would disappear into a rest room or someplace until it was gone."

There was a pause with no comment from either one. Dr. Bailey waited in sympathetic silence for him to continue. Mr. Laird seemed ready to speak but was weighing his next words trying to decide whether to continue in the same vein or not.

"I did some pretty crazy things."

"What?"

"Well, one day—I don't know why—but one day I didn't go to work. I just rented a room at the hotel in town and sat in it all day long. I didn't do anything. I just sat there."

"Your boss knew about it?"

"Yes, and he didn't like it very much. Things just kept getting worse and worse. I was taking 10 or 12 tablets a day and 3 weeks ago I saw the company doc again and he asked how I was doing. I told him how depressed I felt and he told me to quit taking the pills. I've been feeling better since then. I think the pills made me depressed."

Dr. Bailey now had the essential information about the situation Mr. Laird was in. He needed eventually to know more about the marital difficulties leading Mrs. Laird to seek a divorce 6 months before, but he thought this could wait a while. Right now he wanted some background information to help him understand a little better just what sort of person Mr. Laird was. He wanted, therefore, to know about his family background and his earlier experiences in life. He made the transition quickly and simply, using the information Mr. Laird had given during the interview.

"You say you and your wife both came from poor farm families?"

"Yes."

"What was it like back then on a farm?"

"Oh, like life on any other farm I guess. Lots of hard work. My father worked awfully hard. My older brother and I worked with him on the farm. He was pretty strict. He wouldn't take *no* argument from *no*body." The repeated negatives were used knowingly and for emphasis. A slight shake of the head as he spoke added further vigor to his statement. Even 40 or more years later he was still obviously responding emotionally to how strict his father had been. "I guess that's why my brother ran away when he was 14. But dad was fair. He punished us often, usually with a switch, but only when we deserved it. And he sure wouldn't let anybody talk back to him. I never did it. Wouldn't even have considered it. He brought us up right."

"What about your mother?"

"My real mother died when I was born. My father married again when I was about 2 years old. She was very high tempered, but a good woman. They were happy, though he often told me that my mother had been the best woman ever and if anyone ever got to heaven she would."

"Were your parents warm and affectionate?"

"Not particularly. They didn't have time to be affectionate. I think they probably loved us as much as any parents but just were too busy. There's an awful lot of work on a farm, you know."

"Your brother ran away from home. What about you?"

"No, I stayed at home and helped with the work. There were six children younger than me and I was needed. I didn't leave home until I got married. That was when I was 20. We had two children and then my wife died. I always wanted an education. After her death I went back to school. My parents raised the children. I finally got a college degree. Without it I couldn't be doing the work I'm doing now."

"Do you think some of these things that happened earlier in your life could affect your reactions now?"

"Yes, I guess so. Psychiatrists say they do. How could it help but affect what a person is later on?"

Though Mr. Laird had said repeatedly that he did not know the reason for his nervousness, he nevertheless gave a very adequate account of the factors which contributed to it. He said he could not function under pressure. For 6 months he had been under great pressure at home. He did not make enough money to meet his bills; his wife told him that a man should. She had no respect for the work he did and let him know she thought him much less of a man than her first husband was. The primary stress, therefore, seemed to be at home.

It had been reflected in his work, however, causing increasing pressures to be applied there until this, too, became a major area of stress. As the situation deteriorated he felt more hopeless and helpless. He began to have crying spells and tried to withdraw; but there was no way to withdraw. At work or at home he was in the midst of it. So he retired to a hotel room, only to get into more trouble because of this.

If such a formulation was correct, then solving the problem at home should decrease his nervousness. Was the home situation correctable? His wife had been trying to force him to be more aggressive, more masculine. Four times in this brief interview he referred to the proper duties of the "man of the house" indicating that he accepted the obligations as proper but was inadequate to discharge them. Nor had he ever been very aggressive. When someone argued with him he trembled and left. But even without altering this part of his personality there was a chance of improving the situation. His wife apparently did not plan to proceed with the divorce even though things were far worse than when she first discussed it with her attorney. Their plans for the future left much to be settled and would not be so easy to accomplish as they seemed to feel. It would be hard for her to revise her standard of living downward voluntarily without some feelings of resentment toward him. A little outside help during this phase of adjustment might make the process a little easier.

The immediate situation may be alterable; but what about the personality problem? Not just with his wife did he have trouble being aggressive. He could not take an aggressive position with anyone. The problem was a major one for him, with ramifications in all areas in his life. And what was the nature of the trouble? A hypothesis that seems to fit the facts would be that in situations where anger was aroused he reacted with anxiety and depression. The subordinate who argued, the boss who criticized, and the wife who put pressure on him for more than he could give were all setting up situations which might arouse anger. His statement that if comparisons between himself and his wife's first husband were made frequently he "couldn't stand that" suggests that the feelings were quite close to the surface. And the background for such a reaction was present in his childhood. His father was a strict and severe disciplinarian who would not tolerate any back talk. Anger, the desire to lash back verbally, therefore aroused the fear of punishment, anxiety. As a child Mr. Laird accepted this as just and proper, incorporating this value system and the punishment within his own make-up. He would not "talk back." The urge to do so aroused feelings of guilt and unworthiness which he experienced as depression.

This interview illustrates the flow of conversation as a physician seeks information about stressful situations pertinent to a patient's complaints. The tone of the conversation was set immediately, before the chief complaint had been stated, by the mien of the patient. The physician responded to this by expressing his interest and concern in his manner of speaking. Such nonverbal communication is an essential part of interviewing and determines how smoothly the interview will go. Questions were kept meaningful to the patient by framing all of them in the context of the patient's own statements, following clues that appeared, and using material given by the patient to move from one area of interest to another. Open-ended questions and specific questions were interspersed as seemed indicated. Recurrent references to a topic, statements and expressions of emotions, key words, and physical manifestations were noted and integrated with factual material given verbally to give increased understanding of the bare facts elaborated. In this way the free flow of conversation was never interrupted, yet the interview was directed into pertinent areas so that essential information could be gathered rapidly.

Not all areas of importance were explored during this sample interview. The physician allowed many significant statements to pass without comment. This is commonly the case, particularly in an initial interview. But you must make mental note of potentially important areas so that you can return to them at a later interview. In this instance, for example, one would like to know more about the death of Mr. Laird's mother and his reaction to it. His father seemed to feel the loss deeply. Feelings of guilt over his mother's death might well have contributed to Mr. Laird's acceptance of his father's discipline as "just" when his brother reacted by rebelling and running away. It could be closely linked emotionally to the problem currently disturbing Mr. Laird and therefore needs to be discussed in some detail. Had Dr. Bailey wished, this could have been investigated when it was first mentioned. He chose instead to note the fact and discuss it later.

But this interview illustrates a more basic point than these—the importance of the doctor-patient relationship in interviewing. At the beginning of this interview, Mr. Laird was on guard, not certain how Dr. Bailey would react to a discussion of his symptoms. Without knowing what was wrong, Dr. Bailey recognized the need for an attitude of serious concern before Mr. Laird had spoken. He continued to indicate his concern and capacity for understanding by directing questions warmly and uncritically toward the emotional problems. Mr. Laird watched the physician's reactions to what he said, testing him out before talking freely. This was seen when, early in the interview, he hesitantly admitted that sometimes he "felt like" hiding from people. Later, it became evident that he had actually run away and hidden. But it is unlikely he would have revealed this "crazy" action had the physician not made him feel safe from ridicule by his reaction to the earlier admission. Dr. Bailey's communication of respect and interest at a nonverbal level made the verbal flow of information possible. The process of gathering information is markedly dependent on the nature of the doctor-patient relationship.

Chapter 9

Doctor-Patient Relationship

WHEN Mrs. Bertrand (p. 26) was referred to a neurosurgical clinic to be evaluated for sympathectomy, she was advised to have surgery. The physician was brusque and impersonal, taking no cognizance of her anxiety about her condition or about surgery. He was not aware that another physician had advised against surgery nor of the factors in her situation which militated against it. He was, however, aware of her hesitation. He tried to motivate her by arousing anxiety, the anxiety of dying in 2 years if she did not have surgery. Mobilizing anxiety can be an effective means to motivate patients when lack of action is related to complacency. But Mrs. Bertrand was already anxious and concerned. Anxiety was increased and resentment aroused as well, but the physician could not offer reasons for surgery sufficiently cogent to induce her to accept it. At this point he told her to "diet or die."

She therefore approached her next physician with some trepidation. She needed to discuss surgery, ventilate her feelings of anger and anxiety, and seek reassurance about the decision she had made. This physician repeated history, physical examination, and indicated laboratory tests. He then took time to explain to her some of the facts she needed to know about obesity, hypertension, and coronary disease and their treatment. He reassured her in realistic terms which recognized the severity of her illnesses but was also optimistic for the immediate future. At first he saw her at fairly frequent intervals, giving his moral support to her efforts to adhere to a stringent diet which seemed to eliminate most of the foods she particularly enjoyed eating.

He discussed her husband's blindness and his resistance to accepting it or making concrete plans for the future. Together they formulated a plan to overcome this resistance. The plan succeeded, and her husband became a happier person with new satisfactions in life when he

204

joined in the activities of the Guild for the Blind. The physician also encouraged her to try light work, since this was physically feasible, economically desirable, and a source of satisfaction. When she met with racial discrimination, he was there to hear her story, express interest and sympathy, and encourage her to try again. As the 2 years approached an end, her symptoms became much more severe and frequent. He re-evaluated her condition from all points of view and repeated chest film, electrocardiogram, and various renal studies. He was then able to reassure her that, despite increasing symptoms, there was no appreciable objective change. This and a discussion of her fear of death as a possible reason for the increasing symptoms was so reassuring that her angina promptly subsided and she felt much better physically.

These are not unusual activities for a physician, but they emphasize the many ways in which he may help a patient. He must be ready to teach a patient about his illness, listen to his problems sympathetically, give moral support in times of adversity, help motivate to appropriate action, give insight into emotional problems, and allay anxiety. The power for good in the doctor-patient relationship when it performs these functions and its ability to arouse anger or anxiety when it fails to deserves serious thought and attention, for it is the crux of medical practice. From what does the doctor-patient relationship draw its strength?

BACKGROUNDS

A basic factor in this relationship is the position of a physician in his community, which is ordinarily one of prestige. He is recognized as having knowledge and skills which make him an authority. He devotes his life to the care of the ill. A community's respect for a physician, for his skills, and for him as a healer are most important in establishing a therapeutic atmosphere. When these are lacking, the relationship will be altered accordingly.

In certain superficial ways, the physician's position in the community is not unlike that of a father in his own home. The father of a household also has prestige, knowledge, and skills above those of his children and cares for them when they are in need of help. It is in part because of these similarities that patients' conflicts in their relationship with their parents may be activated in their contacts with a physician. The doctor-patient relationship, therefore, becomes one in which conflicts may be mobilized, to be intensified or alleviated depending on the way they are handled by the physician. In dealing with such conflicts, the relation between a doctor and his patient is often more significant to the outcome of treatment than the specific material discussed or any conscious insights obtained.

A physician's position of authority carries with it certain responsibilities. Just as society believes that parents have an obligation to care for their children, it believes that physicians have responsibilities to patients. Patients who strongly identify you, the physician, with a parent figure, consciously or unconsciously, are apt to feel strongly about your obligations and to be very sensitive to occasions when you seem not to be meeting them. Such patients expect you to be constantly available and to meet all demands, just as they wished this to be true of their parents earlier in life. They are also very conscious of the amount of time spent with them and the amount of interest shown. To establish a strong relationship with such a patient, you must accept and meet your obligations. This does not mean that you must accede to all demands. It does mean that you must respect the demands and meet those which will benefit the patient. When meeting a patient's demands would not be to his best interests, you should offer some explanation and express your concern for his welfare, despite refusal to meet the specific request. Ordinarily this will strengthen, not weaken, the relationship.

Whether the relationship is strong or weak, highly sexualized or impersonal, your awareness of its nature may contribute more to an understanding of the patient's personality problems than any specific statements made. To analyze the relationship and use the information intelligently, you must be aware of your contribution to the relationship as well as the patient's contribution. Your inferences will then be valid and useful both in understanding the patient and in treating him. The alert physician can make effective use of himself in therapy through appropriate manipulation of relationship. To do so requires that he have some understanding of the factors which operate to strengthen a relationship or to weaken it.

CONFLICTS EXPRESSED IN RELATIONSHIP

Your position of authority and the need for a close working relation between you and the patient may activate conflicts which disrupt the relationship or render it less than optimal for therapeutic goals. Expression of these conflicts may take many forms, some subtle, others obvious even to a casual observer. A study of the relationship as viewed by patients with hypertension and peptic ulcer disclosed that the hypertensive patient saw his relationships with significant people as potentially hostile and threatening, while the patient with peptic ulcer did not.[89] Hypertensive patients usually avoided close relationships and seemed particularly sensitive to acts or words which might suggest hostility or derision. The passive role in relation to authority was itself a threat and a source of hostility, but this hostility was well controlled in an effort to maintain "emotional insulation." Patients with peptic ulcer, on the other hand, were more apt to seek a dependent relationship, particularly if the physician was able to satisfy these needs. Passivity in the doctor-patient relationship was not itself a threat, though any disruption of the dependent relationship was and might result in a hostile outburst. Thus the two groups tended to seek different types of relationships, to find different sources of threat in it, and to react to the physician in different ways.

Usually the relation between physician and patient is formed gradually as a result of complex interpersonal reactions between them. Occasionally, however, the conflicts are so urgent that a patient seeks to impose a specific type of relationship at the outset. At such times the area of conflict may be obvious upon first meeting the patient if you correctly evaluate what you observe. His general appearance, dress, manner of speaking, gait, and behavior may all express conflict.

A 19 year old boy with a congenital heart lesion was referred to a physician for evaluation before vocational training and job placement. He arrived late for his appointment. As he entered the office, a number of conflicting impressions were made almost immediately. He had rather soft, delicate features and a carefully nurtured wave in his hair. However, he was dressed with studied carelessness. A dirty and wrinkled shirt with sleeves removed at the shoulders topped faded working pants. He slouched and walked with a rolling gait. He smiled politely as he shook hands, but as he did so he announced that his time was limited; he would have to leave in half an hour. His speech throughout the interview remained superficially polite and friendly, but hostility was obviously close to the surface. His appearance suggested possible conflict about masculinity, and his manner of speaking indicated a need to be independent and to avoid a close relationship. He was trying to establish a relationship in which he could maintain command.

During the half hour which he had set as the time he would devote to the evaluation requested, a substantial amount of pertinent information was elicited. It not only confirmed the original impression but gave some possible reasons for his appearance and behavior. He was one of several children, and the others were strong and healthy. He could engage in any physical activity without developing symptoms, but, because of his heart condition, his parents had severely restricted his activities. They had treated him as a "heart case" without consideration for him as a person. As he became more rebellious at their restrictions, they became increasingly rejecting. On five occasions during adolescence, his father, irate at his refusal to obey, had told him to leave the house and not return. Each time he had left for a few days and then returned. He had not completed high school and had no intention of doing so. When asked the reason, he said that classmates had made derogatory comments about his clothes. He didn't care; he would dress any way he wanted to dress. In the 6 months immediately before the interview he had had 6 different jobs. The first was at a service station. He quit this because it paid 85 cents an hour and he was "not going to work for anyone at less than a dollar an hour." He had then worked for a trucking outfit but had trouble with his supervisor. "No one is going to tell *me* what to do" was his comment about this job. He was currently punching cattle with his "buddy," a job which he enjoyed though it paid nothing but room and board. As the end of the half hour neared, he rose and answered questions standing. When he took his leave, it was with a friendly smile and an attitude which seemed to say "I've enjoyed meeting you but I really must be going," though by his own admission he had no place in particular to go.

The conflicts around independence which set the course through life for this boy are fairly obvious. They originated in his relationship with his parents. That they also determined the relationship with his physician is clear. The need to maintain an appearance of complete independence is not always so plain. When present and unrecognized, you may feel puzzled, frustrated, or actually angry at the patient because of your inability to establish good rapport. Recognizing the reason for the poor relationship permits you to deal effectively with it without feeling irritation or anger. But in recognizing the patient's need to appear independent, you should not miss the dependency also there. Though ordered out of the house "permanently" five times, he had never stayed away more than a few days. Though determined to wear whatever he liked, he nevertheless was sufficiently upset by the comments made about his clothes to refuse to return to school. Though many of his comments and actions expressed a basic hostility toward the physician, he maintained a friendly, superficially good manner throughout the interview.

Much more than this was learned in the brief encounter. The physician obtained some insight into this patient's way of meeting potentially stressful situations and handling hostility. He seemed to take aggressive command of new situations, yet it was evident that he withdrew entirely as soon as he felt he was not in control. His smiling belligerence suggested that he denied his hostile feelings insofar as possible, and his statements indicated that when the hostility became conscious he expressed it by taking independent action rather than by actual physical assault.

Such facts give the physician a basis for determining his own course of action. If he wishes to work with this patient, he must permit him some degree of independence. To meet an aggressive approach with an equally aggressive one is to lose the patient, who will withdraw from the situation as he has from others in which he was not in control. To prepare a rigid regimen of therapy and present it in a dogmatic, uncompromising fashion is to invite rebellion and refusal to follow orders. The physician must allow the patient some measure of independence and the appearance, at least, of controlling his own regimen. Anyone working with this patient around vocational planning should anticipate frequent changes of job until some of the conflict around independence has been relieved. To make rigid demands and then reject him for not obeying them is to intensify his conflicts by repeating the pattern established by his parents. Allowing him some control of the situation and using authority only to direct him as he makes decisions should permit you to follow him long enough to establish a better relationship and to help him reach a more satisfactory equilibrium in his conflicts about being dependent on other people.

This case illustrates one of the ways in which a conflict arising in childhood may find expression in the doctor-patient relationship. The act of going to see a physician was sufficient to arouse the conflict and defenses before the physician had an opportunity to indicate how authoritarian he would be or how much independence he would permit. The potential subordination of the patient in a doctor-patient relationship so threatened this boy that he felt he must take measures to protect himself from it before it had a chance to develop. Some patients so need approval from persons in positions of authority that they are fearful of expressing any thought, emotion, or desire which they think might be unacceptable. This may express itself as a denial that there is any such objectionable impulse. On the other hand, if the impulse cannot be denied, the patient may exaggerate it. Both reactions originate from the need for approval. In the first case the patient refuses to acknowledge the undesirable impulse for fear that it will be frowned upon. In the second he talks about nothing except the undesirable impulse to reassure himself that you do not reject him because of it. He may actually flaunt the impulse as though he desired to be punished for it and wanted you to tell him how wicked he is. Both situations demand that you spend your time initially in securing a friendly rapport. The patient must feel that he is respected despite the undesirable impulse.

A problem of this sort was posed by Mrs. Coyle. She was 35 and twice married and came to see her physician because of nervousness and insomnia which had arisen in a setting of conflict with her husband because of her marital infidelity. She was neatly groomed and tastefully dressed. The interview began with an immediate statement of her guilt and unworthiness. Questions were unnecessary. With a continuous flow of tears, she recounted her sins in detail, adding, however, that it was all beyond her comprehension since she was really an idealist and a perfectionist. She had held an excellent job for years, getting nothing but praise for the efficiency with which she had discharged her duties. She and her husband had lived together happily for years and she loved him very much. She had made her savings available to him so that he could start a business of his own. How she could have done the dreadful things she told about, she would never understand.

What sort of relationship was this patient trying to establish with her physician? In her self-accusations and expressions of guilt, one might see a desire to elicit statements of disapproval and possibly a masochistic element in her personality. However, her interjection of statements about her basic worth and capabilities throughout the recital of her wrongs and worthlessness would make it seem more likely that she was pleading for reassurances that she was not guilty of wrong or that she was a fine person despite what she had done. Her general appearance and manner suggested a narcissistic person. Such people need frequent expressions of love and approval from others to maintain their own stores of self-respect. Her way of recounting her misdeeds was well calculated to elicit this type of response.

The background for this way of handling the situation lay again in childhood experiences. Whenever her mother had punished her for wrongdoing, her father had taken her on his knee to console her, telling her not to worry for he still loved her anyway. The doctor-patient relationship she was trying to establish was one in which she would receive similar expressions of affection, sympathy, and approval. Recognition of this fact allowed the physician to handle the situation without widening the rift in her relationship with her husband and without getting personally entangled in the conflict. It also gave a focus for questioning so that he could obtain pertinent background material bearing on this conflict. The type of relationship she was trying to establish was a much clearer expression of the basic problems which had prevented her from finding marital happiness than were any of the verbal statements she made.

Many physicians find it hard to respect a patient with bizarre behavior or unusual impulses which they consider immoral. But it is less difficult to respect such a patient if you remember that he has come to you for help because of these very impulses. There is no need to condone the impulse or behavior. He would not be seeking help if he felt that there was nothing wrong in his behavior or desires. What he wants is to feel that he is accepted despite them and that somebody will help him overcome them. If you respect his capacity to change, it will not be necessary to express approval or disapproval of everything he has done or felt. He will become aware that he is secure in your respect for his potentiality regardless of his past record or his current difficulty.

There are countless patterns of interaction between patient and physician and ways in which conflicts may find expression. Many examples have already been given. Gladys (p. 131), it will be recalled, had deep doubts as to her adequacy and felt it necessary to maintain poise and dignity in all her social relationships. In her relationship to her physician this introduced difficulties both in obtaining a complete history and in treating her symptoms. The young man with acne (p. 186) who had seen a psychiatrist and a dermatologist and had used the formulation of each to disparage the formulation of the other was expressing his conflicts with authority in his relationship with his physicians. In either case, an awareness of the forces at work in shaping the type of relationship is important if the physician wishes to work effectively with these patients. Such awareness makes it possible to focus attention on significant conflicts, to elicit pertinent historical material more rapidly, to avoid entanglement in the emotional conflicts binding the patient, and to utilize the relationship to benefit the patient.

It should be evident that conflicts in the physician's personality will also be expressed in the doctor-patient relationship. A physician may need to appear independent as much as his patient does and may, on occasion, express this as transparently as did the boy with congenital heart disease. Some physicians can brook no criticism, expressed or implied, because it seems to threaten their position of authority. And some need expressions of gratitude and affection from their patients more than others do. This brief mention of conflicts within the physician does not mean that their influence is unimportant.

STRESSES ARISING IN DOCTOR-PATIENT INTERACTIONS

In gathering information about the patient, you must not only make accurate observations but must be able to interpret them correctly. A source of information often neglected is the data which can be gleaned from observing the patient's reaction to stresses arising in his interactions with you. Stress is a highly individual matter. To identify it requires an awareness of the meaning to the patient of what you are and what you have done. But once you have identified an act or word of yours as a threat to the patient, you can learn much by observing the reaction to it. Mr. Grant (p. 70), who had gone from job to job, working 3 to 6 weeks at each and then quitting because of abdominal pain, presented an excellent illustration of this. In his conversations with his physician, he persistently avoided emotion-laden topics. His physician allowed this to continue through several interviews, though noting mentally that emotions seemed to have some threatening significance. He then spent an entire interview questioning the patient about one of the topics which had been avoided. Each digression was promptly turned back to the stressful material, the patient thus being forced to consider and discuss a subject he wished to avoid. The patient was plainly irritated by the physician's persistence but expressed his irritation only in his facial expressions. His tone of voice maintained its calm, level quality, and no words expressed his feeling. Instead, he suddenly said he would have to leave because he was having an attack of abdominal pain.

He did not ask for medication to relieve the pain but felt impelled to get out of the uncomfortable situation just as he had for years past in other stressful situations. This episode was used to help the patient understand himself more fully and to learn new devices by which to meet unpleasant situations.

RELATIONSHIP AND TREATMENT

Patients ordinarily come to you with a feeling that they are consulting an expert for help with their problems, whatever these may be. They are, in effect, seeking the aid of a powerful ally who can ease pain, set a leg, cure asthma, or allay anxiety. The act of coming can therefore be a potent force in decreasing stress. But you can destroy this force. The patient who seeks help and meets a superficial, cursory, or disinterested physician may leave worse than he came. He has asked for help and the person capable of giving that help has not been sufficiently concerned to do so. The patient may feel panic-stricken as a result. If the only person who can help him in his trouble refuses to do so, then he is indeed left entirely on his own. If he cannot cope with the situation unaided, he may feel intense anxiety and have an exacerbation of symptoms. The patient who obviously exaggerates the severity of his complaints may only be trying to overcome this feeling and to ensure that you take his problem seriously. You may be tempted to ignore symptoms which appear to be exaggerated. If you recognize that the exaggeration arises from anxiety and is a plea for help, you will be less inclined to treat it lightly and will thereby establish a better relationship and effect a better therapeutic result.

The importance of the patient's confidence in his physician cannot be overemphasized. Many factors contribute to this confidence or lack of it. The physician's ability to accept his authoritative position without engendering anger and rebellion is important. The nonverbal communication between physician and patient adds its part. And the confidence of the physician in himself and his therapy contributes significantly to the confidence of the patient in the physician and his remedies.

Confidence in the ability of the physician to cure is important for the security it affords the patient. The magical charms and incantations of medicine men have been followed by loss of symptoms. Patent medicines, perhaps harmless but also useless so far as their intrinsic pharmacologic action is concerned, have been reported to effect cures.

Whether a magical charm or a useless drug, these prescriptions have value in the security they confer on those who have faith in them. A ritual has been established which, if followed carefully, will bring relief. Thus, both physician and patient have done what is necessary and can relax, secure in that knowledge.

Modern physicians and patients need this sense of security just as much as did their forebears. Your confidence in what you offer, whether advice or medication, is communicated to the patient. The insistence of patients on receiving some type of medication or some therapeutic regimen, regardless of its intrinsic value, is only an expression of their desire for security. The need to do something, anything, rather than sit idly by while someone is suffering can be very powerful at times. You may feel this need and may find security in prescriptions even when you know that they do not meet the real needs of the patient. The plea of medical students for specific dosage schedules and of practicing physicians for specific medications of wide applicability are also expressions of the sense of security these impart to their users. Some therapy has little value apart from this.

The importance of security is most dramatic during states of extreme anxiety, where feelings of insecurity are intense. Much of the value of narcotics in such situations lies in the physician's confidence in them and the security the patient feels as a result. Narcotics are frequently misused in the treatment of headache and asthma, for example, in which anxiety may be marked. The need for using narcotics in such a situation decreases in direct proportion to the confidence you have in other therapeutic measures. If you have learned that you can allay anxiety by talking with the patient, you will need narcotics less often and will make active and directed use of the doctor-patient relationship to give the needed feeling of security. These remarks are not intended to minimize the value of narcotic agents but to emphasize that other measures are available to allay anxiety.

A physician may try to communicate confidence in his capacity to treat illness by expressing himself in a dogmatic, uncompromising, authoritarian manner. This manner offers security to many patients. It also fosters a dependent relationship, which may be good, bad, or indifferent, depending on the aims in therapy. In patients who find it hard to be submissive toward authority, it engenders anger or rebellion, an emotional state which usually interferes with therapy. In patients who need someone on whom to be dependent, it encourages dependency and may lead to endless demands. The physician who is aware of the meaning of his relationship with the patient can alter it to meet the needs of changing circumstances.

The importance of the doctor-patient relationship in therapy has been documented in recent studies evaluating the effectiveness of therapeutic agents. In a study of hypertensive patients, it was found that the response of the patient to a drug increased with the degree of the physician's interest in the patient or in the drug being used. [90] This was true whether the agent was a placebo or a drug with pronounced pharmacologic action. This observation has been made so generally in recent years that drug evaluations are now considered suspect unless carried out as a "double-blind" procedure, in which neither physician nor patient know when the test agent is given.

Relationship is important in affecting response to surgical treatment as well. Patients come to one general practitioner from considerable distances for surgery in preference to surgical specialists living closer to them. Though he is not particularly skilled in surgical techniques, his percentage of postoperative complications is low and the length of hospitalization for his patients is shorter than for those of his surgical colleagues. His patients are devoted to him personally and have great confidence in him as a physician and as a surgeon. Before surgery, he explains to his patients what he plans to do at the time of operation. He gives them some idea of the results anticipated and what the immediate postoperative period is likely to bring. It matters little whether he actually does precisely what he has indicated will be done. He has given his patients a feeling that he knows what he is about, that he is a warm and friendly person interested in their well-being. He makes them feel that he respects them. He takes time to allay apprehension about the operation itself and its immediate aftermath. It is probably because of this that he has such an enthusiastic following and achieves such favorable results.

A good doctor-patient relationship has other benefits than improving response to therapy. It can ease the pain of death or the trials of a chronic and disabling disease. The family with confidence in their physician and a feeling that everything possible has been done can accept death or disability with greater equanimity than the family lacking these feelings. The physician's personal interest in his patient and in his patient's family contributes significantly to this security and acceptance.

When a good relationship is lacking, the best of medical care may fail. The patient who thinks that his doctor is not interested in his problems is hard to convince that any treatment suggested is the best one for him. Filled with doubts, he is apt to wander from doctor to doctor and to carry out instructions irregularly. Even if he does not change physicians and follows instructions carefully, he is apt to be overly aware of symptoms or of residua of symptoms which have not completely disappeared. Associated with this attitude of doubt and skepticism, symptoms may flare up anew despite adequate symptomatic therapy.

THE PHYSIOLOGY OF THE DOCTOR-PATIENT RELATIONSHIP

Little work has been done to elucidate the mechanisms by which a favorable doctor-patient relationship enhances the effectiveness of drugs, increases the capacity to withstand the stress of surgery, or accelerates recovery from illness. Much emphasis has been put on the security which a patient finds in a good relationship. It is known that young animals react less to stressful circumstances if the mother is with them[91] and that children likewise are less anxious in a stressful situation when the mother is present, if this relationship is a secure one. But what is the physiology of security? Much of the answer to this question must be phrased in terms of the absence of the physiologic changes associated with insecurity when it has aroused feelings of anxiety, anger, tension, or depression. A few specific observations are available.

In a study of renal excretion in association with stressful situations,[30] the effect of the doctor-patient relationship became strikingly evident. A 34 year old nurse, familiar with laboratory procedures, agreed to be an experimental subject. Her personal physician had told her he would be present during the study, but when she arrived at the laboratory he was not there. She knew that the studies were connected in some way with behavior and emotions and did not wish to discuss personal topics with a strange doctor. During the first hour she sat quietly in the laboratory while an unfamiliar physician walked in and out about his duties. She said later that she felt "alert" and "on guard" during this part of the study lest something be "put over" on her. After specimens had been collected, her own physician came into the room. "When I saw him I felt a wave of relief," she said later and both she and the observers were aware that she relaxed at this point. She continued to sit during the second hour without stress.

Though she had had no fluid for more than 12 hours before the experiment, urine volume increased strikingly during the hour of relaxation in the presence of a familiar physician (Table 5).

Though the changes in renal excretion in this experiment were striking, their real pertinence to recovery from disease is not immediately apparent, for the subject was essentially healthy. The significance becomes clearer when the changes are related to patients who retain fluid and sodium as patients with cardiac disease may do.

TABLE 5.—DOCTOR-PATIENT RELATIONSHIP AND RENAL EXCRETION

TIME	VOL. cc./min.	NA μEq./min.	K μEq./min.	CL μEq./min.	SITUATION
9-10 A.M.	0.56	18	10	25	With unfamiliar physician
10-11 A.M.	4.98	71	42	139	With familiar physician

Barnes,[50] in studying patients who had had episodes of congestive failure, found similar changes when the physician took a reassuring attitude. In a hypertensive patient on a low-sodium regimen, tension engendered by concern over his illness was associated with water and sodium retention. When reassured about his cardiac disease, he showed a prompt diuresis (Table 6). Similar observations were made on other patients in this series.

Other effects than diuresis were noted in the nurse. When a familiar physician with whom she felt secure entered the laboratory, she relaxed visibly. The effects of doctor-patient relationship on muscle tone

TABLE 6.—EFFECT OF REASSURANCE ON RENAL EXCRETION
IN A CARDIAC PATIENT

CIRCUMSTANCE	OBSERVATIONS	VOL. cc./min.	NA μEq./min.	K μEq./min.
Tension	2	0.66	23	55
Reassurance	2	1.03	80	75

have been studied.[92] It has been reported that reassurance and praise decrease muscle tension in both the investigator giving the praise and the subject receiving it. This decrease occurs rapidly. Criticism, on the other hand, increases muscle tension. The doctor-patient relationship may therefore be used to affect symptoms related to muscle tension.

The same report included interesting data on heart rate. The rate was more rapid after criticism than after praise. It was also more rapid on days which the investigator felt had been "bad" ones for him than on days which had been "good," though the procedure was carried out in an identical way on all days. Review of recordings made of the experimental sessions suggested that his voice may have been somewhat higher in pitch on "bad" days but no other difference was noted. This again emphasizes the importance of nonverbal communication as a part of the doctor-patient relationship; furthermore, it demonstrates that nonverbal communication may have physiologic repercussions.

The physiology of the doctor-patient relationship is extremely important if we are to understand how relationship affects response to illness and to therapy. Our information at present is sketchy, to say the least. Further studies are needed and should be rewarding.

SOME THERAPEUTIC ROLES

Physicians must assume multiple roles to do their job effectively. You may act as a teacher, educating the patient on the facts of health and disease. You may be a confidant or confessor, encouraging the patient to express ideas and feelings ordinarily kept secret. You may be a friend, giving support and encouragement through adversity and helping the patient change his attitudes or behavior. And you may act as a sort of private detective, investigating the patient's problems and past experience, seeking cause and effect, and helping him achieve a fuller understanding of his actions and motivations. You may do any one of these things or each of them in rapid succession, all as a part of your professional duties. Each requires a different type of relationship if it is to be effective. Relationship is not constant and invariable. The skillful physician can alter it to suit the needs of the moment. And if the relationship is not handled smoothly, he will not be able to supply what is needed even though he may understand the need and wish to fill it.

If you understand the action of drugs, the mechanism by which they act, and the difficulties to be anticipated in their use, you use drugs more intelligently and more effectively. The same is true of relationship. Intuition and sensitivity in interpersonal relations will always be important in patient care. But if you are aware of your activities as functions of relationship, you will be able to adjust your words and actions to fit the needs of your patients and will handle them more skillfully and effectively. You will be able to select your approach to the patient with logic and reason and to change it as circumstances require.

TEACHER

Education is the simplest form of treatment, useful whenever distress is caused by ignorance or misunderstanding. It is an effective way of expressing your personal concern for the patient's welfare and in many illnesses an indispensable therapeutic tool. To patients with diabetes or heart disease, for example, explanation is essential for intelligent cooperation. It is a form of psychotherapy as well. When a parent is distraught because her child does not speak though past the age of 12 months, or upset at finding her 5 year old son masturbating, or disturbed because her 8 year old daughter giggles constantly, simple explanation of normal behavior patterns and stages of development constitutes psychotherapy. The parent has come to you anxious, angry, or depressed, and factual information allays this emotional reaction and prevents it from engendering disturbances in others. Thus simple explanation may at once be educational, psychotherapeutic, and preventive.

For this type of therapy to be effective, your relationship with the patient must be such that he accepts you as an authority by virtue of your knowledge. If the patient does not respect your superior knowledge, explanations may well be rejected. Even though superior knowledge is accepted, if the patient is unable to accept an authoritarian relationship he may not benefit from the information transmitted.

A young man of 18 who had diabetes mellitus and a duodenal ulcer was recurrently in trouble with one or the other. In childhood he had had considerable difficulty with parental restrictions, to which he responded with anger and rebellion. Though he wanted to maintain good health, he was unable to accept the rigid restrictions imposed by one physician after another in their efforts to control both ailments at once. These restrictions were imposed by an authority. Despite his desire to be healthy and his awareness that the restrictions were for his own good, the boy reacted to them in the same way he had reacted to parental restrictions. He followed no regimen for long and seemed to oscillate between diabetic acidosis and hemorrhage from his ulcer. Such a person requires an understanding of his emotional problems in addition to explanation of the therapeutic regimen. This does not lessen the importance of education in treatment but emphasizes its limitations when the relationship between physician and patient is not conducive to its effective use.

One way in which you may help patients whose illness is linked with stressful situations is by reorienting them to their environment so that they gain a better perspective on their circumstances and responses. Reorientation is particularly important to patients who feel they are "trapped" in situations they cannot meet successfully or in situations in which pertinent relationships are vague or confused. You try to help a patient see alternative solutions, new relationships, or new resources within himself or his immediate environment which will enable him to cope with the situation effectively. By asking questions in the proper order, by bringing together bits of information volunteered by the patient, you help him to gain new perspectives. Much of this is education and explanation.

An example of the efficiency of this process in treatment has already been given in the instance of the young man (p. 66) who suffered from episodic urticaria that always occurred at work, usually within a short time after his supervisor had come to inspect his work. Leading him to discover the relationship between criticism of his work, his anger, and the appearance of hives was all the treatment he required. As a result, he asked to be changed to another shift at work and had no more recurrences of hives.

A calm discussion of the physiologic mechanisms producing a symptom may sometimes help a patient. Even though he does not fully understand it, it can be reassuring to feel that someone understands and knows what is wrong whether the patient does or not. A patient with tachycardia may sometimes be reassured by being told how it is produced, provided the explanation allays his fears of serious heart disease or sudden death. A person who becomes weak and dizzy as a result of hyperventilation may be reassured by explanations and demonstrations of the mechanisms producing the dizziness, especially if he thereby learns that the symptoms are at least partially under his control. One patient with a breast cancer which had metastasized expressed great relief when her physician assured her that the mestastases were "only" in her bones.

But patient education is more than explanation of the facts of life or the mechanisms of disease or symptom formation. Education plays a part in all forms of psychotherapy, for the patient is learning both about himself and about his relations with other people. One of the most important lessons he learns may be gained without any conscious attention to it by either therapist or patient, for in most continuing therapeutic relationships the patient is learning how to relate to others through the process of doing so. Thus he is being reeducated in interpersonal relations.

CONFESSOR, CONFIDANT

Quite a different relationship is needed when you want the patient to express his feelings freely. In this relationship you are viewed as confessor or confidant with whom the patient feels assured of acceptance personally and of secrecy for whatever he reveals. Such a relationship is most advantageous for patients who have suppressed their frustrations and irritations in life, whether because of feelings of guilt for having such reactions or because of fear that those about them would not understand or sympathize with their feelings. Often the relationship in which free expression of such emotions is possible without arousing argument or rejection is an entirely new experience for the patient. "I've never talked to anyone like this before" is not an uncommon statement. Whether you are directive or nondirective in this relationship, the free atmosphere is beneficial. One great benefit is the patient's growing understanding that there is someone who can hear his inmost thoughts and desires without being repelled or recoiling in disgust.

The important feature of expressive therapy, therefore, is the patient's ability to ventilate his emotions and desires in an atmosphere of respect and acceptance. You hear the outburst of long pent-up emotions without being emotionally disturbed by it. You hear a confession of sins of commission or desire without rejecting. You listen to descriptions of "impossible" situations without being overwhelmed— indeed, without accepting the situation as impossible. As a result the patient gains in self-respect, is enabled to look at his emotions and desires more objectively, and can see a situation in new perspective and with alternative solutions. All of this may occur without any words from you if the patient feels your calm acceptance and optimism.

Such a relationship is fostered by warm respect on the part of the physician, by his position of authority, and by his tradition of maintaining personal information in strict confidence. It is further stimulated by good listening and appropriate questioning. It is most beneficial when the patient's symptoms are rooted in chronic states of anger and anxiety, particularly when these have been denied adequate expression. Ventilation then allows discharge of the accumulated emotional energy and release of some of the tension associated with control of that emotion. With reassurance that he is accepted despite the emotional outburst, tension decreases further. The physician's position of authority adds significance to his reassurance, and ventilation to a physician is thus more effective therapeutically than ventilation to a peer.

The importance of the doctor-patient relationship is again clearly demonstrated when the proper relationship for this type of therapy has not been established. An example was a young woman referred to me for help with some rather severe sexual problems. She had indulged in both heterosexual and homosexual activities and had tried most of the sexual perversions. Though she knew that I was aware of these activities, she found it impossible to discuss them with me. Her explanation was that I looked to her like a person who would disapprove of what she had done and she therefore could not talk about it. My usefulness to her as a therapist was destroyed by this impression. No efforts succeeded in establishing an appropriate relationship within which to work through her problems, and she was referred to another physician for help.

When the relationship between physician and patient permits free discussion, the benefits may be very dramatic. A young man in his midtwenties came to our hospital because of severe headaches which prevented him from working. He had worked with his father-in-law in a grocery store for several years but had been unable to complete a day's work for several weeks before entering the hospital. The medical resident thought the headaches were related to emotional stress but could not elicit any information which seemed pertinent. However, he had established a good relationship with the patient. I interviewed the patient, asking rather specific questions about his job, his father-in-law, and his wife but got no further than had the resident. A short time after my departure the patient asked if he might talk with the resident again.

In this interview, he managed to talk very freely and to relieve himself of some very intense emotions. He began by apologizing for having "lied" in answer to some of my questions. It was the first time he had met me and he had felt constrained as a result. This statement reflects the need for feelings of security and warmth in the doctor-patient relationship before attempts at expressive therapy can succeed. He then told about some early experiences of his wife. In her teens she had been raped by her own father, who had served a brief prison term as a result. He and his father-in-law worked together and had gotten along fairly well. But a few weeks before, at the time of the onset of his headaches, he had seen his father-in-law stroking his wife's back and arm and patting her affectionately on the buttocks. This had infuriated him and forcefully recalled the incident of rape. He didn't know how to handle the situation—whether to consider it parental affection and remain or an evidence of incestuous desires and take his wife away from her father and establish himself in some other job. His emotions had been so intense he had feared to express them to anyone else or to take any action lest he regret it when he cooled off. Unfortunately, he had never calmed down enough to feel safe in making a decision.

To this revelation, the resident made no response except to express interest and sympathy; he made no suggestions as to what the patient should do. But much of the patient's emotion was relieved by being expressed in words. He could consider the situation more objectively, and he was able to make his own decisions and take action without guidance or support from his physician. He asked for a few days in which to go home and straighten his affairs. When he returned it was to say that he had a new job, that he and his wife were no longer near her father, and that he was no longer having headaches. Such a prompt and dramatic response is unusual, but it illustrates the value of ventilation in an atmosphere of friendly warmth and security.

Friend

At times the patient may need support. Your relationship to a patient should then be that of a strong friend or ally, a person who can offer moral support and strength to see a problem through. There may be no delving into the far reaches of the soul, no deep revelations of things unseen and unheard by other human beings. The crucial fact in this type of therapy is that someone in a position of authority has demonstrated a sympathetic interest, respects the patient and his ability to handle his problems, yet is standing by to help if needed. Sometimes a patient will have tried one thing after another, each one being a bit beyond his capacities. He therefore looks back upon a long succession of failures. If you listen to his recital of failure after failure but respect him for his capacity and for the ambition which led him to overextend himself, he may find considerable support and strength in this relationship.

Respect and reassurance are the basis of most supportive therapy. But reassurance is frequently misunderstood. It does not consist of saying in a hearty voice, "Now just don't worry any more. You're going to be all right!" Nor is it a slap on the back and a cheery "There's nothing the matter with you." Statements such as these are reassuring only when the patient has confidence that you understand what is troubling him. This knowledge is the sum and substance of reassurance. There is no magic formula which can take its place. It is not reassuring to hear "nothing is wrong" from someone who has not taken the time to find out what *is* wrong. Consequently, you should not expect to give specific reassurance the moment you meet a patient. Initially, the most reassuring thing for the patient is the knowledge that his doctor is interested and plans to be thorough in his investigation. After this has been accomplished, the stage is set for more specific reassurance.

Reassurance should be pertinent to the problem disturbing the patient if it is to accomplish its purpose. This should scarcely need mention; yet it is often overlooked. A middle-aged woman with moderately severe rheumatic heart disease visited her physician with mild congestive failure; she was in a state of obvious anxiety. The physician wished to relieve her anxiety. He assumed that she was worrying about her heart condition and therefore spent his time "reassuring" her that she could anticipate a prompt recovery and need not fear a stroke from embolization since this was statistically uncommon. Her anxiety, however, was not about her physical condition but about a very unsatisfactory marital situation. The difficulties which had arisen in her marriage were pertinent both to her anxiety and to her episode of cardiac decompensation. The physician's "reassuring" comments about a stroke only added a new worry about something she had not even thought of.

At times it may be wise to suppress disturbing material. Suppression is usually combined with strong supportive measures. Thus, in a patient whose succession of failures was overwhelming him and threatening to produce panic or disorganization, the best therapy may be to concentrate on the positive aspects of the patient's past to reinforce his self-respect. Suppressive therapy is used when the material is so threatening as to produce disorganization or when it is something which the patient can neither alter nor accept. Latent homosexuality may sometimes be better handled by suppression than by expression, at least temporarily. Judgment is required in making this decision, however, and you must consider the pros and cons of both methods of treatment before undertaking either.

Suppressive treatment is used rather commonly in another type of situation. The patient who has lost a member of his family may be told to "go back to work and get your mind on something else." This is suppressing a prolonged grief reaction by concentrating on other things. Obviously, advice such as this can succeed only when grief is not overwhelming, even as suppression of homosexual tendencies can succeed only when the controlling forces mobilized are stronger than the drive. The physician must assess the relative strengths of these contending forces before determining his course of action.

Physicians spend much of their time working with patient's attitudes, often without being aware of the nature of their activities. Giving a diabetic information about how he can control the manifestations of his disease changes his feelings about being a diabetic. Giving a mother information about the usual "phases" of development may change her attitude toward her children. Adequate premarital counsel may alter a person's attitude toward sexual relations. Information is effective in changing attitudes when the physician is accepted as authoritative and when the emotional determinants of the attitude are not rigidly fixed or strong. Acceptance of the physician as authoritative involves more than knowing that he possesses factual knowledge. He must know the patient and his situation so that the patient is assured not only that what is said is generally true but also that it applies specifically to him in his particular circumstances. Short of this it is not authoritative.

The physician must likewise, on occasion, be ready to help patients and their families accept illness or specific therapeutic procedures. This is also working to alter attitudes and motivations. The patient who feels ashamed because he has epilepsy needs reeducation and reorienting of his attitudes toward epilepsy. The patient who does not follow a therapeutic regimen because he distrusts or rebels against his physician must learn that the physician is trustworthy and understanding. The family that thinks one of its members is malingering needs help in accepting the illness as genuine and in understanding the emotional factors which have led them to accuse the person falsely. And the person who rejects necessary major surgery needs help in overcoming this resistance.

Many patients have difficulty in accepting an emotional basis for physical complaints. Despite the commonplace expressions "he's a pain in the neck" or "it makes me sick to my stomach," which implicitly state a relation between emotions and symptoms, there is a tendency to feel that attributing a physical complaint to an emotional state implies there is nothing physically wrong. Expression of interest by the doctor in the emotional circumstances surrounding a complaint then implies that he does not believe the complaint to be real. When the block to acceptance of the relation between emotions and symptoms is based on ignorance of the physiologic facts, dealing with the problem is fairly easy. The process is then an educational one.

It is not necessary that every patient with a psychophysiologic complaint recognize the association between emotions and symptoms. Relief may be achieved without this. But the patient who accepts and understands the association is in a better position to prevent recurrences and to accept the limitations of physical measures in treatment. It sometimes becomes desirable, therefore, to explain this association, avoiding any implication that the complaint is imaginary and that nothing is physically wrong. Part of this is educational, but it may also entail detective work by the physician, ventilation from the patient, and strong reassurance before it is effective.

In explaining the relation between stress, emotions, and symptoms, it is useful to start out with common phenomena with which everyone is acquainted. The physician may mention, for example, that it is common to see people blush when they are embarrassed. An angry person may turn white and his muscles become tense. It is possible to tell by looking at him that he is angry. Similarly, a person may be visibly depressed. In all these instances, physical changes have occurred in association with an emotion, and these changes are so specific that another person can recognize the embarrassment, anger, or depression.

Once a patient has accepted this association of physical changes with emotional states, it is usually not too difficult to explain that things less easily seen by the eye are also associated with emotions. With a patient with peptic ulcer, you can proceed from a description of blushing with anger and embarrassment to a description of emotionally caused changes in the state of the vessels within the stomach. Changes in gastric motility and acidity in association with emotions are an easy step from this point. You then proceed to situations which have given rise to the pertinent emotional state.

Acceptance of an emotional basis for a physical symptom may be blocked by the threatening nature of this idea itself. A patient may refuse to accept an obvious connection simply because to him the statement that a symptom is emotional in origin means that it is psychiatric in nature, and he does not wish to consider himself "crazy." One young girl had recurrent headaches for 6 months before she was willing to accept the relation of her headaches to the emotional strains under which she was living. She recognized the emotional strains. She certainly was very much aware of the headaches. But she refused to accept any connection between the two until the evidence was irrefutable. One reason for this was her feeling that anyone who became ill as a result of stress should be locked up in an "insane asylum." This was strengthened somewhat by the fact that institutionalization had been discussed for one of her relatives who was emotionally disturbed. She was afraid to admit that her symptoms might be a result of stresses in her life lest she too be committed to a psychiatric hospital.

A more difficult problem is presented by the patient who defends himself against recognizing the connection between emotions and symptoms by stating that he has no emotions. In such a person, questions about emotional feelings become, in effect, a statement of disbelief. If he has no emotions, then questions concerning his emotions are completely out of place. It is difficult to break through this barrier when a patient is determined to maintain it, but it is possible to do so with patience. If you discuss the circumstances in which a symptom arose or the circumstances of his life in general, emotional tones are bound to enter into the description sooner or later. You cannot use these immediately or you will cut off any further statements of emotions. You must listen carefully for emotional undercurrents, keep them clearly in mind, and be ready to bring them up at an appropriate time days or weeks later. To such a patient, recognition of emotional reactions is threatening. Your job is to find out why emotions represent such a threat and to help him accept them as a normal and desirable part of living.

Physicians must also affect patients' motivations, particularly for therapeutic procedures, such as surgery or formal psychiatric care, and for return to productive activity. Generally, you are trying to increase the motivation for some specific action but at times just the opposite is required. A patient who is driving and ambitious and does not want to stop work, even temporarily, may require a good deal of your time before he will take the prescribed rest or go to the hospital. Physicians who take time to deal with this situation often succeed. Motivation is not a unitary force but the result of many forces affecting the desire to work. By increasing a patient's awareness of the need for relaxation you decrease his drive to incessant activity. It is equally possible to alter the balance of forces in favor of return to work. In this case you must minimize factors which decrease the drive toward work or emphasize those which increase it. To accomplish this, you should avoid pessimistic prognoses. You should not, ordinarily, tell a patient that he will never return to work, though you may have to tell him that his ideas about the kind of work he can do must be revised. You should not be contemptuous of the patient with little desire to work, since only interest in the reasons for this lack of desire can correct it. A positive orientation to work must be maintained from the start of treatment. The patient's attention should be directed toward the type of work he will do when he recovers, not toward whether he will work or not. In doing this, you exert pressure to return to work just as parents and friends did with their question "What are you going to do when you grow up?" The most powerful force in motivating a patient to return to work is a strong relationship in which he wishes to please his physician and receive his approval.

Much of this affects the patient's concept of himself. Few people are able to undertake all types of work. Not everyone can be a musician, a mathematician, a physician, a lawyer, a physicist, or, for that matter, a common laborer. There are gradations in all capacities. Illness accentuates gradation but seldom eliminates the potential for work. This should be kept clearly in mind. When a physician says, "you will never be able to work again," he may only mean that the patient will never be able to return to his previous type of work. But if he gives no indication that some work is possible, the patient may take the statement at its face value. The actual capacity of a person to work is less important than his evaluation of that capacity. It is the patient's concept of his own adequacy which is undermined when he is told that he will not be able to work again. His basic physical capacity for work is not affected, but his attempts to return to work may be destroyed.

A more specialized function of the physician is helping the patient gain insight into the needs and drives which motivate his behavior. Though insight may be gained in the process of ventilation with little help, it may at times require a good deal of discreet activity on your part. Associations and similarities between actions taken at different times or between relationships of the patient with different people may be pointed out. Connections between present problems and past experiences may need to be mentioned quite specifically. For example, a patient complaining of marital difficulties may not see what he contributes to the conflict without recognizing similarities between his relationship with his wife and his relationship with his mother. Seeing these similarities and understanding their significance may lead to a fuller understanding of the marital problem and set the stage for dealing with it realistically. Such interpretations, however, should seldom be given early in the course of working with a patient. Using them effectively requires training and judgment. The physician without psychiatric training should use them cautiously or not at all.

Whatever the approach to the patient, the most important ingredient for a good doctor-patient relationship is genuine, warm respect. You cannot help an individual overcome feelings of inadequacy and inferiority if your manner tells him that you do indeed consider him inadequate and inferior. Nor can you help a person become mature and independent by expressing contempt for his immaturity and dependence. You cannot help a patient learn to deal with anger and hostility if you yourself consider anger to be base and undesirable in a mature person. You cannot establish a good relationship with a patient who is fearful or rebellious unless you respect him despite his fear or his rebellion. You cannot give the patient a feeling of security while rejecting him as unworthy of careful attention. Respect for the person despite his weaknesses; respect for his capacity to change; and respect for his desire to improve as expressed in his seeking help are essential. A good doctor-patient relationship is the most powerful force at a physician's command in attaining therapeutic success.

Chapter 10

Dealing with Emotions

EMOTIONS occupy a central position in psychophysiologic formulations. Since the psychic and physiologic manifestations of an emotion are two facets of a single experience, recognition of the emotional state of the patient is an important first step in understanding these phenomena. Frequently the emotional state of the patient may be evident the moment he enters your office. Even when less obvious, it can often be determined during a brief interview. It can serve as a guidepost to the types of questions that should be asked. In addition, the patient's emotional state gives a convenient starting point for treatment, one which can be used effectively even before you learn the details of the illness, the circumstances of its onset, the nature of the stress, or the reasons for the patient's response.

The importance of dealing with the emotional state early in treatment is emphasized by the potential effect of emotions on thought and behavior. Since emotions affect both the perception and the meaning of stimuli, they influence what a person finds threatening in his environment and the way in which he reacts. Since they may impair memory, they may affect the history which is given. Since some emotions increase the intensity of drives, they may change the quality or direction of behavior and render it inappropriate as judged by an observer. Since emotions may arouse fresh conflicts, they may increase the confusion or emotional turmoil of the patient. Since they affect evaluation and judgment, they may interfere with therapy, leading to irrational decisions or premature action. Marked emotional disturbance must be dealt with first if treatment is to be effective. When emotional disturbance is mild, you may wish to attend to other matters first.

Stress is individual and subjective. Some people are seldom threatened by situations; others feel threatened repeatedly every day. Many situations are threatening largely because of the attitudes which the person brings to them. For example, one student may respond to examinations with exhilaration at the challenge, while another is bored and sees no challenge whatever; one student may be apprehensive, another depressed. These emotions express the person's evaluation of the situation and of his relation to it. The person who is exhilarated has evaluated the examination situation differently than has the person who is bored. He has a different level of motivation and a different concept of himself. People must face many tests in life. As you learn what types of situations are challenging or threatening to your patient and explore the reasons for his reaction to these situations, you begin to understand his value system, his goals in life, and his self-concept. The more clearly you understand these, the more points of attack you will have in helping him.

At times the quality of the emotional response will seem quite natural. "Anyone would get angry if he had to live with a spouse like that!" may be your feeling. You may then wonder what can be done to help, since trying to change the quality of the emotional reaction would, in a sense, be trying to make the patient abnormal. Before deciding that an emotional reaction has been normal, however, its intensity and duration should be evaluated. Though "anyone might get angry" in a similar situation, they might not get *that* angry. If, with calm reflection, you decide that the emotional response should be considered "normal" in quality, intensity, and duration, much can still be done to help the patient and relieve his symptoms. Instead of altering the reaction to the stimulus itself you may try to relieve its intensity between occurrences, may help the patient find new defenses to handle the emotion or the situation, or may, on rare occasions, alter the situation or its frequency. Your goal is not the ultimate elimination of emotions because some of them may be associated with symptoms. The goal is to eliminate the symptoms and leave the patient warmly responsive to his environment without illness.

ANGER

Anger is an outgoing emotion which is dissipated by free expression. Therefore, when unexpressed anger or resentment are prominent features of a patient's illness, ventilation is appropriate therapy. This can start as you take the history. History taking can itself be therapeutic if anger finds adequate expression in the process. Listen carefully for any indications of anger or for situations which might have aroused anger. When these are noted, direct questions into these areas and encourage expression of the anger by continued questioning. You need not call the patient's attention to his anger. Indeed, some patients become self-conscious when anger is pointed out, and their expression of it becomes inhibited and inadequate.

Most people with symptoms associated with anger or resentment are in situations which constantly renew these feelings. The relief obtained by expressing them is transient and offers little or no protection against renewal, but the temporary nature of the relief should not lead you to underestimate its value. It is a necessary first step. Only with dissipation of the anger can the patient think clearly and constructively about the situation which has aroused it and about the forces within himself which contribute to the reaction.

With this goal of relieving the emotional reaction clearly in mind, it becomes obvious that further anger should not be aroused during this phase of treatment. Anger may be aroused by any barrier in the path of gratification, by deprivation of something the patient desires or thinks is deserved, or by a conflict of principles or drives. Cutting the patient short not only prevents adequate expression but may engender fresh anger if he feels he deserves to be heard. Criticism, expressed or implied, may also arouse anger and should be avoided. You should not become angry and fan the flames of hostility with aggressive argument. Nor should you show anger at the persons or events which have angered the patient. Aggressive agreement can also increase anger. Your part is to elicit more and more information as the anger is expressed more fully, keeping your mind on the problem of analyzing objectively what has happened. The combination of sympathetic interest and objective analysis may be difficult to achieve at times but should be your aim. Sympathetic interest fosters free communication. An objective, analytic frame of mind gradually impresses the patient and has important benefits in reducing the intensity of anger and fostering a thoughtful, constructive approach on his part. It benefits you too, for it prevents your reaction to the patient from becoming overly emotional. Your primary responsibility is to help the patient. You will do this more effectively if you remain objective.

It should be emphasized that a major factor in the benefit derived from ventilation lies in the way you respond to the expression of anger. The question has been asked, "Isn't it harmful to allow a patient to express his anger freely? You simply make him aware of how

angry he is. Aren't you making matters worse rather than better?"
You can indeed make the patient worse if you arouse fresh anger;
but encouraging expression of anger does not intensify symptoms.
You should not engender hostility toward yourself when dealing with
a patient whose symptoms are related to anger.

As an example, consider the patient with ulcerative colitis who may
appear excessively passive and dependent. Beneath the surface there
may be a great deal of hostility that is unexpressed because the patient is afraid to express it, particularly if it is aroused by parents
or parent substitutes. It may seem obvious that such a patient needs to
learn effective ways of expressing anger. But if you try to arouse anger
to demonstrate that no harm comes from expressing anger, the patient is more apt to have an exacerbation of his illness than to get
outwardly angry. At such times you may say that the patient is show-
ing resistance. He is. You are trying to get him to express his anger
verbally; he resists this and his bloody diarrhea increases. Unfortunately, many physicians have concluded from reactions of this sort that
the patient should not be encouraged to express anger. One might
better conclude that the physician should not add to the anger already
present. It should also be added that expressions of anger should not
be precipitated until the fear of disrupting an important relationship
has been at least partly allayed.

The problem of inadequately expressed anger is sometimes met
with the advice, "Let yourself go. If you get mad, blow up. It's better
than letting yourself get sick over it." The aim of this advice is similar
to the aim of the physician who taunts his patient in order to provoke an open expression of anger. With many patients, the advice is
wasted; years of self-discipline make "blowing up" virtually impossible. It is doubtful that such advice is ever appropriate. The screaming, hitting, or throwing of objects which may be a part of losing one's
temper are not far removed from a childish temper tantrum. Are you
helping a patient mature when you encourage this type of expression of anger? There are adult ways of expressing anger and of dealing with situations which arouse anger. These should be encouraged
in preference to "blowing up." Part of your responsibility is to reduce
the intensity of accumulated hostility to manageable proportions before asking the patient to act on his feelings in the situation which has
aroused anger. If he loses control of himself and feels guilty as a result, little has been gained.

In addition to making sure that the anger is within the capacity of the patient to control, you should assess the situation which has aroused it. You need to know what the effect of expressing anger will be. If it will destroy a relationship which is important to the patient, advice should be given cautiously. It may be far better for the patient to express his anger only to you and then to discuss other ways of handling the problem than expressing anger directly to the person who has provoked it.

The benefit from expressing anger to you can be materially increased by appropriate direction. Adequate expression of anger should be encouraged even though it requires repeated discussion of the same events. But you should direct the discussion so that the patient becomes aware of his problems and his contribution to the situation and does not indefinitely reiterate minor irritations which have served to reopen old wounds but are peripheral to the major issue. Expression of anger over trivial incidents should be encouraged, but after a free discussion of each episode, attention should be directed toward the reasons such a trivial episode aroused such an intense reaction.

The initial stages of treatment are similar for all forms of anger, whether the patient comes to you seething with scarcely controllable anger, coldly negative with anger well controlled, warm and friendly but with resentments deeply hidden beneath a pleasant façade, or seemingly indifferent but with anger repressed at an unconscious level. In all these forms, expressive therapy can relieve the immediate emotional tensions and give symptomatic relief.

It should be reemphasized that ventilation is only the initial step in therapy, directed specifically at the emotional reaction itself. While the patient is expressing his feelings and discussing their origins, both he and you are learning what is stressful to him, why it is stressful, and why symptoms develop in this setting. Such information is essential to genuine understanding of the patient, and only when it has been obtained can definitive decisions be made. Except in emergencies, these decisions should be made by the patient, not by you. The processes involved will be considered in more detail in subsequent chapters, but it may be useful to point out the possible lines of action.

One of the first suggestions usually made is for the patient to remove himself from the events which aroused the adverse response. If he can do so, this may be a satisfactory solution, as it proved to be for the patient with headaches who had recognized incestuous desires between his father-in-law and his wife (p. 222). Actually, it is unusual to meet such a state of affairs. Much more frequently, conditions will recur in other circumstances so that no end is served by trying to escape specific situations. Mr. Grant (p. 70) learned this after years of leaving one job for another. He could not tolerate criticism from others or friction among those about him. Leaving his job when friction seemed imminent solved nothing, since the same situation was bound to occur on other jobs. He was trying to run away from himself, from his own feelings of anger and frustration when hostility was displayed by others, and this seldom can be successful.

When the circumstances cannot be avoided, it may be possible for the patient to alter his attitudes so that anger is less intense or no longer aroused. Changing his evaluation of the situation or his interpretation of his relation to it may be effective in altering attitudes and emotional reactions to a threatening situation. If barriers prevent gratification of his desires, he may learn ways to remove them or to circumnavigate them. He may learn to concentrate on long-term goals so that immediate blocks and delays are less frustrating. He may be able to give up anticipated rewards so that he is less disturbed when these are not forthcoming. When anger develops because of opposing drives or disparate value systems, he may be able to work out an effective compromise. On occasion, no effort is made to avoid or alter the reaction of anger, and attention is focused instead on learning new ways of dealing with the anger so that symptoms do not develop. Some situations require that the patient achieve a more realistic self-concept and more realistic expectations of others.

This does not mean that you decide which path is best for the patient and then lead him over it. Indeed, such disregard for a patient's feelings and goals is apt to evoke fresh anger. Instead you and the patient discuss the various alternatives and you help him make an appropriate and satisfying decision from among them. You offer support and help to the patient as he tries to put his decision into action, even though his course may not seem ideal to you.

Frequently a patient needs to learn new ways to relate to other people, particularly to those in positions of authority. You may then try to help him understand his reactions to people in authority and the origins of these reactions. You make every effort, as well, to establish a relation between you and the patient in which new feelings can be learned and new patterns of interaction can develop. The relationship is far more important than intellectual understanding. Many people have achieved satisfactory levels of adjustment in adult life despite unfavorable childhood relationships with parental figures.

New generalizations about authority have been accomplished through association with other figures of authority, such as teachers, ministers, relatives, or adult acquaintances. No understanding of how this has been accomplished is necessary for it to happen. On the other hand, many patients have become so deeply enmeshed in conflicts aroused in childhood that a reassessment has not been possible, despite opportunities in their life experiences. You can help them by increasing their understanding of their problems and by establishing a relationship in which they may learn a more satisfactory social adjustment.

ANXIETY

The treatment of anxiety may, on occasion, be much like the treatment of anger. When the anxiety is aroused by an identifiable situation in the environment, discussion may be sufficient to ease the emotional reaction. In the course of illness many circumstances arise which may arouse anxiety. Anxiety may be aroused by the fact of illness and the uncertainties commonly associated with it. It may be aroused by the mechanics of taking care of illness—by visits to doctors, diagnostic procedures, venipunctures, x-rays, hospitalization, and surgery, to mention but a few. It may be aroused by the economic problems incident to illness—bills for medical services, caring for the family during illness, loss of income, or concern whether the job will still be available when the illness is over. Or it may be incident to personal problems raised by illness—the reaction of friends and relatives, feelings of shame for the particular illness, or the need to set a new course in life. In all these situations, anxiety may be aroused because the patient is unfamiliar with the situation and does not know what to expect from it or is unsure of his ability to cope with it.

When unfamiliarity with the situation has occasioned anxiety, explanation may be sufficient to allay it. These discussions remove much of the "unknown" from the situation, making it seem more familiar. The patient then knows what to expect and can judge his ability to handle the situation objectively. Much obviously depends upon the physician's attitude. He cannot instill confidence and give the patient security unless he has it himself. If the situation makes you nervous and anxious, you may well communicate this to the patient and aggravate the anxiety rather than allay it. But physicians are not ordinarily anxious about these matters. Their calmness and confidence can be of great help.

When the patient understands the situation but is not sure of his ability to meet it adequately, a discussion balancing the demands against his resources to meet them may be reassuring. Decreasing the standards of conduct which he demands of himself may be helpful, for example, letting the patient know that he may complain freely if a procedure is painful. Discussion in this area is not always effective in allaying anxiety, however, and you must then make full use of the forces present in a good doctor-patient relationship. Your presence may allay apprehension if the patient has confidence in you and feels security in the relationship. Like the child who can adjust to new and frightening experiences more easily when his mother is with him, the adult patient gains security from the presence of a friend and powerful ally. Many patients, for example, feel more at ease about a surgical procedure if they know that *their* physician will be present, even though they are fully aware that he is not doing the operation.

The origins of anxiety may be more complex than these examples suggest. When the degree of anxiety is out of proportion to the threat present in the situation, when anxiety is not allayed by explanation or by reassurance, you should consider the possibility that the fear is related more to factors within the patient than to factors within the situation. This is always true of "free-floating" anxiety, an anxiety attached to no object or situation but pervading the person's being with a sense of impending disaster. It is also true of the anxiety present in chronic anxiety states, in hypochondriasis, and in the so-called organ neuroses. Anxiety at such times offers a more difficult problem since its origin will not become apparent in direct questioning.

A male nurse from a children's ward was referred for examination because of "nervousness." He said that he liked children and got along well with them but for some reason they were inclined to tease him a great deal. He was afraid to go back to work. He felt that he had a great deal of responsibility in his job. He sometimes turned oxygen tanks on and off. He was afraid he might turn the valve the wrong way or might drop the oxygen tank and thus harm somebody. He also feared that he might drop one of the children when helping him on or off a bed pan. This fear had become so overpowering that it was impossible for him to return to work and he had requested a vacation to recover from his "nervousness."

These matters would not arouse anxiety in most nurses. He was aware of this and could not understand why he had such fears. However, it is apparent that all of them concern harming someone else. Where there is no possibility of harm, there should be no fear of it. One might logically deduce therefore that where there is so much fear there must be some possibility, if only as a desire. But the patient has not told us that he has any desire to harm another. In fact, he would deny it were it suggested to him. This is not something he has said but an interpretation which has been made. It is important to keep this distinction in mind. The hostile impulses have been repressed in the setting where they should be expected to come to the fore, but the fact of hostility is clearly evident in all of the things which he fears he will do. He can remain unaware of his basic hostility because he views his preoccupations as a concern for the patient's welfare. It matters little how one reassures such a person that he will not harm patients. His fear essentially is of his own hostile impulses and he needs help in learning how to handle these adequately.

The patient himself is unaware of the sources of his anxiety, yet he must discuss them before he will be free of the anxiety. This obviously poses a problem. If you tell him bluntly that his anxiety is due to feelings of hostility, he will look within himself and, because of his defenses, will find nothing there to corroborate the statement. On the contrary, he is so filled with love that he spends his waking hours concerned lest he harm someone. Stating the matter to him bluntly has added nothing to his understanding of himself and may even rouse doubts as to your understanding. You cannot proceed so directly nor so rapidly. Explanations or interpretations of the anxiety must wait. In some way, you must help the patient find the sources of his anxiety by himself.

There are many ways to proceed. One would be to discuss any source of anger or irritation he was able to recognize until he felt at ease in discussing his anger. This part of treatment would then be spent in making him feel at ease and helping him learn that you will not be disturbed by hearing expressions of anger. You might ask about childhood experiences that had aroused anger, since these are usually so remote that they do not threaten the patient on retelling. Questions about his relationship with brothers, sisters, and peers during childhood would be pertinent, as well as his parents' response to arguments and signs of friction within the family. You might ask about experiences with teasing during childhood, why children tease one another and why the reaction tends to be anger. Only when the patient seems comfortable in discussing these matters would you try to get him to relate them directly to the situation which aroused anxiety.

It is obvious that the atmosphere of the therapeutic session is extremely important. The freer the patient feels to discuss his inner feelings and thoughts, the easier it will be for him to overcome his defenses against disturbing material. Much of a psychiatrist's attention is focused on providing such a favorable atmosphere for therapy. If the patient knows the physician is not going to react with censure, it is easier for him to discuss material freely. His defenses can be less active. In addition, it is reassuring to find that he can divulge thoughts which have been horrifying to him and see that they are not horrifying to his physician. Emotions or drives which might be overwhelming if they became conscious in the situations that aroused them may find their way to consciousness fairly readily in the physician's office where there is no danger that the patient will lose control of himself and little fear of the consequences if he does. To discuss such problems freely, however, the patient must feel secure with his physician.

Another way of approaching hostile or sexual desires which are unacceptable to the patient yet responsible for anxiety is through dreams. When a person is asleep his defenses against disturbing material may be weak. Consequently, ideas may be expressed in dreams which would not otherwise be expressed. The dreams of an anxious patient may be a fruitful source of information. People do not consider themselves responsible for the content of their dreams in quite the same way they feel responsible for their thoughts and ideas during their waking hours. Nevertheless, dreams are peculiarly personal and do have meaning to the person who has had them.

You can start by asking the patient to recount his dreams and make associations to their content. This may be a long or a short procedure depending on the productivity of the patient. The more that he can say in relation to a dream, the more material you have to work with. No specific interpretation is necessary. You may merely listen for hostile or sexual implications and never give the patient a formulation. The important gain in this procedure does not lie in the specific interpretation by either you or the patient of the dream as such. But the dream is an entering wedge into areas which need discussion and thus serves as a start for a discussion of impulses unacceptable to the patient. He and you may see symbolic meaning in various parts of the dream. It matters little whether these symbolic meanings are "true" or "false" in any absolute sense. The important point is not whether the interpretation is true but whether it allows the patient to view his own emotions and drives with some equanimity. If it does, it has been successful therapy regardless of its basic truth.

One patient recounted a dream which had produced a state of panic so severe that he had jumped out of bed and, while still asleep, had run to the second-story window to jump out of it. The dream was of a vast expanse of asphalt in the middle of which was a tiny blade of grass. At one side of the dream, almost out of sight, was a pillar holding up the front porch of a house. This was all there was to the dream but it precipitated panic. When asked what came to his mind as he pictured the dream, he mentioned that the pillar looked like a huge penis. His physician can then ask him what this brings to mind, what memories it awakens, or can continue having him give other associations. In the course of the discussions, a great many of his ideas about sexuality should come to the foreground. By using a neutral source of material, a dream, the physician has entered a field which is anything but neutral. Since the dream is something over which the patient has no control, it is permissible for something in it to have sexual connotations. At the same time, the fact that he has dreamt about it makes it personally meaningful so that he sees some point to discussing it.

When there is no adequate way of expressing irritations, they may build up sufficient energy to seem overpowering. When first expressed they may take the extreme form of a desire for the death of oneself or another. That such feelings actually exist is known both from talking to patients who have such feelings and from reading newspaper accounts of such acts. However, you ordinarily need not be afraid to bring these feelings into consciousness nor to discuss them with patients. You need only remember that they are accumulations of day-to-day irritations and that, once the feeling is out in the open where it can be viewed coolly and the sources of it discovered, the patient will find that these feelings can be controlled. The intense desire to kill is an accumulation of anger, unexpressed, to the point where only a violent act seems adequate to discharge the accumulated energy. Fortunately this is not necessary. Discussion of these "murderous impulses" dissipates them. Since the anxiety has been aroused by the fear of inability to control these impulses, bringing them into consciousness and viewing them dispassionately reduces the anxiety. The patient finds that he can control them from the mere fact of discussing them without succumbing to them. He also finds, eventually, that these feelings are not nearly so strong as he originally thought. As the anger is dissipated, he can relax and become a more effective person.

The same holds true for sexual impulses. When repressed, with no outlet permitted them and with constant sources of stimulation for them, they build up energy until only the wildest sexual orgies seem adequate to express the drive properly. Again this may be rooted in many day-to-day accumulations of sexual desire. The sexual drive need not be stronger than average, and the sexual needs may be no different from those of other people. However, the initial expression of them may take an extreme form.

To handle situations of this sort, you must be able to view hostile and sexual impulses calmly. If you are frightened or horrified by what is said, you make the patient more frightened than he was before. If you meet the patient's first statements with "Oh, you can't feel that way. It's ridiculous" or if in some other way you reject his confidences you tell him in effect that these impulses are disturbing and unacceptable to you. He is already anxious and upset because of these feelings and to find them rejected by the first person to whom he tells them can only increase his anxiety. Acceptance of the patient, however, does not mean that you must encourage putting into action the first wild expressions of his impulses. He is frightened by his own feelings; he knows that they are not socially acceptable in the intense form in which he feels them. Your role is not to make him feel that the intense expression of them is acceptable when it is not but to make him feel that he can handle them and that their basic sources are acceptable and normal. Every normal person has aggressive impulses and sexual desires. No one need set complete passivity or asexuality as a personal goal. He needs to find, however, some socially acceptable way of expressing these impulses, either directly or in a sublimated form.

It is possible to proceed too rapidly in uncovering sources of anxiety. The danger signals are those of panic, disorganization, and depression. These dangers can usually be avoided. If you use only material given by the patient and point out connections between statements which he has not seen before or ask questions for clarification of things that have been said, material will ordinarily not come forth too rapidly. You should avoid making your own interpretations too early in the course of treatment. If you wish to suggest to the patient that something he has said may have other meanings than those he has given it, the suggestion should be in a form which allows the patient a loophole of escape if he is not ready for this new view. And, always, you must find ways of reassuring him that he is acceptable despite the destructive or sexual impulses he is expressing.

One of the potential dangers of free expression in a patient with acute anxiety is the development of panic. If you are aware of the possibility, this danger can usually be avoided. Acute anxiety ordinarily implies the presence of strong drives which the patient fears he cannot control. As these are first expressed, the intense feelings which occasioned this fear may seem overwhelming, and the fear of losing control seems to be becoming an actuality. Another aspect of the anxiety attack is fear that expression of the drives will evoke disapproval and make the patient unacceptable to those about him. This fear, too, may become overwhelming as he first begins to face the problems within himself. Consequently, when panic seems to be developing, reassurance is much needed, not the reassurance of a verbal statement that you understand but the reassurance of an accepting attitude and manner. Acceptance of this sort is the most powerful force in allaying anxiety aroused by hostile or sexual desires.

If anxiety seems to be mounting despite your accepting attitude, it may be expedient to halt the flow of words gently. This must be done in such a way that the patient has no feeling of being rejected. "I think we have gone far enough for today. Let's leave part of the story for another time," may be one way of stopping the discussion. The interview should not end abruptly here, however. A few minutes, at least, should be spent reassuring the patient that the impulses which frighten him are basically normal and that their intensity will decrease as treatment continues. Such simple statements lend objectivity to the discussion but, more importantly, they also reassure the patient that you are not disturbed by what he has said. In addition, a prompt return appointment is further assurance of your acceptance and willingness to help.

While probing into the emotional problems of the patient, you should also be alert to evidences of disorganization, which may be manifest in speech or behavior. If speech becomes incoherent, the connection between statements being remote or illogical, or if behavior becomes bizarre and inappropriate, further probing should wait. Discussion should be directed away from the disturbing material to immediate and specific problems; and these should be discussed in realistic, down-to-earth terms. When disorganization has appeared imminent in response to discussion of anxiety-laden problems, you should seriously consider giving support and reassurance without further exploration. If continued explorations seems necessary, it should be undertaken with caution and preceded by extended efforts to strengthen the patient's mechanisms for handling the disturbing material when it is uncovered and to reduce the intensity of the forces before they become fully conscious.

Occasionally in the course of working with one of these patients a rather puzzling situation arises. You may think that the patient has discussed significant material, for example, hostile impulses toward some member of his family, and learned that he can control the impulses. He discusses his difficulties freely in your office, but when he goes home all his previous difficulties reappear and the anxiety is once more present in its old intensity. It appears that he has received no benefit at all from his discussions. This is often related to the atmosphere in the office as compared to the atmosphere in the home. While with you his defenses are lowered because his anger toward some member of the family is not a threat when the person is not present. When he returns home, the other person is near and the anger is again a threat. The same defenses which previously held it in check are therefore called into use again. Irritations are repressed. He is unaware that they exist, but a vague uneasiness begins to overcome him and gradually his anxiety mounts. It is important to be understanding at such times and to realize that this is a phase of recovery which will pass in time if the patient can find an adequate way of handling his anger.

In treating patients with anxiety it should be remembered that anxiety is useful to the patient. It is distressing and serves as a powerful motivation for change. Physical pain serves as a stimulus to patients to do something to relieve that pain. Anxiety may be looked upon as mental pain. The more intense the anxiety, the more intensely the patient desires help. A patient who has no anxiety about his symptoms is extremely difficult to treat. At such times, his doctor may wish to provoke anxiety in order to use it as a motivation for therapy.

The presence of anxiety, therefore, is not alarming and should not arouse anxiety in you. Its presence means that a conflict is going on within the patient. It means that there are drives and emotions which he cannot admit to himself. It means likewise that forces are trying to hold these emotions in check to prevent them from disturbing the patient's equilibrium. You can help the repressive forces win out, if this is what seems most desirable, or bring the feared drives and emotions into consciousness and demonstrate to the patient that they can be controlled. Whether you strengthen the defenses or lessen the drive, you have helped the patient. The more beneficial approach, usually, is to bring the drives and emotions into consciousness and demonstrate that they are not beyond his powers of control. This removes the source of the difficulty and the need for repression. The physician who tries to strengthen the repressive defenses is undertaking a more difficult job, ordinarily, since the presence of overt anxiety demonstrates that the repressive forces are not sufficient to control the intensity of drive with which the patient is forced to cope.

The discussion thus far has emphasized acute anxiety states. These are often dramatic and respond very well to brief psychotherapy. But one should be alert to the many conditions in which mild anxiety is chronically present. The same general principles of treatment apply but may require patience and ingenuity. The symptoms of which such a patient may complain bitterly are useful to him in decreasing the intensity of his anxiety. Relieving such symptoms without relieving the underlying anxiety leaves the patient with "free-floating" anxiety which may immediately attach itself to a new symptom. To treat such a patient successfully requires adequate handling of the anxiety, which usually means consideration of the unacceptable impulses at the base of the trouble.

Not all patients with anxiety give immediate evidence of it. Physicians sometimes think that if a patient is not obviously nervous and jittery, emotionally labile, or apprehenisve he is not anxious. But anxiety underlies the complete indifference of the patient with conversion hysteria. It may be abundantly present in the perfectly poised and socially active woman with headaches. It may be present in the ambitious patient with a duodenal ulcer, who claims to have no emotions whatever. It is always a major factor in the hypochondriacal patient. Anxiety, through its physiologic concomitants, can precipitate coma in a diabetic patient. It can contribute to angina in the patient with coronary artery disease. It can initiate an asthmatic attack. It can intensify joint pain in a patient with rheumatoid arthritis. It may aggravate the cramping pain and bloody diarrhea of a patient with ulcerative colitis. It can appear under many guises. The physician who ignores it is missing one of the most important problems that patients bring to him. Relieving anxiety may be the key to controlling the disease from which the patient is suffering.

Chronic anxiety is easily overlooked when it is associated with multiple physical complaints. That symptoms decrease the intensity of overt anxiety is recognized. That hypochondriasis is related to anxiety is also known. Yet these facts are often forgotten in dealing with individual patients; they need forceful reemphasis. It is easy to be misled by such a patient and to agree with him that his anxiety is the result of his symptoms, since we are all aware that symptoms can and do arouse anxiety. It is not uncommon, moreover, to meet physicians who feel they should not make psychiatric diagnoses so long as some nameable disease is present. Yet many hypochondriacal patients have readily identifiable diseases. In fact, people with chronic anxiety commonly have many other medical difficulties as well. Adequate therapy requires a complete evaluation. Neglect of emotional factors in patients with multiple diagnoses can lead to gross mishandling. The anxiety markedly influences the patient's attitudes toward his complaints, his physician, and the treatment given. It cannot properly be ignored.

Mrs. Winn (p. 16) was such a patient. She was 41 years old and gave as her chief complaint recurrent urinary tract infections for the previous 10 years. But she was equally disturbed by intermittent attacks of right lower quadrant pain which she had had for 27 years, since the onset of her menses at 14. She complained bitterly of frequent, severe headaches from which she had received no relief despite careful adherence to medical therapy. She suffered from chronic constipation and fatigue. She had frequent upper respiratory infections and recurrent "sinusitis." Her physicians had never given adequate treatment for these, she felt, since they continued to recur. At times she had dyspnea on exertion and occasionally even at rest, often accompanied by dizziness, faintness, and numbness and tingling in her extremities. As she related these symptoms, she commented with some heat that one physician had suggested that these symptoms might be related to worry. This was ridiculous since she had no reason to worry; she had a fine husband and daughter; they owned their own home; and she lived as she had always wanted to live. Anyway, more important than the dyspnea and its associated symptoms, a sharp, burning pain kept recurring in her right shoulder without any apparent reason. And she hurried to add a list of sensitivities which had been discovered in the course of her many treatments. She was sensitive to all laxatives and all sedatives, could not tolerate aspirin, got sick on any medicine containing atropine, had experienced a reaction to penicillin, and could eat few foods with impunity, milk being the worst offender. In addition, she had had seven operations: a tonsillectomy when 9, an appendectomy when 16, a plastic operation on her nose when 26, a uterine suspension when 34, a dilatation and curettage when 36, a hysterectomy when 39, and an exploratory laparotomy when 40. Because of her multiple complaints she had been seen by specialists in cardiology, urology, and gynecology. All three had rendered the same opinion—the findings were not sufficient to explain her symptoms.

A thorough history, physical examination, and laboratory workup made a number of diagnoses quite certain. She had chronic cystitis with persistent infection with Proteus vulgaris and a staphylococcus. She also had a cystocele and rectocele with a small cul-de-sac hernia. A Pseudomonas vaginitis was discovered, and she had hemorrhoids. In addition, it seemed clear that she suffered intermittently from vascular headaches, allergic rhinitis, and urticaria. She had had toxemia of pregnancy with a spontaneous abortion when 37 years old. She gave a convincing history of rheumatic fever when 15, though there were no demonstrable residua. One brother died of rheumatic heart disease and two sisters had the disease.

This patient had multiple complaints and multiple diagnoses. She had some hostility toward physicians but carried out their instructions carefully, often, apparently, to her own detriment since she was "allergic" to so many things. Despite frequent reactions to medications and at best little or no relief from her symptoms, she had continued going from doctor to doctor seeking relief. She had little overt anxiety, unless you consider her concern over her symptoms to be overt anxiety. Certainly she was vociferous in denying any worries, suggesting this possibility herself but doing so only to denounce it as absurd. Such a case offers many difficulties to a physician, as evidenced by the many physicians she had seen without obtaining satisfaction. Despite the obvious complexities of this case, the essential background information can be summarized fairly briefly.

Mrs. Winn had been the eighth of 11 children. Her father had been a house painter and her mother had kept a paint store. Mrs. Winn considered her father to have been a mild, kindly, hard working but rather ineffectual man who, unfortunately, had seldom been at home. She looked upon her mother as a mean and aggressive woman who dominated her husband and was always too busy in the store to pay any attention to her many children. Because of this, the patient had been raised by two older sisters who disliked the chore assigned them and made her life miserable. Because of her dark complexion, they taunted her with being a Negro and not really their sister. They made her feel unwanted and excluded her from their play with friends. She was raised believing she was ugly to look at, stupid, and of a mean disposition. She described herself as always "sickly" but noted that she was healthier when away from home. She ascribed this to her "allergy to paint" and the fact that the paint store was at the front of the house. She seemed to accept the judgment that she was ugly, stupid, and mean and constantly strove to overcome this.

She was the only one of the 11 children to complete 4 years of college. She went beyond this and received a master's degree in accounting, putting herself through school. At 26 she had a plastic operation on her nose in an effort to become more attractive, though she felt she was too big-boned to be really attractive anyway. She learned to be witty and humorous rather than to express her anger openly. She nevertheless had a very deep concern over her basic worth, doubting that anyone could love her or that she could rely wholeheartedly upon anyone. When 31, she married a fellow accountant who was "just like my father"—mild, kindly, hard working, but not too effectual. He had had renal disease before their marriage. A few months afterward he had a right nephrectomy. Her own urinary troubles had begun at the time of this operation, though there was no question whatever of the infectious nature of her urinary disease. Her symptoms had multiplied rapidly thereafter.

It is evident that this woman had considerable difficulties with feelings of hostility. The vein of hostility, however, ran far deeper than the superficial expressions of it toward physicians. It would hardly be possible for a person to have been raised in the setting from which she came without developing deep feelings of resentment and distrust of people about her. As such feelings become evident in the course of interviews, the physician should encourage their expression since this helps to decrease their intensity.

It is also evident that Mrs. Winn had a major personality conflict around dependence. This conflict was manifested by her drive to be independent and self-sufficient. At the same time she was seeking approval from others and looking for someone on whom she could depend. More will be said about this type of conflict and how to deal with it.

The core of her problem, however, seems to lie in basic anxieties about herself that centered around feelings of personal inadequacy and insecurity. She was obviously concerned about her basic physical, intellectual, and emotional endowments. She needed to prove to herself over and over again that she was adequate. Therefore she was extremely sensitive to any comments or any events which seemed to reflect to her disadvantage.

These things were expressed in her symptoms and in her attitudes toward them. Earlier in life her anxiety was concentrated on physical appearance—her complexion and her nose. But she had anxieties about her physical endowment apart from superficial appearances. Her symptoms expressed this feeling of physical inadequacy in a way which she could comprehend and which was acceptable to her. It was easy enough for her to feel that if she were free of pain and constant fatigue she would be adequate physically. But the basic feeling of something being wrong with her body would still be there even though the symptoms were cleared. To serve their purpose the symptoms had to have their origin in a physical disease which could be eradicated. Then cure of the symptoms with medications would leave her a person adequate in her own eyes. If she accepted the idea that the symptoms were related to her reaction to stresses and strains in her life or to worry, then she accepted an additional inadequacy which would not be cured simply by receiving medications from physicians.

Her feelings of emotional inadequacy centered around anger and expressions of it, since she had been raised by her sisters to believe that she had a "mean disposition." She had a great deal of resentment within herself and was aware of it. Its presence was a constant reminder that some truth lay in the comments. She spent much of her time trying to prevent expression of anger. One of the defenses she chose was wit.

Her feelings of inadequacy also had repercussions in her illness. She went from doctor to doctor seeking help for her symptoms. None of the medications gave her any marked degree of relief. These constant failures frustrated her and aroused hostility toward the physicians who had promised to cure her and had not succeeded. Any rebellious act was, to her, an expression of anger and evidence that she had a mean disposition. To refuse to follow a physician's instructions was, in a sense, rebelling against what he had asked her to do. Consequently, she felt compelled to follow instructions faithfully whether cure resulted or not, in order to avoid feelings of guilt. Yet the anger had not been dissipated simply because she held it in check.

Another potent source of anxiety was the deep insecurity of her background. She was not permitted to feel that she belonged to her own family. She was ignored, if not actually rejected, by her mother and certainly was actively rejected by her sisters, who excluded her from their group activities as well as from their play with each other. Through most of her childhood there was no one on whom she could depend for care and sympathy and no one who gave her a feeling of personal security or a sense of belonging. She had felt more acceptance from her father than from anyone else, though this had not been adequate to meet her emotional needs. She married a man who was much like her father, including the fact that he was not a strong, effective person. In addition, within a few months of their marriage, he had an illness which was life threatening and required major surgery. He offered only a limited amount of security, which she prized highly, but it was insufficient. One of the things which she was seeking most urgently was someone, some physician, on whom she could depend completely. She was seeking someone who could give her the security she lacked. Her symptoms were of considerable importance, for their presence gave her a means whereby she might constantly test whether people understood, sympathized, and would care for her. It was important to her, therefore, that the symptoms not be cured until she found someone who was dependable and gave her feelings of security and adequacy.

How should a physician handle such a patient? There is no one answer to this question. Some physicians will prefer not to deal at all with the emotional factors and the basic anxieties. If the physician has a strong personality and effects a good relationship with such a patient, he may be able to satisfy enough of the needs for security to allow the patient to function adequately despite occasional recurring symptoms. This is the way many physicians handle such patients. It is sometimes effective but always has one potential danger. It is a relationship in which the patient is entirely dependent on the physician, and it fosters dependency. Such patients have considerable conflicts around dependency and wish to be as independent as possible, superficially at least. Therefore, if awareness of dependency is forced upon such a patient, considerable hostility may be engendered. This destroys the effectiveness of the relationship. In establishing such a relationship, the doctor is dealing directly with the basic anxieties of the patient, but through relationship entirely rather than by helping the patient understand the source of the difficulties.

If the physician chooses instead to help the patient by discussing the background for the difficulties and by trying to help him gain an understanding of the nature of his problems, the job will be difficult but ultimately may be much more rewarding. He should allow, in fact encourage, expression of hostility when this is discovered. He should try to help the patient recognize intense feelings of inadequacy. If the physician has genuine respect for the patient's capacities to overcome his troubles and respect for his basic adequacy despite feelings of inadequacy, this discussion can be accomplished without leading to panic or disorganization. If the physician feels that people with such problems are actually inadequate, then a discussion of this nature should not be initiated at all. Finally, the physician should help the patient achieve an independence based on feelings of personal adequacy and security rather than a display of independence which arises from the need to deny inadequacies and insecurities.

TENSION

Tension arises when a person is exercising control. The first question which must be answered, therefore, is what requires control? Though the circumstances in which tension arises give the precipitating external stressful stimuli, they do not explain the origin of tension rather than some other response. Certain types of behavior commonly accompany anger, anxiety, and depression. A person may be exerting control over his behavior to prevent aggressive action, flight, or tears. The emotion itself may be threatening, and the tension may be an effort to suppress it directly. And, of course, both may seem to the patient to require control. Behavior patterns and emotional reactions are the two things most commonly pertinent to tension states. You need to know which is pertinent to the particular patient with whom you are dealing. Investigating this question is in fact defining the nature of the stress.

You also need to know why the emotion or behavior is threatening to the patient. Does he look upon the emotion as "sinful" or as a sign of a "weak character"? Must the behavior be controlled lest it disrupt some important relationship, as with a parent, spouse, friend, or boss? Or must it be controlled in order to maintain a standard of conduct consistent with the person's concept of himself or with the role he wishes to play? The answers to these questions need to be clarified in the patient's mind if he is to find a solution free of symptoms.

Having answered these questions, you must then help the patient decide whether the controlling forces are appropriate to the situation or not, how to relax them if this seems desirable, and how to avoid symptoms if controls must be continued. If the behavior being controlled could prevent achievement of an important goal in life, the controlling forces may be entirely appropriate. In this regard it should be remembered that symptoms arise in part from the intensity and duration of tension. It is not necessary, therefore, to set as a goal the abolition of all controls in order to achieve symptomatic relief. Decreasing either the intensity or the duration of the response may be all that is necessary. Often such a plan will relieve symptoms without precipitating fresh difficulties in the patient's life.

In view of these considerations, three bits of advice that are frequently given patients with symptoms resulting from emotional stresses and strains become patently absurd for patients with tension states. The advice "get control of yourself" is exactly what these patients do not need. Their symptoms arise from the fact that they are exerting too much control. If the emotional forces are so intense as to be disrupting, this control is necessary until something has been done to alleviate the intensity of the emotions. The advice to exert more control, or the attempt on the part of the patient to do so, can only result in an intensification of symptoms.

Similarly, the advice to "take a vacation" is not always appropriate. True, a vacation may result in relief of the symptoms, but unless the situation or responses of the patient are changed, the symptoms will reappear upon his return. Carrying this advice to its logical conclusion would mean advising the patient to take a permanent vacation to get relief from his symptoms.

The advice "relax" would be fine if the patient could relax simply by being told to do so. Before the advice can be appropriate, you must have some idea of what is being controlled. Having discovered this, you must help the patient deal with the reasons for tension so that controls can be relaxed without undesirable consequences. Without such help the advice is apt to prove worthless.

To disregard the reasons of the ward clerk (p. 194) for controlling her activities and to tell her that it was ridiculous to exercise so much control as to result in headaches, to tell her in effect to do sloppy work, to be carefree about her job and not to worry about turning in a good performance, would not be intelligent therapy. True enough, she might get over her headaches, but she might also lose her job and, therefore, much of her satisfaction in life. With her aspirations and satisfactions on the job, it is not likely she would be able to carry out the advice anyway. It is not necessary for her to become carefree and careless in her work to get over the headaches. As the job becomes routinized, control becomes less necessary. Rest periods during the day could also be effective.

Treatment of tension states thus begins with an evaluation of the realities of the situation, the factors affecting the patient's response to that situation, and the reasons for control being of such intensity and duration as to lead to the appearance of symptoms. If control is being exerted to suppress an emotional reaction which seems undesirable to the patient, then expressive therapy for that emotion is the first step in treatment. Before the patient is advised to express this emotion outside your office, the reasons for controlling it must be evaluated. Ordinarily the patient controls the emotion lest it interfere with some important relationship, prevent him from achieving his goals or aims in life, or seems to him to be sinful or evidence of weakness. In the situation in which the emotion is aroused, he feels it necessary to control it, and his evaluation may be entirely correct. In your office, however, control is no longer important unless the emotion is considered sinful or a sign of weakness. Anger aroused in a marital relationship does not threaten the marriage when the anger is expressed to you. Therefore the patient can often express his feelings quite freely and adequately to you, and in doing so he decreases the intensity of the feeling. With the feeling less intense, the controlling mechanisms need not be so strong and the tension is temporarily relieved. It may be aroused again, however, immediately upon returning home. Other measures must be taken if the effects are to be lasting. To prevent recurrence requires consideration of the reasons such an intense emotion has been evoked and treatment designed to deal with these adequately.

Similar considerations are pertinent if it is behavior that is being controlled. Again you need to understand why behavior must be controlled so carefully—whether it is to achieve some goal in life or to preserve an important relationship. If the patient is controlling his behavior to achieve a goal, considerations of how appropriate that goal is for him and whether that degree of tension is necessary to attain it become pertinent. If control is being exercised in order to preserve a relationship, it becomes pertinent to consider the type of relationship and what drives lead the patient to desire it so strongly.

With an understanding of these backgrounds for tension, you can direct your attention to decreasing the duration or the intensity of the controls which led him to seek medical aid.

Situations arise in which the controlling forces need to be strong and prolonged if the patient is to achieve his aims or preserve an essential relationship. In such a situation neither the intensity nor the duration of tension may be alterable. This does not mean that you can do nothing, but your goals will necessarily be limited. It may be helpful to discuss this with the patient so that he understands why his symptoms are not relieved. You can still give your support and whatever relief medications can afford. You should not withdraw completely just because the tension is realistic. Knowing that an ally is present and ready to help is a source of strength to most people and makes adversity more tolerable. The patient should know, not so much by words as by actions, that you are ready to give as much help and symptomatic relief as you can.

DEPRESSION

Depressive reactions which require medical attention are frequently intermixed with anger and anxiety. The anger is often turned upon the patient's self, being expressed as feelings of unworthiness and self-reproach; these intensify the depression and give it a dynamic, forceful quality lacking in simple depression. Mr. Earl, who was 48, had had ulcerative colitis for 20 years. Despite frequent exacerbations, he had maintained his weight quite well and seemed to be doing satisfactorily. He came in unexpectedly one day saying that he was having 40 or 50 bowel movements a day. He could not understand why. He feared he might have cancer and had told his family that it would be a good thing if he did. He was a burden to them; they would be better off if he were not living. He appeared to be depressed but showed no overt evidences of anger or anxiety. Investigation revealed that these feelings were clearly present and quite close to the surface, though only after several interviews could he discuss them.

Some background information is essential to understanding this exacerbation of colitis. He described his father as a strict, hard-working man who mistreated his mother. He had been the oldest of nine children in a farm family and had been forced to quit school at an early age to help his father on the farm. He resented this strongly but did as he was told. He had been very close to his mother and could not tolerate the slightest expression of disapproval from her. If she criticized anything he did or said, he broke into tears. When he married in his early twenties his mother made him promise on his wedding night that he would never mistreat his wife the way his father had mistreated her. He promised that he would not.

The first 5 years of his marriage were very difficult ones. He worked hard on his farm and got little in return. His wife was unprepared for hardships and expressed her dissatisfaction openly. A local minister visited in his home frequently. His wife played the piano and the minister and she sang songs. This happened with increasing frequency while he was working in the fields. One day when he returned home his wife told him that the minister had tried to seduce her. This was a great shock to him. Thereafter, while working in the fields, he was constantly wondering what was happening at home. At this time his diarrhea began. Interestingly enough, it was also at this time that he and his wife finally made a "satisfactory adjustment" in their marriage. Not a harsh word passed between them from that day on.

Successive crop failures forced them to sell their farm. He then worked in a machine shop. Despite continuing diarrhea, he did so well that within a few months he was offered a position in the regional office in Kansas City. He went there with high hopes, but his wife did not like life in a large city so he gave up this job. Through succeeding years he felt that he had lost his one big chance to be a success because his wife had been unable to adjust to life in Kansas City. He opened a machine shop of his own. Just as he was getting on his feet financially, the shop burned down. With the help of friends it was rebuilt and the debts paid off. But with the beginning of the war he was unable to get adequate help. Since he could not turn out enough work to keep the shop going by himself, he was forced to sell it. He began to feel that fate was against him.

In the years which followed they raised five children, and he did farm work. Diarrhea was almost constant, though its severity waxed and waned. Since he was unable to control bowel movements, his wife was constantly washing clothing and bed linen. Painful hemorrhoids required surgery, and healing was slow and associated with considerable scarring so that a rectal stricture developed and even more difficulty in bowel control resulted.

During the following years crops were good, and Mr. Earl was able to buy his own home and farm. This had been a lifelong ambition. Despite the considerable financial obligation which this entailed, everything seemed favorable. He bought the farm but with some mis-givings that failure might continue to dog his footsteps. Things did go wrong. The first crop failed. A bean crop which his son raised on and rented from Mr. Earl's sister was harvested and sold without payments to Mr. Earl or his son. A visit to the sister to get payments for the crop only resulted in an argument. "Its our land and any-thing raised on it belongs to us," was her statement. Mr. Earl and his sister were not on speaking terms after this. A chance to sell some wood failed to materialize. His oldest son went to a nearby city hoping to get a good job. He was unable to get what he wanted and accepted work which barely paid his living expenses. Mr. Earl could see himself falling short of another one of his goals in life.

However, the financial situation disturbed him less than his wife's lack of enthusiasm for her new home. She took no interest in the farm or the crops. She found it hard to keep up with the daily house-hold routine, and the meals she prepared were adequate for herself but scarcely sufficient for working men. She seemed always to be tired. One day when he confronted her with her lack of interest and general weariness she told him that she certainly was tired. He should expect her to be since she had had six children to raise. Even the recollection of this comment brought tears to his eyes. They had only five children; he was the sixth. He tried to defend himself, saying that it was not his fault that he had colitis. She answered that it might not be his fault but he was as much work to care for as any child had ever been. He resented her attitude. He had given up his goals in life to please her; her lack of gratitude disappointed him greatly. He recognized that he had been a burden, through no fault of his own, but was not prepared for her to tire of caring for him. If he was not wanted in his own home, what was there for him? It was this that led to his statement that he would be better off dead. His fear of cancer was as much a wish as a fear.

Once the story had unfolded the feelings of depression, resentment and anxiety were clear enough. The question then was: How does one treat such a patient?

The depressed person is, in a sense, immobilized. Completely ab-sorbed in himself and his problems, he has little interest in people around him (except as they contribute to his depressed state) or in ordinary daily activity. The deeper the depression, the more complete the self-absorption and lack of interest in outside things become. Activ-ties hold no interest, appetite is lost, sleep habits change, friendships are forgotten, the person withdraws from social contacts and may even resist conversation.

Perhaps the strongest force to break into this state of denial that the world, cruel place, exists is a strong personal relationship. The more severe the depression, however, the harder this is to establish. But the process of establishing a good relationship acts to decrease the depression. A good relationship requires an interest in someone besides oneself. This is an early step toward socialization and an externalization of interests. A good relationship means that someone else is interested in one's welfare and the problems one must face. I brings renewed self-respect and restores some of the lost stores of approval and social esteem. It is a powerful force for recovery.

Establishing such a relationship may be difficult. It may require great patience and certainly requires sincerity on the part of the physician. Repeated expressions of interest and of the desire to help may be needed; when the patient is ready to speak, he must be heard through in an unhurried way. Reassurance cannot be given until the problems facing the patient are understood. First expressions of the problem may, as with Mr. Earl, dwell on peripheral issues which add to the depression but are not the crux of the problem. They need to be known, but the successive failures, shortcomings, or rejection by others, which give the patient the feelings of futility and hopelessness constituting a depression, should not be permitted endless repetition. The physician cannot dismiss these events and reactions as unimportant; neither can he accept them as beyond solution. Sympathetic interest must be combined with a optimistic outlook for the future.

Once a good relationship exists, reassurance can be given with benefit. Reassurance must be directed properly. Mr. Earl discussed his financial problems first because they were the easiest for him to discuss. Initially it was the only problem he admitted. Reassurance was useful in indicating the physician's interest, and was limited to the financial problems with no implication that the patient's overall situation was solved simply by finding ways to handle the financial difficulties.

Mr. Earl then discussed troubles with his brothers and sisters. This was harder for him since he was getting nearer to matters which touched on his feelings about himself. He considered that resentment toward members of his family was bad or unchristian. Reassurance that his brothers and sisters probably did not dislike him as much as

e feared would have seemed indicated by the way in which he pre-
ented the material, since his emphasis was on their dislike of him. The
hysician is not in a position to give reassurance about attitudes of
iblings unless evidence indicates that the patient's evaluation is in
rror. Sibling attitudes were not the important issue here, in any
ise. The reassurance most needed was about himself, that he was
ot rejected by the physician because he resented the injustices to
hich his brothers and sisters had subjected him. Reassurance that
ie physician accepted him despite his feelings of resentment toward
is brothers and sisters was a necessary preliminary to the next step
f the discussion.

The last thing Mr. Earl discussed with his physician was the diffi-
ulty with his wife. This was the hardest for him to discuss. He felt
uilty about his resentment of her, but the feelings were intense and
ould not really be denied. Discussion at this time touched upon his
vife's realistic reasons for being tired of the constant washing and care
nd the possibility that she loved him even though she was tired of
ie work. He needed to hear this even though basically he was aware
f it all the time. What he needed even more was to know that the
eelings of anger toward the person closest and nearest to him did
ot occasion censure from the physician. He needed, in addition, to
iscuss his attitudes toward anger and the origin of these attitudes.
Iis feelings toward his parents and their marital relationship, his
oals in his own marriage, and the promise given his mother on his
vedding night were all pertinent to helping him understand his
eactions to events and to the emotions aroused by these events. More
olerance for his resentment and less fear that it would disrupt his
narriage had to develop gradually. His suicidal preoccupations would
hen decrease.

People whose depression has resulted in a lack of interest in outside
ctivities need to have their attention directed to these again. This is
est done with a positive approach rather than an attempt to suppress
he patient's ruminations about himself. The advice "go back to work"
r "forget it" may be given in an attempt to externalize interests. In
ffect, however, it is suppressive therapy, which has a useful place in
reating mild depressions. The milder the depression, the more likely
s suppressive therapy to be of value. But if depression is intense, the
atient cannot carry out such advice, and another failure may ac-
ually increase the depression, especially if he anticipates rejection for
is failure. Advice of this sort should be given only when you are

reasonably certain that the patient can follow it with some success

For mild or moderate situational depressions, superficial psycho
therapy can be quite valuable. The interviews need not be long. In
terviews of 15 or 30 minutes once or twice a week often relieve symp
toms. During these interviews, there is no need to prod deeply into
personality conflicts. Instead, one should concentrate on day-to-day
problems and help the patient meet these as they arise. Sometimes it
is useful to help him plan his daily activities so that a definite sched
ule is set. In any event, the presence of someone who is interested in
him, who can reassure him with authority about his physical com
plaints and direct his attention to people and events about him is a
source of strength and a vital force for recovery.

Chapter 11

Defenses in Treatment

EMOTIONAL disturbances are not always obvious nor can they invariably be approached directly. Even when of major importance their expression may be grossly altered by mental defense mechanisms. These defense mechanisms may prevent you, initially at least, from getting at the basic difficulty. When they prevent a direct approach to the difficulty you must be able to recognize the defenses and deal with them before you can work with the emotional state.

Knowing how to deal with defense mechanisms is important at all stages of treatment. A basic cause of psychosomatic symptoms lies in the defense mechanisms by which the patient meets stressful situations in his life. To overcome the symptoms the patient may need help in learning new mechanisms to handle the problems. Thus it becomes necessary to understand not only what the mechanisms are, how they affect body physiology, and what they accomplish for the patient but also why they are utilized and how you can help a patient learn new mechanisms when old ones are failing him.

MEANING OF DEFENSES

The mental mechanisms discussed in Chapter 3 are ways in which people deal with stressful situations. They are essential to normal development and behavior. A person without defenses would be helpless and unable to deal with the troublesome circumstances which arise in the lives of all. Most people have many defense mechanisms and use whichever seems most appropriate. Most people develop patterns of reaction for familiar situations rather than make a conscious decision of what is appropriate for each set of conditions that arises. Since these patterns have developed through social interactions in which they were at least partially successful, they usually serve well in situations like the original one. When generalized to different circumstances they may serve less well but be used anyway. The person is generally unaware of what he is doing, since no conscious decision has been made.

As a consequence of this process, mechanisms may be utilized repeatedly, despite their failure to achieve the ends desired and despite the availability of other defenses. Mr. Grant (p. 70) withdrew from situations in which irritation was expressed or aggressive action was about to be taken. This defense had been satisfactory in childhood and he continued to use it as an adult although its use militated against his long-term goals of advancement at work. It was used habitually and for situations which did not require it. It seemed almost to be a "way of life" for him, even though he used other defense mechanisms for other types of situations.

The importance of successful defenses is clear enough, but defenses are important even when they fail. Their presence gives strength and security, and even poor defenses are better than none. A person who characteristically withdraws from stressful situations as Mr. Grant did may feel helpless when he cannot withdraw unless he knows some other way of handling the situation appropriately. Preventing withdrawal when the patient sees no other way of handling the situation may lead to severe anxiety or even panic. You cannot attack a defense directly without due consideration for what the patient will do without it. New defenses cannot develop overnight.

Defenses are important in other ways than for the security they afford when successful or the anxiety aroused when they fail or are attacked. They strikingly affect the physiologic processes associated with emotions, both to increase or prolong them and to decrease or eliminate them. Successful repression may eliminate the physiologic concomitants of anger and anxiety. Suppression, when stronger than the suppressed emotion, may decrease the intensity of the response markedly. When emotions and controlling mechanisms are evenly matched the effects of suppression on the intensity of the physiologic response may be less certain, but the response may be significantly prolonged, and symptoms may develop. In addition, suppression may add new physiologic responses if a significant degree of tension is developed. These physiologic manifestations of the defense mechanism may combine with manifestations of emotions and increase the intensity of response, may oppose the manifestations and decrease the intensity of response, or may be unrelated and give rise to new manifestations. Thus the individual symptoms of anxiety, for example, may be decreased, increased, or changed in quality when tension is added. The physiologic results of the interaction between emotions and the defenses against them is determined by a complex of factors which is not reducible to a simple one-to-one expression.

DANGERS IN ATTACKING DEFENSES

An awareness of the importance of defenses in maintaining interpersonal relations, affording emotional security, and affecting body physiology should make the physician cautious in his attacks on them. Removal of a defense when no substitute is available may arouse anxiety and increase the intensity of physiologic manifestations. Substitution of a new defense may not only alter the patient's patterns of behavior but also foster new symptoms. It is often difficult to predict the social, psychiatric, or physiologic effect of altering the defenses.

A psychotic episode in a 30 year old man with acute thyrotoxicosis has been reported.[93] The episode was apparently a response simply to divulging important information about himself. His history and his approach to the physician treating him indicated that his relationship with people in authority was extremely important to him and that he was dependent on their approval. During the eighth interview, the psychiatrist commented, "Often we find that a sudden shock precipitates hyperthyroidism. There doesn't appear to be any such shock in your case." The report continues "This comment produced a profoundly dramatic effect upon the patient. He suddenly changed from a relaxed position into one of fright. The visible pulsation of his goiter increased markedly. His respiration became rapid and shallow. Perspiration dotted his forehead. For a long moment he stared at the therapist.

"In a strangled, harsh voice the patient finally spoke. 'There is something I haven't told you. I've never told anyone . . .' With great affect, he then revealed his secret. Two weeks prior to his marriage the patient had met his wife after her weekly appointment with her physician. In a public conveyance she confessed to him that she was being treated for syphilis. 'My world was shattered. In little pieces all around me. I couldn't believe it. I couldn't believe it. My Sarah. My sweet little Sarah. She had syphilis.'

"The patient now cried openly. 'I couldn't let her know what a shock this was. I had to pick up the pieces. I had to smile and tell her it made no difference . . . and it didn't, it didn't. She was still the same lovely person.' "

The following morning the patient requested an extra hour from his therapist; this was denied since it was not in the original schedule. During the interview on the next day the patient seemed depressed and diffident, and within a few hours a psychotic reaction developed in which he was negativistic and mute.

Some of the patients mentioned earlier also responded adversely to the attempt to break through defenses. The adolescent boy who had a reaction-formation in regard to his younger brother (p. 77) had many schizophrenic tendencies. When encouraged to express his sexual and aggressive impulses verbally, he became increasingly disorganized as he did so. His thinking became illogical and his behavior more bizarre, even to the point of physical violence. His defenses were necessary to continued socially acceptable behavior. Removing them left inadequate controls. Mr. Miller (p. 75) the patient with neurodermatitis, is another case in point. He reacted to attempts to break through his defenses with a flare-up in his dermatitis and an abortive suicidal gesture. The attempt to destroy his defenses of suppressing outward expression of anger and turning it in upon himself did not succeed. Instead these defenses were intensified.

The plea for caution is not a mandate for inaction, however. The patient is ill because his way of meeting stressful situations gives rise to physical alterations which are disturbing to him. To alleviate the symptoms, the patient's way of meeting stresses needs careful consideration. What is stressful? Why is it stressful? What is the patient's reaction emotionally, defensively, physiologically? Unless some feature of the situation or the patient's reaction to it is altered symptomatic relief cannot be given. Defenses must be dealt with and often must be changed.

At times you can proceed directly and attack the defense mechanism. At other times such a frontal attack may precipitate an exacerbation of symptoms, psychotic confusion, a severe depression, or a suicidal gesture. Indirect approaches, using more subtle means, may also be either beneficial or detrimental. How then are you to proceed? Are there any general principles by which to judge a given situation and patient to determine the best approach?

In working with emotional problems the physician's immediate goal is the acquisition of basic information about the patient and the formation of a doctor-patient relationship appropriate for the patient.

As you begin to understand the patient's problem you formulate goals of treatment, at least in a broad sense, and direct your attention to helping him find a more satisfactory adjustment to the troublesome circumstances of his life. You are most apt to become aware of defenses as they hinder his progress. You will become aware of defenses the patient uses to prevent you from getting information which he considers prejudicial. You will have to differentiate defenses used for this purpose from those used to protect himself from viewing a threatening impulse too closely. You will become aware of defenses used to prevent development of certain types of relationship or to assure formation of another type of relationship and of defenses which block recovery by opposing change. Your job will then be to evaluate these defenses and assess the effects of removing or changing them. You must then decide what approach is most apt to benefit the patient.

DEFENSES AGAINST DIVULGING INFORMATION

When you are fairly certain that a patient has significant information about himself which he is not divulging, you should look for the explanation first in the doctor-patient relationship. A common reason for failure to divulge information is that the patient fears disapproval or outright rejection. A simple form of this was seen when Mr. Laird (p. 253) told Dr. Bailey that he sometimes felt like running away to hide but withheld the fact that he had actually done so until he felt fairly certain of Dr. Bailey's ability to understand and to accept such behavior. The patient may likewise fear exposure to others who are unknown and whose reactions are therefore not predictable. The defense against divulging information serves a "social" function of protecting himself against disapproval from others. At such times the obvious solution is to establish a friendly, permissive relationship in which the patient feels free to talk about himself without the usual social restrictions. When such a relationship is established the information is usually forthcoming.

That these defenses are used for "social" purposes should not lead you to underestimate their significance to the patient. It is true that he is aware of the information, so being confronted by it does not come as a revelation to him. He knows and tolerates it himself, though perhaps with considerable psychic unrest and many physiologic manifestations. Nevertheless, divulging it to another person may be a great stress. A large part of this stress is the fear of disapproval or rejection by the person to whom the information has been divulged

The need for defense against divulging information varies greatly among patients and depends to a considerable degree on the type of doctor-patient relationship and the meaning of that relationship to the patient. An authoritative relationship means one thing to a patient who expects people in authority to be kindly and understanding, another to one who expects people in authority to be punitive but to stand by during adverse times, and still another to one who expects people in authority to reject and abandon him when they disapprove. The third expectation engenders considerable anxiety. A friendly relationship of equality and comradeship has different meanings to people who have experienced friends as people who are supportive despite circumstances and to people who expect to be abandoned by friends when they dislike something that has been done. The meaning of friendship is also affected by numbers. Though most people have experienced two major authority relationships during formative years, the number of meaningful friendships may vary from none to many. With few friends, the loss of one becomes more threatening.

Whether the relationship is one of authority or equality, the sequence of disapproval-rejection-isolation is potent. Social isolation, loneliness, can at times be more distressing than anxiety. The fear of social isolation powerfully influences behavior at any age and under diverse circumstances.

Clarence, a young college student, was seen because of recurrent feelings of depression and scholastic difficulty. The setting of discussions with his physician was friendly and permissive, and questions were posed in an open-ended fashion so that he could answer freely or evasively. During these discussions the problem of homosexuality seemed suggested by his statements about his relationships with his friends, both male and female. It was not at all clear that he recognized this as a problem, and the physician approached the matter cautiously, discussing his friendship without reference to sexuality while trying to evaluate the extent of the problem and his awareness of it. Questions directed at his emotional feelings for his friends were answered in vague, noncommital terms. At times these questions were ignored except for a shrug of the shoulders and some irrelevant comment that distracted the conversation. The problem was brought in focus one day when the patient mentioned that he was considering joining the Catholic Church. The reason he gave was the emotional satisfaction he found in Catholicism. When asked about his introduction to the Catholic faith he named a close male friend who had taken him to church only a few Sundays before. The physician tried to find out how much of the emotional satisfaction lay in the religion, as such, and how much in this friendship. The questions which might have elicited an answer were deflected by long monologues on theological doctrine, and the emotional meaning of dogma and ritual. When discussions came uncomfortably close to the relationship with his friend, they were terminated by his giving up Catholicism "because my parents won't permit it." This deflected the discussions back to his relationship with his parents, an area of trouble but an easier one for him to discuss.

His inability to discuss frankly the relationship with his friend suggested that the hypothesis of homosexuality might be correct and that the subject aroused anxiety. The physician allowed time to elapse before probing further, hoping to establish a relationship in which a discussion of homosexuality could be introduced without arousing undue anxiety. The occasion arose again during discussions of roommates he had had during his college life. Questions about the roommates obviously made the patient uncomfortable but he successfully avoided the primary issue by evasive answers. The discussions came close enough to the primary issue, however, for the physician to learn that one roommate, a close friend of the patient, had quite violently expressed disapproval of relationships with any hint of homosexuality in them. At this point the student began having frequent sexual relations with a girl he had dated often. Their prior relationship had been one of brother-sister companionship and he had had no previous interest in her physically. He introduced the subject of heterosexual activity at the beginning of the following interview, keeping the entire discussion in the realm of heterosexuality. Suggestion that his activities might have other meanings than he was ascribing to them were ignored during the interview but the student temporarily stopped treatment. Later it was learned that his sexual activity also stopped at this time.

He returned to the physician shortly, however, to discuss numerous other problems which still disturbed him. Many of these related indirectly to his sexual difficulty so that discussions always came back to this central theme even though they might begin with his father, his teachers, his difficulty in learning, his feelings of depression, or his inability to set a meaningful goal for himself in life. As pressures mounted toward a discussion of the anxiety-laden subject of homosexuality, the word still never mentioned, epigastric pain suddenly developed. An upper gastrointestinal series disclosed a duodenal ulcer. He greeted this news with some relief and happily went off to see an internist, again terminating psychotherapy temporarily, despite its pertinence to his physical complaint.

It was some months before he returned and when he did he had been married. Again his chief complaint was depression and unsatisfactory scholastic achievement. On this occasion the physician forcefully altered the doctor-patient relationship. The discussion was no longer an amiable and permissive one with a friend. The physician took an authoritative attitude and told him that he had not been discussing his problems freely and that no progress could be anticipated until he did so. He assured him that there were more adequate solutions for handling his problem than he had found but that he would have to face them frankly and honestly. Thus the immediate atmosphere of the interview was an earnest one, sharply focused for the patient, and with no permissiveness.

The student met this situation by saying "I guess I'm not being honest with myself then, because I don't know what the problem is."

The physician shrugged his shoulders, suggesting some doubt. "You've never discussed it with me, at any rate. I suggest you sit down and think for awhile and see if you come up with the answer."

To this the student said "Good" and started to leave. The physician stopped him briefly, commenting that finding an answer was extremely important to him since for several years he had been having recurrent feelings of depression and difficulty with his school work far beyond what would have been anticipated from one of his intellectual capacity. He had every reason, therefore, to put some effort into solving his problem.

The student answered "Well, I do have a sexual problem but I don't see how that would affect it."

To this the physician answered "I agree. I think if you sit down, starting with the problem you know about and follow it wherever logic takes you, you will find your answer."

The student then said, "Well," (there was a prolonged pause before he continued) "I think my major problem is in my relationships with other males."

The physician answered, "And so do I. If your problem *is* homosexuality it needs to be faced as such if you are ever to do anything about it."

Actually this approach—directly confronting the patient with the information that the physician knew of his homosexual tendencies— cleared the air and set the tone for a subsequent serious discussion of them. The student had been aware of his difficulties in his relationship with men but had been afraid to discuss them for fear of the reaction of the person to whom he was speaking. This fear was not allayed by a friendly, permissive atmosphere; for the student knew very well that his former roommate, who had been a close friend, would not have tolerated exposure of homosexual impulses no matter how friendly or permissive he had seemed to be in leading up to such a discussion. Finding that the physician knew about it and could use the word without being disturbed or upset was a source of relief to the patient. The feeling of depression with which he had entered the physician's office was, at least temporarily, dispelled, and he went away with renewed hope and encouragement.

One should note the diversity of defenses which this patient used during discussions probing a problem of which he was aware but was afraid to talk. He tried to avoid discussing homosexuality by ignoring questions or by giving evasive answers which told only part of the story. At times he attempted to divert the conversation by displacing interest from one subject to another. His discussions of Catholicism were of this nature. When the diversion failed he gave up a change of religion, using a spurious reason for doing so. Pressures for discussing this topic subsequently were met by an episode of "acting out" during which he attempted to document his heterosexuality and divert attention in this way from the problem of homosexuality, which had been implied in questions though never stated frankly. His marriage was intended as a forceful denial of homosexuality but did not succeed in disproving it either to him or to the physician. Consequently when the subject came up again, evasion, displacement, and denial by acting out were no longer acceptable solutions. He had no way of handling the mounting anxiety and frustration in the interview situation, and his emotions were manifest in epigastric pain. All of these defenses served the purpose of avoiding discussion of a topic which aroused anxiety. Yet confrontation with the fact of homosexuality did not arouse panic or a psychotic episode. On the contrary, it relieved much of his anxiety and depression and set the stage for profitable later discussions.

It seems evident that it is not the defense mechanism itself but the purpose which it serves that is important. In the patient with thyroid disease and the student who was depressed and doing unsatisfactorily in school, the defenses served a purpose to maintain interpersonal relations. When such defenses are weakened so that the information is given, you should be aware that the information has been withheld to protect a relationship. A major therapeutic function must therefore be to reassure the patient that a favorable relationship still exists. You cannot remain noncommittal at such a time, though the reassurance need not be personalized or verbal. It is not necessary to say explicitly "I don't condemn you for this," but an intense, well defined relationship is necessary. A weak and ill defined relationship is not one in which strong emotional reassurance can be given. When a strong and well defined relationship can be established, direct confrontation can be used to attack defenses which have served a social purpose. With such a relationship, strong reassurance can be given immediately to allay the anxiety aroused by having disclosed something which is intensely threatening to the patient in terms of his relation with others.

Social defenses should not always be attacked directly. The gain to the patient of a frontal attack must be considered. An example of this was given earlier in the case of a woman who had had three cerebrovascular accidents and an episode of cardiac decompensation (p. 166). Verbally she denied that she was able to do any physical work whatever, though it seemed plain from her comments that she was aware that she was capable of more than she was doing. The physician could have attacked this problem directly had he so desired. It probably would have done little harm, since she was aware that she could do more. It would also have done little good, since she would be risking the loss of a very important relationship if she worked. Neither she nor her husband wanted her to do more. Had physical activity seemed essential to treatment, her physician would have had to deal with her husband's attitudes and the blocks they posed in treatment of the patient.

DEFENSES AGAINST THREATENING IMPULSES

Defenses may be used to prevent the patient himself from becoming aware of threatening impulses which he cannot tolerate. Since he has no awareness of the problem he has never faced the necessity of incorporating it into his concept of himself and is unprepared for any realization that it exists within him. If suddenly confronted with this unacceptable impulse as an integral part of his own make-up, he may become panic-stricken and be unable to handle the impulse at all. In addition, if it becomes obvious to him in the presence of another person, such as a physician, he has also to face interpersonal anxiety. Such a situation requires considerable caution, therefore, and the patient should not be forced to face the impulse prematurely. Much preparation may be necessary. Interpretations should be withheld until it is plain that the patient has become aware of the problem himself and is seeking clarification of it.

An instructive example of both personal and interpersonal anxiety in a patient who suddenly became aware of homosexual tendencies within himself was afforded by another young college student, Lloyd. He went to his physician one day in great distress, and as he sat in the office his face alternately flushed and paled, his mouth was constantly engaged in nervous movements, and his hands clutched the arms of his chair violently. He seemed totally unable to speak. When asked what had brought him, he opened his mouth but no words came forth. He seemed to be in a panic and gave the impression that he wished he had not come and would like to flee. He managed finally to say in an unnatural voice which cracked that he could not talk. After a long and agitated silence he added that it was utterly impossible for him to tell the physician about his problem; he should not have come. It was suggested that the problem might be sexual. He nodded. It was further suggested that it might be homosexual. He clenched his teeth and gave no response. Eventually, with a good deal of help from the physician, he was able to tell what had happened. For 2 years he had been living with a roommate with no awareness of any feelings except friendship. A few weeks before the visit he had become aware of jealousy of his roommate's girl friends, a reaction which disturbed and puzzled him. Then, the night before the visit, he had become suddenly and acutely aware of a strong physical attraction toward his roommate and a desire for actual physical contact with him. This horrified him and precipitated the acute anxiety which had led him to seek help. Seeking help aroused the further anxiety of rejection, which made discussion of his problem temporarily impossible. The physician must be prepared to deal with both types of anxiety and to help the patient form a new and acceptable self-concept which includes these impulses.

A state of panic may occur, either spontaneously or during a therapeutic interview, with sudden awareness of any unacceptable component of the self. It occurs most commonly when the unacceptable component is sexual, whether normal or aberrant, or when it is a hostile impulse directed at some close relative. Hostile and sexual impulses are normal; a person devoid of either would be considered abnormal. Why, then, should the discovery of such impulses within oneself occasion panic, disorganization, or depression?

Part of the answer lies in the self-concept and its importance in affecting the meaning of stimuli. The self-concept gives order and stability to personality, determines what will be stressful, forms the basis for behavior, and helps to give purpose and meaning to life. Developed over a period of many years, it represents a fusion of a person's ideas about himself—his physique, his intellect, his emotional resources, his stability, his value systems, his social interactions. It is his evaluation of all these elements compared with those of other people and with his ideal of what he would like to be. The personal investment in this concept of self varies from person to person both in intensity and in particular emphasis. However, the exclusion of any impulse, the need for repression or denial, is evidence of the importance which the person has assigned to freedom from such impulses.

When unacceptable sexual or hostile impulses are suddenly recognized, disorganization may develop. If one is not the sort of person he has always considered himself to be, then what is he? Can he be sure of anything if not of himself? Can he cope with these impulses, at least so that others will not know of them? Having no prior experience with them, he has no basis for answering these questions. But the mere fact of recognizing the presence of these desires affects his feelings of adequacy, requires reassessment of the roles he plays in life and the way in which he plays them. They are contrary to his value system, his moral code, or they would not have been repressed. He must alter his code or find some way of fitting the impulse into the code without doing violence to it. In addition, there may be a loss of prior satisfactions. Lloyd had enjoyed his friendship with his roommate while it remained a friendship. With the discovery of a sexual basis for it, all friendships became suspect, and new awakening of warmth in this one occasioned anxiety and guilt.

The intensity of the response therefore depends on how important the area involved is to self-esteem, on the strength of the person's moral code, on the degree of security he obtains from knowing how he will react, on the intensity of his effort to live up to an ideal self, on satisfactions lost, on anticipations of disapproval from others and the effect this will have on self-esteem, and on substitute satisfactions and remaining sources of self-respect. This emphasizes again the need for caution and full understanding of the patient before offering interpretations which confront him with a new fact about himself.

When material has been excluded from consciousness, treatment is often prolonged and may require patience and skill. The traditional, passive role of the psychotherapist is most important. If the physician who first hears these thoughts expressed reacts to them emotionally, defense mechanisms may be reinvoked and prevent further exploration, or considerable anxiety may be aroused. Discussion of childhood experiences, fantasies, dreams, abstract discussions of anger, sex, or other appropriate subjects serve to prepare the patient for learning about himself. When anger or sex is the objectionable material, discussions of minor expressions of these impulses or sublimations which render them acceptable may pave the way for acceptance of the basic impulses. Through such discussions, the patient learns to view the impulse with less anxiety, learns that a calm attitude is possible, and knows that the physician will not be disturbed by admission of hostile or sexual desires. It is then easier for him to integrate these impulses into his concept of himself when he becomes conscious of them.

The most potent mechanisms for excluding material from consciousness seem to be repression and denial. When successful, these mechanisms protect the patient from awareness of the threatening impulse though the physician may be aware of them by inference. A brief illustration should clarify this. Phil was a college student who went to his physician because of nervousness and a tremor which had been present for some years. He had had one acute episode which he called a "nervous breakdown" a year before, when one of his girl friends thought she was pregnant and insisted on marriage. He had had sexual relations with many girls and enjoyed it. No warmth or lasting relationship developed with any of them, however, and he did not wish to get married. His disinterest in marriage was the reason he gave for his "nervous breakdown," but the reaction he described seemed rather intense to have developed from "disinterest." He had, in fact, become panic-stricken at the thought and had fled several thousand miles to be with his mother. He had never told her what was wrong but took to his bed at home, trembling violently, and had no interest in food or companionship. His anxiety decreased gradually when he learned his girl friend had had a normal menstrual period and no longer insisted on marriage. Since then his nervousness had been mild but he had occasional outbursts of anger and an almost constant tremulousness. His most violent anger usually went unexpressed, however, for it was aroused by circumstances which would have made it incomprehensible to others. Whenever one of his friends came up to him and grabbed him by the sleeve or slapped him on the back with a friendly "Hi, Phil, how's it going?" he felt an intense desire to strike back in anger. He explained this as due to his distaste for physicial contact with others. When asked why he should dislike friendly physical contact, his answer was "I don't know why. It's just the way I am." Though perhaps inconclusive, these facts suggested that homosexual impulses might underlie the nervousness and the intense emotional reactions. Phil was unaware of any homosexual tendencies, however, and would, in all sincerity, have denied them categorically if asked.

Three examples of homosexuality have been used because their similarities and differences bring into clearer focus the importance of evaluating defenses and what they accomplish. All three students were young males with homosexual tendencies; the basic problem was therefore similar. But they came to their physicians with very different levels of awareness of their problem and used defense mechanisms differently. A physician's approach must be adjusted to differences in defenses. Clarence denied the problem verbally but had been aware of his homosexual tendencies long enough to find ways, however inadequate, of dealing with them. Though disturbed by their presence, he was able to inhibit any expression of them, and his major concern was that no one should learn about them. He had never allowed himself to face the problem frankly. The physician needed to break through the denial so that the problem could be dealt with more effectively, not through overt expression but by coming to terms with the impulses as a part of what he himself was. Lloyd had repressed his homosexual impulses until they became too strong to be excluded from consciousness. He had developed no defenses, and the impulses threatened to overwhelm him. Complete mutism and inactivity were his only means of coping with the problem, and he could not accept the impulses as a part of his make-up. Alleviation of his anxiety was needed. He needed help in finding mechanisms to handle the impulses and help in integrating them into his self-concept. Phil's repressive mechanisms were adequate to prevent his awareness of homosexual impulses but inadequate to prevent emotional outbursts and chronic "nervousness." Forcing him to face his problem directly might well produce a panic very like that Lloyd experienced. Extensive preparation is needed before awareness can be accomplished in patients like Phil without producing panic, disorganization, or a severe depression. Consequently psychiatric care is advisable.

Though Phil's problem deserves psychiatric care, the principles involved should interest the internist or general practitioner because an understanding of them can facilitate treatment of problems of the sort posed by Clarence and Lloyd. Recognizing the sources from which anxiety may arise when a patient becomes aware of his homosexual impulses, his physician prepares the way by removing or minimizing as many of these sources as possible. He works to establish a strong relationship based on mutual respect. Early discussions may center around recollections of childhood sexual thoughts or activities. Since these are remote in time and meaning and children are not considered responsible for their thoughts and actions in quite the same way adults are, childhood memories can serve as a relatively neutral yet pertinent starting point. Dreams and fantasies may serve the same purpose, with discussions emphasizing obvious or implied sexual material. Adolescent attachments or sexual experiences may also be discussed, emphasizing the normalcy of homosexual attractions during adolescence. He may also discuss the carry-over of childhood and adolescent traits into adulthood. All of these maneuvers tend to increase the acceptability of homosexual tendencies in one's own make-up so that their recognition arouses less anxiety. None of these maneuvers encourages a latent homosexual to become an overt homosexual, since the restraining social forces remain effective. The aim of treatment is to allay enough of the anxiety to permit the patient to cope with the problem adequately. A similar approach is used for other kinds of sexual impulses and for hostile impulses when these have been denied or repressed.

DEFENSES IN RELATIONSHIP

Relationship itself may be so threatening that the patient avoids committing himself to any meaningful relationship or tries to impose a particular type of relationship in order to avoid what is threatening. Several aspects of a close relationship may be stressful. One of these is the element of obligation. In the family setting the parent has an obligation to care for his children and the children have the obligation to respect and obey the parent. Though these obligations are not absolute they have general social acceptance in a broad sense. In the doctor-patient relationship similar expectations are present. The patient may fear the obligations which he anticipates the physician will impose—the expectation that he will do whatever is advised—or he may fear that the physician will not be dependable in fulfilling his obligations. The 19 year old boy with congenital heart disease who made his own rules in seeing the physician (p. 207) fell into the former group. He could not permit an authoritative doctor-patient relationship because of the obligations it might impose upon him. His expectations were a reflection of his relationship with his parents who had been unnecessarily restrictive and had demanded respect and obedience. Fred (p. 56) avoided a close relationship with his physician because he hesitated to depend on the physician. This reflected his relationship with his father, a conspicuously irresponsible man who had deserted the family repeatedly and for prolonged periods.

Another potential threat in a close relationship is the fear that it will end, leaving one with the anguish of separation or abandonment. Marian (p. 62) was beset with this fear in all her close relationships. Though deeply involved emotionally in each while it lasted, she lived in constant fear of its termination. This pattern, established in childhood and adolescence, affected all areas of her life, including relationships with her physicians.

It is evident that the doctor-patient relationship can be stressful of itself. The physician must learn to recognize that a patient is avoiding a meaningful relationship with him. A good relationship is often essential in treatment. When lacking, the reasons should be sought and given careful consideration. In helping patients achieve a satisfying adjustment in life, physicians have several forces available—the anxieties the patient wants relieved, the goals he wants to attain, the strength of the doctor-patient relationship, the desire of the patient for personal approval, and the force of social mores. When relationship is poor and the interpersonal force between doctor and patient is correspondingly weak, a very important factor affecting motivation is missing.

When the relationship is poor because the patient is threatened by it, your first step should ordinarily be to reduce the degree of threat as much as possible. When the potential obligations frighten him, these should be minimized by giving him as much freedom of choice or of decision as the situation permits. When he feels insecure, doubting your dependability, your reactions must be reliable and your care steadfast, offering the patient as much security as the relationship permits. When the patient fears the relationship may be abruptly terminated, you should be understanding, avoiding offense or rejection. You should always seek to understand and to have the patient understand what he fears in the relationship, why he fears it, and what can be done to foster a stronger, more satisfying relationship.

There are many other ways of handling the doctor-patient relationship. For many patients this relationship is seen as stressful only under certain circumstances. They therefore approach a physician by "testing" him in order to find out what sort of person he is, how many restrictions he is apt to impose, and what reactions he is likely to have. This approach often irritates the physician, who should, nevertheless, seek to understand what the testing means.

Some patients test their physicians to assure themselves they are in competent hands. They may offer suggestions about treatment, for example, but not really want them followed. If treatment is left in their hands they feel insecure; what they had hoped for was a strong person who would take the full responsibility upon himself. For such persons, a gentle but firm hand is needed. Their suggestions should neither be discarded categorically nor accepted simply in the hope of "pleasing." They should be given serious consideration but should be put into effect or not according to the physician's judgment of what is best for the patient. The reins of decision are kept in the hands of the physician and the patient is allowed to know this.

Other patients test their physicians to be sure they are in the hands of someone who will be understanding. They also seek security in the relationship. Mr. Laird (p. 196) exemplified this. He could discuss his problems with relative ease once he was assured of sympathetic understanding. One woman in her fifties, hospitalized for multiple complaints that included poor appetite and marked weight loss, greeted each new physician who came to her bedside with "Oh, please go away. I feel *so* sick. I don't think I can talk to anyone now. It hurts so *here*." And she would then indicate some spot, seldom twice the same one, where her pain was great. This, of course, required the physician to remain long enough to ask a few questions and examine the area. If he did so with kindliness she relaxed and became cheerful. If not, she dissolved in tears of pain and suffering. Her greeting was her way of assuring herself that she had doctors who would care for her with sympathy and gentleness. And, though it irritated many of her physicians, it usually succeeded, for she was treated with great care. No one wanted to be the doctor who let his anger prevent him from making a diagnosis.

Sometimes the procedure of testing is continued beyond the initial stages of getting acquainted and becomes a pattern of manipulation. Successful manipulation may give a momentary sense of power over others. It is basically a hostile relationship, and the person who is being manipulated ordinarily resents it when he becomes aware of it. Manipulation, in the long run, robs its user of satisfaction by preventing the development of warm, interpersonal relations. When the physician is being manipulated, he should stop it gently but firmly, without anger or rejection of the patient. In doing so he gives the patient added security and confidence. He may permit himself to be manipulated initially while learning to know the patient well enough to plan his approach; but the patient will not feel secure in his care so long as the pattern is allowed to continue.

Somewhat akin to manipulation is competition with the physician, another defense against an authoritative relationship. It may also begin with testing or with suggestions of proper diagnostic or therapeutic considerations. In psychotherapy it may take the form of anticipating every formulation or interpretation of the physician. One sophisticated patient, who had previously had some psychiatric care, was unable to relax a moment from this mental jousting with his physician. When he mentioned his marriage, he immediately added that he loved his wife because she was such a wonderful mother to him. When he told of adopting a son, his next statement was of hatred and jealousy for the boy because of their rivalry for his wife's affection. He offered a psychiatric interpretation for every fact as he gave it. The physician should not be threatened by such a patient. He should not accept the challenge and try to outdo the patient by finding "deeper" or contrary truths. In doing either, he perpetuates competition, which is not conducive to an effective relationship, whether the purpose is diagnosis and treatment or psychiatric formulations. It is important to learn why the patient feels the need to compete, what he accomplishes by it, and how you can end the competition without terminating the relationship. In this patient, the competition was a continuing effort to best his father, an uneducated man who had had considerable financial success. The patient, a college graduate who liked to consider himself far superior to his father, had never achieved financial or occupational satisfaction. He had moved from one type of work to another, hoping to find wealth and prestige in one of them and growing increasingly bitter because with all his education he could not approach the record of his "ignorant" father. He begrudged any man success, doctors more than most, and spent his life trying to prove to himself that he was really their superior.

DEFENSES AND ILLNESS

SUPPRESSION

Suppression, or inhibition, is a common defense in psychosomatic ailments because it tends to prolong physiologic changes until they become symptoms. There are many reasons for inhibiting an emotion or its behavior pattern. Fear of punishment is a common one. In childhood this may be a fear of physical punishment; in adult life the fear of punishment continues to operate though punishment is no longer physical but more apt to be self-disapproval and feelings of guilt. Suppression may be used to preserve an important relationship or to attain some long-term goal. In one sense, all of these represent fear of punishment, but the nature of the punishment varies greatly.

Recognition of suppression as a mechanism is usually not too difficult. Frequently, the patient himself is aware that he has suppressed his impulses. When a patient reports having felt an emotion without acting upon it, you can surmise that the expected behavior pattern was inhibited. When a patient reports a less intense emotion than the situation seems to justify, you can assume that the emotion was suppressed. The young man in whom urticaria appeared soon after his supervisor criticized his work (p. 66) was aware of the anger and that he had inhibited its expression. The secretary who hated her boss and felt repeatedly that she would like to "hit him over the head" (p. 67) also knew that she was suppressing anger.

The advice "express yourself" is good advice only if expression occurs under appropriate circumstances. Free expression of undesirable impulses should not be recommended without due consideration for the goals of the patient, the relationships which he wishes to preserve, and the possible consequences of expressing himself freely. Expression of impulses to the physician gives partial gratification, may give temporary symptomatic relief, and may reduce their intensity sufficiently for the patient to handle them without symptoms. Partial gratification may thus allow the patient to continue using suppression as a mechanism.

Often it is preferable for the patient to learn some new mechanism of defense to handle the problem causing difficulty. The young man with urticaria asked for a transfer to another shift, worked under another supervisor, and in this way avoided the unpleasant episodes which gave rise to his symptoms. Avoidance or withdrawal from a stressful situation is considered a sign of defeat by many people. There is no reason, however, for the physician or the patient to fear avoidance or withdrawal as a solution if it is a realistic way to handle the situation. Used repeatedly it tends to restrict one's experiences and narrow one's outlook, but if a situation that causes symptoms is an uncommon one which can easily be avoided, there need be no fear of avoidance.

Other mechanisms are also available as alternatives to suppression. The possibility of direct gratification at the time the feelings are aroused has been mentioned, along with certain precautions in recommending this approach. Occasionally displacement will afford sufficient gratification to relieve symptoms. Sports, hobbies, and competitive activities may help discharge some of the feelings, particularly when anger and resentment are prominent. Group activities may also drain off some of the accumulating tensions. Many people find such outlets for themselves without the help of a physician. They are more useful when circumstances arousing the impulse occur infrequently or when the impulse is not too intense.

Suppression as a mechanism should be recognized during evaluation of the patient for treatment. It is fairly common as a source of symptoms and is usually quite easily treated. When the patient's major problems stem from suppression of an undesirable impulse or behavior, the interested internist or general practitioner is well able to treat the patient, and psychiatric referral should not be necessary. The first step in treatment is adequate ventilation, not only of the suppressed impulse but of the circumstances arousing it and the reasons the impulse arises in this setting. Though symptomatic relief may be achieved promptly with ventilation, the physician should look carefully behind the symptom for the personality characteristics responsible for the impulse and the effort to control it.

AVOIDANCE

Avoidance is another common mechanism which may be associated with symptoms. In treatment, the material being avoided must eventually be faced and a decision reached as to whether avoidance is a desirable way of handling the situation. It may be difficult to get the patient to face the problems which have so carefully been avoided. In childhood Mr. Grant (p. 70) handled anger successfully by avoiding situations in which it might be aroused. One of the things which aroused his anger was criticism, and as an adult he tried to avoid it by anticipating it and leaving. By the nature of his work this was difficult to do. In the course of discussions with him, it became plain to the physician that this was a source of trouble to him, but Mr. Grant could not accept it. During one interview, the physician concentrated his efforts on forcing him to recognize his use of avoidance as a defense by repeating questions when he strayed from the point and by telling him in a friendly but direct way that he was avoiding the issue at hand. Mr. Grant suddenly complained that he was having severe abdominal pain and asked that the interview be terminated. The association between the critical nature of the physician's comments and the appearance of pain and its relevance in previous attacks was later discussed. Eventually he was able to see that a connection existed. Seeing the relationship was only the first step in treatment, since avoidance or withdrawal was the only way he knew to handle unpleasant situations. He had to learn new ways of meeting such situations before his symptoms could be relieved.

DENIAL AND REPRESSION

It is probable that more has been written about repression than about any other defense mechanism. When it is successful, the material repressed is lost to awareness and to ordinary memory but still exists as an influence over perception of events and reaction to them. Denial and repression are particularly closely allied to the hysterias among psychiatric disorders. There is sometimes confusion about the so called "hysterical personality" and *"la belle indifference"* of the person with true hysteria. The person with a hysterical personality is quite labile, having violent reactions to what appear to be minor stimuli. The person with a conversion hysteria may be completely unresponsive emotionally to the things that go on about him, particularly those which would be expected to arouse strong emotional reactions. These two grossly dissimilar affective states are related. The emotional instability of the hysterical personality is the first stage in repression of affects, while the indifference of the person with a true hysteria is an emotional rigidity which occurs when the repression has actually succeeded in eliminating the undesirable impulse from the conscious mental life of the individual.

Denial and repression are also used by people without hysteria. You should be alert to the possibility of repression or denial when there seems to be a great disproportion between the affective reactions and the precipitating event. An example of this would be the failure of the death of a very close friend or a relative to elicit an adequate emotional response. One should also think of denial or repression when there are obvious voids in the material presented or when relatively unimportant matters are ruminated upon compulsively and obsessively.

A successful repression is not associated with symptoms. The person who is repressing the affect successfully has none of the physiologic manifestations of that affect. This is well illustrated in the patient with a hysterical personality. Intense anger and anxiety may be present but so long as repression of these emotions is successful there is no physiologic evidence of them and the person appears quiet and unemotional—*la belle indifference*. Psychosomatic symptoms represent a failure of the repressive forces. The nature of the repressed material may be quite clear to a careful listener but remain unclear to the patient. At such times the material may be expressed, but because of its threatening nature a denial of it is immediately given. For example, repressed affects may be allowed voluntary expression if this is accompanied by a ritualistic phrase which negates it. The physician should be alert to recognize such phrases and to understand why the patient is talking in apparent contradictions.

Velda Olson was a woman in her early forties with Raynaud's disease. She came from a large family and felt that as the oldest girl she had occupied a very unfavorable place in it. She also felt that she was the homeliest of the girls; many friends and relatives had made comments about her homely appearance. Her mother had never made such comments; but, she added, this was because she looked exactly like her mother. She felt that her mother did not like her. This feeling was strengthened by an aunt who told her repeatedly how much she loved her and how little her mother cared for her. The aunt had had a child at about the same time that Velda was born but had allowed it to be adopted because "her husband didn't want any children." She apparently tried to make Velda a substitute for her own child and had her with her frequently.

Velda had a sister about 2 years younger who she felt was favored by her mother. The two of them fought constantly throughout child-hood, and Velda was repeatedly reprimanded for the disagreements. She grew up disliking this sister intensely. When reprimanded severely for fighting with her sister she would threaten to live with her aunt. This usually brought forth reassuring statements from her mother that she was wanted at home. But on one occasion when she threat-ened to go to her aunt, her mother told her that if she wanted to go so much she might just as well go. Though it might be expected that this would have confirmed her feelings of being rejected by her mother, she said that she was delighted when told she could go, since this proved that her mother loved her enough to let her do the things that would make her happy. She decided to stay at home, however.

When she was about 18 she decided that she wanted to become a nurse. She had scarcely started nursing training when she was called home by her mother to help take care of a new baby. She resented the fact that her younger sister, then 16, could not help at home, though she added that her sister would not have been of great help anyway. Her younger sister had rebelled against all demands made by the par-ents and had refused to do any of the housework. All of the housework and the raising of successive babies had fallen to Velda. The next year she tried again to take up nursing training but was called home a second time because her mother became ill. This time she decided she would never be able to become a nurse and "gave up" these ambitions. However, at the first opportunity she got a job as a nurses' aide.

Eventually she married and, according to her account, she and her husband had an idyllic life together. The outbreak of war took him overseas, however, and she went to work again as a nurses' aide.

She enjoyed the work and apparently worked hard at it. Though everything seemed to go very well initially, eventually troubles came. She was assigned to a ward where the supervising nurse was Japanese. She looked down upon the Japanese as an inferior group, though she was quick to add that she did not consider this nurse to be inferior. She also said that the nurse disliked all "white people," though "of course, we got along very well together." However the nurse was ex-tremely demanding, would not allow her to take the usual coffee break in the middle of the morning and afternoon, and, though her work was excellent, managed to find many things to complain about. "Asth-ma" developed in this setting. The attacks occurred only when on the ward with the Japanese nurse. They were characterized by a smothering sensation accompanied by dizziness, weakness, blurring of vision, numbness and tingling of the hands, and other evidences of hyperventilation. She also began to have sensations of coldness in her fingers and noticed that this sensation developed during the early morning hours when she was thinking about going to work.

At this time her husband came home from the war and, despite their idyllic relationship, announced that he wanted a divorce. He gave no reasons for wanting the divorce, she said, and was not going with anyone at the time. In this setting her fingers began to ulcerate and the diagnosis of Raynaud's disease was made. Interestingly enough her "asthma" disappeared. Her life following this was a succession of moves. She lived first with relatives, then with friends, and then with other friends. She entered each household jubilant. Each time she left feeling that this relative or friend had rejected her and really didn't care for her after all. Her fingers seemed to improve after each move but each fresh rejection was associated with an exacerbation. When a nurse whom she considered to be a very close friend did not show an appropriate amount of interest and affection, one of her fingers became gangrenous, and she was hospitalized.

Mrs. Olson's story was dramatic, but even more dramatic was the way in which it unfolded. Every mention of her mother was accompanied by a statement about how good, loving, and affectionate she had been, despite the fact that each mention had been a critical one, telling just the opposite. No facts were ever elicited which made her mother sound good, warm, or affectionate. Though she spoke quite freely about her hatred for her sister during childhood, every statement of resentment toward her was accompanied by an avowal that she loved her deeply now and that this had all been "kid stuff." She spoke with a cheery smile about her many difficulties during earlier life and seemed to feel pleasure in martyrdom. She was even able to give a short laugh while talking about suicidal thoughts she had had. Her manner of speaking was a constant denial of the depression she obviously felt. Her expression of love for those who should have been near and dear to her was a repeated denial of the criticisms and resentments to which she gave voice. Denial and repression had been her mechanisms of defense long before any symptoms arose. The symptoms, in fact, did not appear until the material requiring repression was too intense for the repressive forces to control it completely. The resentment she felt toward the world then found voluntary and repeated expression but always in a phrase here or there followed

uickly by a denial that this really meant anything to her. She herself
as not aware that she had more resentment than others nor that she
lt rejected by her friends and relatives.

When denial and repression are a patient's major defense mech-
nisms, treatment is apt to be quite prolonged and to require great pa-
ence. One approach to treatment has been outlined in discussing
hil's problem (p. 271). Whatever the approach, you must not push
ɔ uncover material faster than the patient can give it easily. You must
lso refrain from making interpretations to the patient which carry
im beyond material of which he is already aware. Judgment is re-
uired in deciding how rapidly to proceed and when to offer your
wn formulations to the patient. In addition, expression of the threat-
ning material, though it may temporarily relieve the patient of some
f his anxiety, is accompanied by fresh denials and repressions until
herapy is complete. All of these things should warn the internist or
eneral practitioner to proceed cautiously in treating such patients,
ut they do not preclude his helping the patient if circumstances re-
uire that he rather than a trained psychiatrist do it.

If you decide to treat such a patient you should be prepared for
ong-continued treatment. You should do a minimum of talking and
great deal of careful listening. If you recognize the denials as a ritual
vhich makes it permissible for the patient to talk about the threaten-
ng material, you will not criticize him for denying obvious facts
bout his emotional life. In fact, pertinent material will come more
apidly if you also use the ritualistic phrases of the patient, saying such
hings as, "I'm sure you do love your mother; and she loves you. But
t must have been very disappointing to have to give up nursing train-
ng twice in succession." However, you should not forget that, though
he patient may love her mother and resent her simultaneously, the
mportant part of this (in terms of the symptoms) is the resentment,
ɩot the love.

Mrs. Olson had a private room just off an open ward. She com-
ɔlained to her physicians that other patients came in to visit and that
his made her very nervous. When they left, her hands hurt more
han they did before. She hurried to add that she loved to talk with
ɔeople and wouldn't for the world have a "No visitors" sign put on
ɩer door. After all, it was necessary that one get along with others and
he felt it was an important part of her treatment. It was important
or her physician to recognize that this was a double request: first,
hat a "No visitors" sign be put on her door and second, that she be

absolved of all responsibility for this sign. Recognizing this he could deal with it appropriately, either by deciding that it was better for her not to be disturbed by visitors and putting up the sign or by deciding that it was better that people see her occasionally even though it made her nervous. In either case her statement was pertinent to the problem which brought her into the hospital and deserved careful consideration. Why did visitors affect the pain in her fingers and her nervousness? Why was her request phrased in so contradictory a way? Discussions of such matters, however, should be free, allowing a patient an opportunity to discuss them with no attempt to force the development of insight. Insight will come eventually with prolonged contact and repeated discussions. The aim is to make the repressions unnecessary, but procedure toward this goal must be cautious.

DISPLACEMENT

Another mechanism commonly met in the treatment of psychosomatic disorders is displacement. Its features are quite different from those of denial and repression. One is alerted to displacement by a response of greater intensity than would be expected; impulses aroused in another situation are discharged in some trifling incident. The emotion may be appropriate or inappropriate to the circumstances but its intensity is excessive. Inhibition and postponement ordinarily precede displacement. The postponement may be momentary or it may be for hours, days, or weeks. In dealing with displacement, it is important to recognize whether the initial feeling has been suppressed or repressed. Suppression preceding displacement is a favorable sign, since if the initial episode is known to the patient and expression of his emotions has simply been inhibited at the time, the difficulty is much more easily attacked than if the connecting link between the initial arousal and the final gratification has been lost because of repression. The treatment is again ventilation, helping the patient understand why he acted as he did and helping him learn new mechanisms for dealing with similar situations.

INTELLECTUALIZATION

When intellectualization is used as a mechanism of defense an undesirable affect or impulse is converted into a problem in logic, and the patient develops mastery over the impulse a little at a time. The partial mastery attained is the source of pleasure to be found in philosophical ruminations about free will, love, beauty, and other abstractions. Such intellectualizations are common in adolescence, particularly if there is conflict about independence or sexuality. The obsessive quality of some of these ruminations is an index of the intensity of the drive or emotion. By converting the problem into one in logic, a person defends himself against recognizing the drives or emotions on which it is based. Some people carry this to the point of denying any significant place in life to emotions and attempt to deal with all problems at an intellectual level. When the attempt fails and the person seeks your help, the first focus of attention must be the nature of the threatening drive or emotion. You then introduce this as a necessary consideration before any solution can be reached. As the patient gives drives and emotions a more important place in his life and learns to view them as normal and desirable rather than threatening, he will usually be able to solve his problem for himself.

GRATIFICATION

Gratification is not ordinarily looked upon as a defense, though the expression "the best defense is a good offense" is common in our language. Occasionally we meet patients, like Marian, who gratify their impulses freely but feel guilty about it later. How should this be handled? When the patient is a child, limits may be set gently but firmly with no transgressions permitted. Security may be gained by knowing that these limits exist. In adults, limits may also be set but it may not be possible to prevent transgressions. You may also allow a patient to "act out" freely. When transgressions occur or when he "acts out," each episode is discussed objectively. The patient is forced to consider the reasons for and the desirability of his actions. Discussions concern what he wished to gain and whether his actions succeeded when other actions would have failed. For example, Marian became enraged when rejected by other people. What she obviously wanted most was to be liked by others. Getting angry and kicking her friends and the landlord in no way achieved her basic desire of winning friends. Actually she was well aware that she was defeating her own ends before discussions were started, and the discussions concerned themselves largely with why she should behave so illogically. This meant discussing her childhood, her attitudes toward her parents, and the interplay between them. She had to understand herself first and then to learn new ways of handling situations so that she would not antagonize the people she wanted most to please. Put in logical terms it sounded simple. In actuality, it was difficult to accomplish.

DEFENSES AND REACTION TO ILLNESS

Illnesses are often threatening to patients. They give rise to emotional responses and are met with defensive reactions just as are other stresses in life. A middle-aged man with cardiovascular disease, a devoted husband and active church member, reacted with shame and guilt to learning that his cardiovascular ailment was syphilitic in origin. He had acquired syphilis as a young adult on the single occasion of infidelity to his wife. He avoided telling her the nature of his heart disease as long as his conscience would allow and remained tense and inhibited in her presence until she knew. Shame and guilt are not infrequent with venereal disease, nor is avoidance of discussion of the disease. Similar reactions are also common with mental disease and with epilepsy. In all these, both the emotional and the defensive reaction are strongly conditioned by social factors. Coronary disease often arouses apprehension and may be denied until pain makes further denial impossible. Acceptance of the diagnosis carries with it an implied threat to life itself; it is not surprising that acceptance is sometimes slow to come. Illnesses may threaten values, goals, or life, and reactions to them are diverse. One cannot treat the patient adequately if these reactions are neglected.

Mr. Boyer was a 34 year old diabetic who found it hard to accept his illness; he denied its presence and refused to follow dietary instructions lest someone learn of his disease. When seen 7 years after the diagnosis had first been made, he was in acidosis and had early vascular complications. He had never followed a diet and said he neither could nor would. He did take insulin fairly regularly but never checked his urine for sugar, though he had been given adequate instructions. He did not deny that he had diabetes when talking to his physician, but he wanted no one else to know about it. Eliciting his cooperation in the management of his illness seemed virtually impossible; several physicians had tried and failed. The first step toward success with this patient was to know and to understand him—to discover the reasons for his attitudes, the gains to him of denying his illness to others, his goals in life, and the forces which motivated him, so that these could be used to overcome his resistances.

The essential points in his story were these. He felt his father had been a "penny-pincher," overly critical, and very restrictive in raising him. His mother, on the other hand, had been indulgent, giving him whatever he wanted. His description of their relation to each other was epitomized by his statement that whenever his father punished or criticized him, his mother gave him a large piece of cake for consolation. From adolescence on, he noted that his appetite was always greater when those around him were critical or unfriendly. Late in his childhood, his mother had diabetes. This was never discussed at home, being considered a "purely personal matter," so that he did not ask questions nor learn about the disease until she died in diabetic coma 8 years after the diagnosis had been established. He left home soon after this and was first in the Navy and then in one job after another, never remaining on a job more than a few months. About 2 years after discharge from the Navy weight loss, fatigue, increased appetite, and thirst led him to seek medical advice. He was told he had diabetes, was given a diet and insulin and told he would require insulin for the rest of his life. He found the restrictions onerous and resented having a disease which made him different from his friends. He told no one about the diabetes and ignored the diet. A year later, difficulties in regulating the diabetes resulted in hospitalization. He found the staff unfriendly. When he complained that he was not getting enough food, he was told that he was diabetic and would have to remain on an 1800 calorie diet whether it seemed ideal to him or not. His appetite became ravenous and when he finally left the hospital, it was to go straight to a restaurant where he ate heavily, indulging himself in all his favorite foods.

The following years were difficult. He failed to get one job he wanted because he had misrepresented himself as healthy and the prospective employer learned of his hospitalization for diabetes. He left several other jobs as soon as someone at work learned of his illness. He resented the questions, the comments about his eating habits, the concern about his insulin or his care in regulating the disease. He wanted to appear perfectly normal. He wanted to be free and independent, answering to no one for his actions. He therefore became irritated and resentful even though he knew his friends were expressing a normal interest and were not trying to run his life. As a result he moved from place to place and formed few friendships, none of them close or lasting. When symptoms reappeared and he learned he was in diabetic acidosis, he chose to be hospitalized several hundred miles from his friends and from the town in which he worked.

Upon entering the hospital, he almost immediately antagonized his physicians by his indifference to his disease and to its control. He said it was impossible to adhere to a diet. His physician told him it would be easy; he could eat whatever he liked and it would be covered with insulin. But what he said he would like to eat daily was so great that a compromise was made and he was started on a 3200 calorie diet and 110 units of insulin daily. Diabetes was not well controlled on this regimen. Though minimal restrictions were imposed, he felt the physician was basically unfriendly and belittled the problem of adhering to a diet when he had to eat in restaurants and with friends. The doctor had never had to do it so of course it sounded easy to him. He was resentful and his craving for food was not appeased even by the liberal diet.

A change in physicians brought with it a great change in his attitude toward his disease and toward its management. The new physician had been a diabetic for 9 years, understood his problems and could still say that adherence to the regimen was possible. She was deeply interested in him and in why he felt as he did. She did not belittle or criticize; neither did she indulge him. He was put on a 2100 calorie diet and 60 units of insulin daily. The change in diet was not made as a punitive gesture, and he was told that adjustments would be made if necessary but only after an adequate trial. Restrictions had been reimposed but he was given detailed instructions about deviations from the diet, their occasional necessity in his case, how to adjust his insulin to meet them, and in general was made to feel that he would be in control of his own regimen. The greatest difference, however, was in the warm, friendly, sympathetic doctor-patient relationship. His appetite decreased so that 2100 calories seemed to him adequate. His diabetes was well controlled, with only an occasional faint spilling of sugar into the urine. He was able to discuss his diabetes freely and to make plans for returning to work, even though his employer had discovered that he was diabetic. Efforts were made to help him overcome his sensitivity to questions about his disease. The importance of controlling his diabetes in order to achieve his goals of independence and normalcy was emphasized, and the necessary safeguards were presented not as restrictions imposed by a physician but as simple means to reach his goals. The forces motivating him were redirected so that they no longer acted as resistances to treatment but reinforced treatment.

SUMMARY

People frequently use the same defense mechanism repeatedly as though a defense useful in some particular situation should therefore e useful in all situations. A person who is ill because he suppresses is emotions or avoids unpleasant situations is apt to suppress or avoid the same things in his relations with a physician. A patient who denies things when talking with his physician is apt to deny them to himself.

patient who fears emotional involvement in the doctor-patient relationship is apt to fear it in other relationships. Actually, this is useful in treatment, because it allows reeducation in the controllable nvironment of the physician's office. The strongest motive for giving up an old defense or habit is the knowledge that it is not and cannot be effective in achieving one's goals. The best motive for using new one is to find that it works. The physician has a structured situation in which he can, within limits, see that the patient has successful experiences in establishing new ways of meeting his environment. In dealing with the defenses used in the doctor-patient relationship he is facilitating the use of new measures in life outside his office. The patient needs more than one defense if he is to be adaptable in meeting the problems of life. Adaptability in turn allows a greater chance of success. Teaching new defenses is therefore an important art of treatment.

To help a patient learn new defenses, the physician must first recognize the defense which is being used. He must understand why it is being used, what it accomplishes, and what it fails to accomplish. If the defense serves to protect the patient from the possibility of ensure by the physician, it can be attacked directly but *only* if a good doctor-patient relationship based on mutual respect exists. It should not be attacked if the relationship is weak or one in which strong interpersonal reassurance cannot be given. If the defense serves to protect the patient from recognizing unacceptable impulses within imself, it should be approached cautiously. The more successful the mechanism is in preventing recognition of the impulse and the more unacceptable the impulse to the patient, the greater is the need for a trained person, usually a psychiatrist, to assume responsibility in treatment. Defenses are needed for effective adaptation. They should not be attacked unless some other way of dealing with the problem is available to the patient.

The physician must, therefore, evaluate defenses as well as emotional reactions. If the defenses are inadequate for the purposes the are meant to serve, as was true for Lloyd (p. 269) and for Mrs. Olson (p. 280), new defenses may be needed. Repression was no longer effective for either of these patients. Part of the treatment was to decrease the stressful significance of the repressed material so that i was less threatening; part was to teach new defensive maneuvers, fo example, suppression of overt expression of the sexual or hostile impulses to keep them within socially acceptable limits or sublimation of these impulses into some satisfying form of expression. If the defenses are inappropriate, as was true for Mr. Grant (p. 70) and Mr. Boyer (p. 286), similar measures may be used, decreasing the stressful significance of the situation so that defenses become unnecessary or finding a substitute defense which is more appropriate. Defenses may be adequate and appropriate and still lead to symptoms as was true for the ward clerk whose concentration on her duties resulted in headaches. The defenses may need to be altered or the tension aroused in association with them may need to be decreased in intensit or duration. These changes may be quite difficult for patients to accomplish. In all instances, success is more likely to be achieved in the presence of a good doctor-patient relationship.

Chapter 12

Social Forces and Conflicts

AFTER you have obtained details about the patient's symptoms, social information becomes the major focus of interest and provides the material used in treatment. Whether dealing with interpersonal actions, social events, attitudes toward work, or financial problems, you are dealing with social forces in the patient's life. In treating a patient these must be interpreted in terms of that person. Listen for the emotions aroused, the defenses utilized, the values by which these events are judged, and the conflicts which seem to be pertinent to them, remembering that emotions, defenses, values, and conflicts are molded by social and cultural forces and are expressed in a social context. You may treat a patient without considering these social phenomena as such, but their recognition will indicate areas of difficulty, will point questions into areas that need discussion, and will help the patient see himself and his problem in a broader perspective.

The experiences to which people are subjected differ markedly from one social or religious group to another. The values by which these experiences are judged differ from one group to another. The reactions to them—both the emotions aroused and the defenses used in trying to cope with them—vary with the values by which experiences are judged. You cannot know the social factors at work in a patient's life or his personal idiosyncrasies unless he is allowed to discuss them at length. This is interviewing focused upon understanding the patient. You must discuss his background, views, and reactions until these are understood; only then can treatment properly proceed. Understanding the patient means understanding a composite of constitutional endowment, social forces, individual experiences, emotions, defenses, values, and conflicts. The social history is the backbone of therapy for psychosomatic disorders.

INADEQUACY

A common problem in patients with psychosomatic disorders is a feeling of inadequacy. Feelings of inadequacy depend upon a person's attitude toward his own basic endowment as related to the demands made upon him by himself and by his environment. The child who finds demands far in excess of what he is capable of doing is apt to withdraw or rebel. The child who is subjected to demands which are within his capacity only if he is alert is apt to react to these with striving and tension. Adults react in the same way. The ward clerk who wanted to turn in a perfect performance on her job (p. 194) thought that with extreme care she could do so. She reacted with striving and feelings of tension.

Treatment is directed first at the emotional reaction of the patient and his defenses in handling the troubling situation. But in addition to this the basic conflict requires attention since it is crucial in determining the emotion and the defense. If he is actually more adequate than he thinks, your job is to help him reach a more realistic evaluation of his capacities. If he is inadequate for the goals and activities which he is pursuing, you try to decrease the demands he makes upon himself so that they become more nearly consistent with his capacities. This must be done carefully and gently so that you do not tell the patient, in subtle ways, that you think him an inadequate person. The problem can sometimes be approached by attacking the goals as unrealistic or undesirable and helping the patient see that more happiness can be obtained if his goals are reformulated. Thus the patient's attitudes and value systems are altered so that he makes more realistic demands upon himself. You must be careful when appraising the patient's capabilities, however, remembering that removal of blocks and resistances to adequate performance will make a striking difference in performance, though the basic capacity may be unchanged. As in all other areas of psychotherapy the relationship between physician and patient is of crucial importance.

William James [94] has expressed the problem of adequacy colorfully: "So we have the paradox of a man shamed to death because he is only the second pugilist or the second oarsman in the world. That he is able to beat the whole population of the globe minus one is nothing; he has 'pitted' himself to beat that one; and as long as he doesn't do that nothing else counts. He is to his own regard as if he were not, indeed he *is* not.

"Yonder puny fellow, however, whom everyone can beat, suffers no chagrin about it, for he has long ago abandoned the attempt to 'carry that line', as the merchants say, of self at all. With no attempt there can be no failure; with no failure no humiliation. So our self-feeling in this world depends entirely on what we *back* ourselves to be and do. It is determined by the ratio of our actualities to our supposed potentialities; a fraction of which our pretensions are the denominator and the numerator our success: thus, Self-esteem $= \dfrac{\text{Success}}{\text{Pretensions}}$. Such a fraction may be increased as well by diminishing the denominator as by increasing the numerator. To give up pretensions is as blessed a relief as to get them gratified . . ."

How can one proceed in helping a person reformulate his goals and values and find satisfaction in more realistic aims? A specific illustration should help clarify this. Gladys (p. 131) wanted to be just a little bit better than her friends and neighbors. She wanted her husband to be a little bit better as a husband and her young son a little bit better as a son. There are many ways of attacking this problem, but one should start with a part of it which has real meaning to the patient. One of Gladys's immediate complaints to her physician was that her husband was far too lenient with her son. He refused to spank him, saying that he was already the best little boy in the neighborhood and there was no need to spank him. She felt that if he were not spanked he would not continue to be the best boy in the neighborhood. She gave her son a small allowance from which he was expected to save a little each month. When he had spent the money his father would often buy him candy bars. She thought this poor training for the handling of money later in life. She reacted with anger to his refusal to spank and to his buying candy, but she suppressed the emotion, insofar as she could because she felt it was not proper for a wife to get angry at her husband. When she did burst forth in anger she felt guilty and inadequate. At such times she usually had a vascular headache. Initially in treatment you would encourage free expression of this anger, asking questions which would elicit as much feeling as possible. This should decrease the intensity of anger. It also should reduce the degree of suppression required for control and the physiologic effects of suppression.

You do more than simply encourage free expression of anger and ventilation of all the irritations which contribute to it. You listen carefully to what is said, noting anything which helps to clarify why the situation arose and why the patient reacted in this manner. These facts are stored away for use at the appropriate time—later in the same interview or weeks later, depending upon circumstances. Ultimately you want more than just a free expression of anger. Despite the value of this, preventing renewed attacks ordinarily requires more than simple ventilation. Further treatment is constructed from the details of social information given by the patient.

There is no set pathway through this maze. There are many points of attack and the way chosen will depend largely on the order in which the patient unfolds his story and how threatening various aspects of it seem to be. When the story unfolds freely and easily you may begin the task of reconstructing the background in the patient's mind immediately. If emotions are intense or defenses strong, you may want to listen quietly for some time without suggesting associations between facts which the patient has recounted but has not related to each other. There is no standard attitude for you to take except to be interested and want to help. A slightly jesting approach may be effective with one patient but intense seriousness may be best with another. A display of warm emotion or a very impersonal, detached air may be indicated. The variations depend on the physician as well as the patient, upon the immediate circumstances of the interview, and upon the relationship between physician and patient. Thus an approach which is successful for one physician may fail when used by another with the same patient.

Why should her husband's refusal to spank their son anger Gladys? Her answer to this question was that he ought to uphold her in her discipline and that he ought to want his son to be the best-behaved boy in the neighborhood. These reasons introduce the problem of role definition—what a husband and a father should be like—and the question of values and goals. Where did she get her ideas about roles? What gave this aspect of life such importance to her? Her story about her childhood gave some of the answers. Her parents had no arguments in front of her; her mother seemed to make the decisions about her rearing and her father went along with them. She was an adopted child, expected to be better behaved than other children to make up to her foster mother for not being her own. To be better, she had to have her role as daughter well defined; to carry this over into other relationships required that her role in these relationships be equally well defined. Some of this came by imitation, by watching what her parents did and by their comments about marriage and family life.

art of the intensity of her need to be better came from the fact that
o fail in this reflected on her mother's adequacy as well as her own.
Obviously she accepted her mother as authority, identified with her,
nd desired her approval. This made conformance all the more important.

Had she ever stopped to consider how competitive life became with
her goal set at being a little bit better. Was this really so desirable,
always to be striving to outdo others? Why not set another goal and
be happy in achieving it without making every act and gesture a competition—to have a better husband, a better son, a better house, in a
better neighborhood, with better friends, meeting them with more
poise and greater composure?

Accepting that she wished to be better, why the emphasis on behavior? She could just as well concentrate on being more intelligent,
more industrious, more creative, or just happier. Why not these? The
goal was set by her mother, partly to meet her mother's needs but also
to meet society's demands that children be socialized. To a certain degree, the goal was desirable but the way of reaching it need not have
been competitive. Any discussion of it, however, only emphasized
Gladys's desire to be a good daughter. In the framework of her family
she was using her husband and her son to help her be a good daughter.

Her husband, unfortunately, shared neither her goal nor her desire
to be better than others. He wanted to make a good living and to live
comfortably; but compete—why? His background was pertinent to his
attitude toward life. He was the son of a miner. His father had lived
in a company town with little opportunity to better himself, living
from day to day, trying not to think about the morrow since he had
little control over it and only hoping that fate would not be unkind.
His pleasures were immediate and carnal. Gladys viewed him with
contempt—"common as pig tracks" was her evaluation of him. Her
husband had had little affection from his parents and much punishment. He wanted to give his own son just the opposite, much affection
and little punishment.

With such contempt for his background and such a different attitude toward life, why had she married him? The question needs to
be considered for it is a part of her problem and the answer highlights
another facet of her conflict. She married him after dropping out of
college, and her reason for dropping out was her "failure" to get into
the right sorority and her "failure" to get all A's. In short, she had not
lived up to her mother's goals for her, had therefore not been a good

daughter. She felt inadequate, worthless, depressed. She wanted some
one to love her for herself; she wanted security without demands. Sh
married her husband because he was not demanding and loved he
whether she was better than others or not. As time passed after th
marriage some of her self-esteem returned, and she once again took u
the old competitive goals, this time with renewed vigor, trying to wip
out the failures and the sense of inadequacy they had engendered

The background for her problems was reconstructed by posin
questions or interjecting occasional comments as she talked to direc
her attention to the pattern into which her life had fallen and to th
forces at work in producing that pattern. Part of her conflict la
within herself and part of it between her and her husband. She ha
definite ideas about how the roles of husband and father should b
played and these were not in accord with her husband's ideas on th
subject. Her ideas were based largely on what she thought would pleas
her mother. She wanted both her mother's love and her husband'
love. The desire for her mother's love made her insist that he conform
to her picture of the perfect husband and father. Her desire for his
love tempered this insistence. But at the time she first came to the
physician, there was little doubt as to which seemed more importan
to her. Her husband, obviously, should conform and love her too; then
she would have no conflict. But her husband had his own problems.
To conform to her demands required accepting an attitude toward
life which was foreign to him, put him in a position he felt was inappropriate for a husband, and made of him a type of father he could
not tolerate to be. The stalemate they had reached was the source
of her symptoms.

How can you help a patient in such a situation? It is done essentially by helping her get a clearer picture of what is happening to her
and by having her reevaluate the situation in terms of this new
point of view. You try to reduce the satisfactions gained by the pattern
associated with physical symptoms and increase the satisfactions to be
gained by alternate ways of handling the problems. To do this, you
use motivating forces already present whenever possible. With Gladys,
you would emphasize her desire to be a good wife and mother and the
satisfactions to be attained from a smooth marital relationship. You
might even try to direct her energies to having a better marriage than
others as an expression of being a good daughter. For her own adjustment, it would be better, however, to decrease her dependence on her
mother for approval.

How do you put these ideas into action? Pointing out to her that her striving is basically an attempt to be a good daughter puts striving in a new perspective, gives it less status than it had as an absolute virtue. Helping her to see her problem partly as a conflict of roles allows this aspect of it to be reexamined with more objectivity. When the friction between herself and her husband is seen not as a conflict between what is "right" and a recalcitrant human who refuses to accept the "right" but as a difference in definition of roles, it becomes of an entirely different order of magnitude. Indicating to Gladys that she is imposing upon her son the same pattern of life which has led to her inability to find happiness—indeed, one which has contributed to her illness, may make her hesitate and take thought. Is she using her son for her own needs or doing what is best for him? Will he accept the demands or rebel against them? Will her actions cement their relationship with love and affection or will he sense that he is being used to bolster her feelings of adequacy and therefore feel that she has little genuine interest in him? She is asking her husband to be more punitive and less indulgent in the hope that this will make her son strive to be best in all things; yet this pattern was used on her husband in his childhood and had a very different effect. And what about her husband? She wants his love and affection. Is this the best way to get it? Which does she really want the more—his love or the feeling she has satisfied her mother's goals?

Questions such as these are seldom posed directly. You would not make up a list of questions and ask them in sequence but would encourage her to talk about her problems in detail. When she mentions her mother, you are interested in their relationship. When she mentions her husband, you ask about his background and his attitudes toward whatever is being discussed. When she mentions dropping out of school, you show an interest in her reasons for doing so. When she expresses dissatisfaction with her marriage, you try to draw out her reasons for getting married. This obviously must take a good many interviews, and the rapidity with which you progress is determined by the patient. You act as a catalyst to speed the process, for the most part, though on occasion you may serve as an additional reactant to shift the equilibrium in a specific direction. Over many interviews of this sort, however, a coherent picture slowly begins to form in the patient's mind as the connections between isolated facts become clear.

When asked whether she wanted her husband's love or the satisfaction of achieving her mother's goal for her, Gladys might have retorted, "Why can't I have both?" Such an answer only means that you have proceeded too rapidly and the import of the discussions has been missed. In the abstract, both may be possible; in the flesh, they are not. That she is still considering them abstractly may be because you introduced the ideas yourself rather than drawing them from her, and they were thus dry, relatively meaningless intellectualizations. Or you may have proceeded as soon as you understood each facet of the problem without waiting for similar understanding from her. At such a time, turn the question back to the patient—"Why not?"—and help her find the answers. She demands a good deal of herself. When she fails to live up to her ideals she is angry at herself or depressed. Making similar demands on others, trying to force them to live up to her standards, is apt to arouse similar feelings, and these get in the way of love and affection.

These discussions are but an extension of history taking. No attempt is made to fix blame, to decide who is "right" or "wrong." As with the situation which Gladys faced, it is usual to find no right or wrong, only two conflicting viewpoints or attitudes toward life, either of which is tenable in the appropriate situation. There are many kinds of fathers and husbands, many kinds of mothers and wives, and no reason to consider variety undesirable. Little good can come from attempts to determine who is to blame. It is far better to focus attention first on understanding the situation and how it developed and then on how it can be improved. What is best for the people involved, should be the question. This is a constructive approach which helps motivate the patient for change.

In trying to understand a patient one focuses his attention first on the emotions and defenses evoked by a situation, then on the goals or value system which has led the individual to react in this way, and then on the sources of these goals and values. One looks for conflicting goals or conflicting values since, when present, these need to be clarified. And one compares the consequences of behavior with the goals presumably set.

The results of this process are manifold. The emotional reaction is decreased in intensity and defense mechanisms are changed. With Gladys, the anger was decreased and suppression became less intense. The threat implied in her husband's behavior was lessened by decreasing the intensity of her striving and reducing the demands made upon him. By clarifying for her that a conflict in values and roles existed, it became possible for her to reevaluate these. She was able to resolve the conflict by reshaping her goals. One of the important changes she made in this regard was to give up her emphasis on being a good daughter. She remained a good daughter but put more emphasis on her roles as wife and mother. These changes resulted in an improved marital relationship in which discussions of areas of disagreement were possible in an atmosphere of tolerance. And all of these factors reduced the likelihood of recurrence of symptoms. Her headaches decreased in intensity and frequency so that she was able to go for months without headache, and when they occurred they were mild and easily controlled.

SEX

Sexual problems are frequently linked with the problem of adequacy. The biologic and social forces which mold sexual behavior are closely intertwined and markedly affect the emotions engendered by sexual activity or its lack. These emotions, again, are most important in the development of symptoms. The overt homosexual, whose only concern is that unsympathetic ears shall not hear of his practices, is not likely to develop somatic symptoms as a result of his sexual deviation, which presents itself only as a psychiatric problem. When anxiety, anger, tension, or depression is associated with homosexual tendencies, physical manifestations are common. Relief of these symptoms, therefore, requires attention primarily to the emotional response and the factors responsible for it.

The problem is not limited, however, to the appearance of emotions as a response to a sexual problem. Emotional responses to nonsexual acts may markedly affect sexual performance. A man who is angry at his wife may become impotent or have premature ejaculations. A woman who is tense may be unable to reach a climax. A person who is depressed may lose sexual desire. Anxiety may be associated with a wide variety of sexual disturbances. These difficulties in sexual performance then arouse a fresh emotional reaction, and a vicious cycle may be initiated. The simultaneous occurrence of sexual problems and emotional reactions carries no implications of which came first. Either may affect the other and the situation must be carefully evaluated.

Conflicts around sexuality are common enough, but it must be remembered that conflicts in other areas may have considerable impact on the meaning of sexual experiences. One cannot judge from his own experience what this meaning will be. It can only be learned by talking with the patient. Frequently the initial description of its meaning by the patient will be misleading, a partial truth, a bit of wishful thinking. You must listen long and well if you wish genuinely to understand.

A young man sought treatment for a peptic ulcer of several years' duration. The symptoms flared up while he was making plans to get married. He was not aware of "stresses"; the two of them got along very well together and he felt happy in contemplating marriage. Interestingly, he recalled that one of his earliest episodes of epigastric pain had been closely associated with a "torrid love affair" during late adolescence. This was the first girl with whom he had had intercourse. He enjoyed physical relations with her and experienced only minimal guilt over his sexual activities, in which he engaged nightly for one memorable month. Near the end of the month ulcer pain developed, and at the end of the month he broke off his relationship with her. Could there have been any association between this sudden burst of heterosexual activity and his epigastric pain or were the two coincidental?

As more information became available about this earlier experience, it became clear that, despite the physical pleasure initially gained, the total experience was stressful. He had strong feelings that the male should be dominant and independent, keeping control of the situation. He found himself going through the act more frequently than he wished, to satisfy her desires rather than his own. He was not really in command of the situation and this aroused his anger. But he also felt that a man should be able to have intercourse nightly with pleasure, should have more desire than a woman. His lack of enthusiasm aroused feelings of inadequacy which distressed him. He continued having intercourse regularly rather than admit this inadequacy. He didn't wish to continue and couldn't bring himself to stop. His inability to reach a decision aroused further feelings of inadequacy and anger at himself. All of these factors combine to make it possible that the ulcer was associated with this "love affair" even as he thought it was. Unravelling the strands responsible for his reaction in this situation gave the starting point for understanding the exacerbation which had brought him to the doctor—again a situation in which he did not feel he was in control or being allowed to make decisions which he should have made.

The sexual problem of a young girl with severe dermatitis also involved more sexual activity than she wished. Her problem was mutual masturbation rather than intercourse, and her reaction to it was primarily of guilt. She did not have orgasm but had learned that she could please her partners by breathing more rapidly and fully after a certain amount of genital stimulation and by certain movements of her body which she thought simulated orgasm. She felt guilty about the sexual activity and inadequate in her response to it. She wanted to be "normal" and rather envied her male partners their ejaculations. She also felt that her physical symptom, dermatitis, was closely related to her sexual problem and to her inability either to enjoy sexual stimulation or to give it up.

Both these patients had sexual problems and in both feelings of inadequacy were prominent. Both presented the problem as one of excessive activity. In the boy, the problem was not primarily sexual, however. His problem lay more in social phenomena than in physical ones. He wished to be independent; he had definite ideas of what the male role should be. He felt inadequate in being unable to assert his independence or to play the male role adequately. Nonsexual conflicts were determining factors in establishing the meaning of his heterosexual relationships. The girl had a sexual problem but in addition had strong feelings of guilt about indulging in masturbation and suffered feelings of inadequacy about her femininity. Her inability to withdraw from a relationship which she described as totally unsatisfying requires explanation. The physician should accept this description cautiously and look with care for other sides to the problem.

Too little sexual activity may also pose problems for patients, whether self-imposed or not. Mr. Stewart was such a patient. Nearing 40, he was a man with long-standing, "burned out" rheumatoid arthritis with fixation of his hips at a 90-degree angle so that he walked facing the ground. His back and hips were ankylosed, his extremities less affected, permitting a fair range of motion. Though sexual desire was not great, it was present. He had fears of attempting intercourse, however, lest he be unsuccessful and shame himself in front of a woman. He managed to overcome these fears with one friend, who seemed sympathetic and willing to try though aware that his physical disability might lead to failure. The attempt *was* a failure and was followed by a severe gastrointestinal upset characterized mainly by nausea, vomiting, and abdominal pain. The experience was devastating to him and left him severely depressed, feeling inadequate as a man and convinced that life could never bring him the happiness of marriage and a home of his own which should be the lot of any man.

Miss Waite was a young woman in her late thirties who had voluntarily denied herself sexual experiences. Her reaction was not one of pride in living up to her code of behavior, however, but one of doubt and uneasiness lest it stem instead from some basic inadequacy in herself. She hesitated to tell her doctor that she had had no sexual experiences, wondering if it might not be better to make one up, since she felt that any normal woman of her age would certainly have had intercourse at least once, if not regularly. Mrs. Lyon, on the other hand, a married woman of about the same age with 10 children felt quite guilty about her sexual relationship with her husband. She told her physician almost plaintively that she did not believe she and her husband were really any worse than other couples but they had "got caught every time."

A young man in his early twenties came to his physician fearful that he had acquired some venereal disease. He had just masturbated for the first time and interpreted the ejaculation as a "urethral discharge." Having never had heterosexual relations, he feared he had picked up some disease from an infected toilet seat. Another young man told his physician that his friends got their sexual pleasure from masturbation or intercourse while he got his from rectal stimulation. He didn't see that it should make much difference and mentioned it only because he had let his toothbrush slip from his grasp and it was up his rectum beyond his reach. A man who had never had intercourse with his wife during 15 years of married life said that it was sufficient joy to be able to look upon her body without defiling it with sexuality. A farmer nearing 40 lost his wife. His sexual needs continued, however, so he told his 17 year old daughter that she would have to take her mother's place in the bedroom as well as in the kitchen. Though aware that his neighbors might disapprove should they learn of this relationship, he gave little evidence of feeling guilty about it himself.

Sexual practices and the attitudes toward them have great variety. You must not assume that the patient will react as you would in a similar situation. An understanding of the patient and his problems can never be acquired unless you keep an open mind and make inquiries freely, allowing the patient a chance to express his own feelings whether they are socially acceptable or not. Neither can you treat these problems lightly. Each patient mentioned had a serious sexual problem that deserved careful consideration and helpful guidance.

There is no one approach to sexual problems. In many instances the major difficulty lies not in the sexual activity itself but in its meaning to the patient in terms of his feelings of adequacy, his ideas about roles, his value systems, and various conflicts such as that of dependency. Therapeutic efforts, therefore, are directed at the forces affecting the meaning of sexuality; the type and intensity of sexual activity are affected secondarily as the meaning is altered. You deal primarily with the emotions and attitudes, the defenses, and the social forces which condition these. Usually, you should work toward a sexual adjustment which is suitable for the social group to which the patient belongs, though exceptions to this statement certainly exist. The adjustment reached should be consistent with the values and moral code of the patient; indeed no adjustment is satisfactory if it is not. This may mean altering values when goals conflict or altering the relative importance of different goals. The process of accomplishing this is the same whether sexual adequacy or social adequacy is the major problem.

Sexuality may be used to express other conflicts. A young woman with asthma who had indulged in a wide variety of sexual activities— heterosexual and homosexual, mutual masturbation, cunnilingus, and fellatio, to mention a few—was using sexuality to express rebellion against her mother. She could not have found a more successful way to express hostility, for her mother was horrified by what she knew and would have been more so had she learned all of what was happening. She had dedicated her life to being a "bad" daughter but felt intense guilt with each episode. A young man who became enraged whenever his wife failed to have an orgasm during intercourse was also using sexual relations as part of a very different conflict. Though he expressed contempt for his father, a violent man who bragged openly to his son about his sexual conquests, he was in competition with him. He could not tolerate being second best to his father. When he had sexual relations with his wife, she *had* to respond so that he would not feel inferior to him. Needless to say, beneath his façade of contempt he greatly admired his father. The ambivalence intensified his reaction. Treatment in instances such as these is not focused directly on the sexual difficulties but on the rebellion or competition which have given rise to the problem.

Sexual impulses may be excluded from consciousness, just as anger may, because they are viewed as sinful no matter what their manner of expression. When sexuality has been suppressed so that the desire remains but gratification is denied, whether by refusal to have intercourse or being so tense and controlled that orgasm is impossible, free discussion of the topic can be very beneficial. Most books dealing with the techniques of intercourse deal also with this problem; their benefit is greatest for those who inhibit sexual expression. When sexuality has been completely excluded from consciousness by repression, no benefit should be expected from superficial discussions of sex no matter how objective or "enlightened" these may be. The factors responsible for the use of repression need to be uncovered and dealt with before any change in sexual behavior can be anticipated.

Another type of sexual problem seen with some frequency is one in which the patient is unable to feel or express affection and physical love for the same person. Mr. Joseph had such a problem. He had recently married for the second time and had become impotent within a week of marriage. His previous marriage had been dissolved because of impotence. For several months before his second marriage, he had dated his second wife, but not exclusively. They had had intercourse frequently and with satisfaction to them both. He told her about his other dates and let her know that his only interest in her was a physical one. Nevertheless, she insisted on marriage, hoping love would eventually come. He finally agreed but almost immediately became impotent with her though continuing to have intercourse with others.

Mrs. Walton had a similar problem. Though she permitted her husband to have intercourse, she never responded to him. She found sex repulsive or boring, depending upon her mood at the moment. Had she had her way, they would never have had sexual relations. She knew intercourse was a normal act, perhaps even desirable in a marriage, but she could not enjoy it no matter how much she tried. Though she was greatly disturbed by her inability to respond to her husband, she was even more upset at the realization that other men sometimes seemed attractive to her. In fantasy, she even thought intercourse with some of these men might be satisfying. The combination of desiring sexual relations but not wanting them with her husband puzzled her and aroused feelings of shame, but the shame did not change her desires.

A common background for this type of reaction to sex is a strong attachment to the parent of the opposite sex, particularly when this relationship has been seductive emotionally but restrictive physically. The seductive quality arouses sexual impulses, but the incest taboo prevents awareness of them. Sex is forbidden though affection is not. Mr. Joseph was deeply attached to his mother who had been seductive without permitting expression of the impulses she aroused. Their relationship emphasized, indeed idealized, affection between mother and son. In later life, whenever feelings of affection were present, sex was automatically forbidden, as though the relationship were again between mother and son. Sexual impulses had been aroused, however, and found free expression with women for whom he felt no affection. In fact, he had to prevent development of warmth in a relationship to retain his potency. For this reason he always dated several women and let each know that he cared little for her as a person.

Treatment must be directed at discovering the origins of these attitudes toward sex and affection. Intellectual explanations, such as that just given, are of little help. The patient must discover the pertinent factors for himself and work through the problem at an emotional level. Psychiatric care is desirable, when available.

It should be emphasized again that interviews are seldom as directive as the discussion of treatment here might indicate. The statements and suggestions are ideas the physician keeps in the back of his mind as possible sources of pertinent information. The interview itself is directive only long enough to center the discussion in the most fruitful area. When this has been accomplished, the patient takes over, as in the sample interview with Mr. Laird (p. 196) the physician nodding or repeating significant words when an important topic has been introduced. The physician cannot do this, however, unless he knows what is important and when it is pertinent to discuss it.

Occasionally patients wish to sexualize the doctor-patient relationship, and you should avoid doing anything which might foster such a development. You can best avoid this by keeping the goals of therapy clearly in mind while talking with the patient. Your interest in the patient is personal and usually warm but should, at the same time, be objective.

A young physician, still in training, once asked, "Why do neurotic women looking for a man always pick on me?" When asked the reason for his query he recounted two episodes within a few weeks of each other. He had seen a middle-aged woman with many complaints which seemed fairly clearly related to emotional difficulties. He described her as very good looking, intelligent, and obviously unhappy. He had also met her husband whom he described as a "real dull character." He listened sympathetically to her troubles and suddenly found that she was offering to get a divorce if he just said the word. At about the same time an 18 year old girl was his patient. She had a boy friend whom he said "followed her around like a puppy dog." He added,

"She's well stacked." She had a bone tumor of the arm and an amputation was scheduled. He was very interested in her and the problems in adjustment which lay ahead of her as a result of the operation. He wanted to help. He had scarcely started his helping when she invited him, instead of her boy friend, whom she was now describing as "a bore," to attend the school dance with her. He felt it strange that both of these patients had misunderstood his professional interest in their emotional problems and had reacted at such a personal level.

It is interesting to consider what he said. In both instances he commented upon how attractive the patients were. He obviously had responded to their physical attractions. His tone as he talked about them was quite intimate, very different from his way of discussing any of his male patients. He had made derogatory evaluations of both the men involved and thought that both women deserved something better. His intimate tone of voice, the personal nature of the topics discussed, and his derogation of the men involved undoubtedly was seductive. If, in addition, his unhappiness in his own marriage was evident to them, their response is not surprising. He had a warm, personal interest in both patients but was thinking more about how attractive they were and how dull the men they were tied to than about how he could best help them find a satisfying adjustment in life.

RELIGION

Religion is a potent force in our society, and its ethical code forms a basis for judging one's own behavior and that of others. Even those who have no formal religious affiliations cannot escape its impact. Actions are judged good or bad whether one thinks this desirable or not, and the judgment depends upon a moral code, which is determined in part by religious beliefs.

When accepted fully, a religious code is usually a stabilizing influence and a positive force in people's lives. Guilt arises when the code is violated. You then try to clarify for the patient his reason for violating the code. Ordinarily this reason will be found in a contrary code, often ill defined, which took precedence for the moment. In helping the patient understand the origins and intensity of the two conflicting codes, you are clarifying the nature of the conflict and the reason for feelings of guilt while preparing the way for a more objective evaluation of the situation which elicited the conflict.

Certain religious practices, such as confession and prayer, play an important role in maintaining the religious codes despite conflicts. When a person recognizes a conflict between codes, he is apt to feel that he must make a decision between the two and live by one while violating the other. The difficulty of such a decision may arouse a great deal of anxiety. At such times, prayer serves to reemphasize the importance of the religious moral code, thus weighting the decision in its favor. When an act contrary to the religious code has been committed, confession and penance reaffirm the importance of the religious code. Since actions usually strengthen the code to which they conform and weaken contrary codes, confession and penance may strengthen a religious code which has been weakened by violation as well as afford emotional relief through ventilation.

Psychotherapy is sometimes considered to be opposed to religion. One reason for this is the need, at times, for a free discussion of hostile or sexual impulses. Another is that psychotherapy is ordinarily directed at the alleviation of anxiety and guilt, even when these have been aroused by violation of a religious code of ethics. But psychotherapy need not destroy faith; it may actually strengthen it. Marian was a Catholic who repeatedly felt guilty because she did not live according to her faith. Removing the conflicts which led her to act as she did made it possible for her to live with her faith and to find more peace and security and less anxiety and guilt in it. Many religious practices are psychotherapeutic: to the believer confession allays guilt and prayer gives security and courage. There need be no conflict between religion and psychotherapy, though they approach human problems from different points of view.

How should you proceed when strong religious beliefs constrain a patient from discussing important hostile and sexual conflicts? Treatment cannot be effective without such a discussion, yet the patient may feel that efforts to encourage ventilation of these impulses are attacks upon his religion. At such times, you should assure the patient by your manner of questioning if not in actual words that you respect religious beliefs and ethical codes. A discussion of religion as a force which prevents him from talking about anger and sex may be helpful, for it gives an opportunity to deal frankly with a portion of his conflict and a chance to reassure him that his faith need not be shattered by free discussion of the problems he meets in life. The key to success lies in working within the framework of the patient's religious beliefs, whatever these may be.

Mrs. Brandvig, a minister's wife, went to her physician because of anxiety and frequent, severe migraine headaches. She had two small daughters. If they were in the kitchen while she was preparing dinner, she could not pick up a knife without thinking, "What if it should slip from my hands and hurt them." This thought filled her with anxiety though it was ridiculous. She had never hurt her children and was sure she never would. And then there was that ominous feeling of impending catastrophe every time her husband gave an especially fine sermon. Why should such a feeling overwhelm her just when all his parishioners were praising him? And then the headaches! They were so severe she was unable to do her housework, care for her children, or attend to those duties which were essential for the minister's wife if the women's activities of the church were to be a success. These were her problems, could the physician help?

The recurrent thoughts seemed to imply hostility behind her anxiety; but she never got angry. Oh, of course, she was frequently irritated at the children but for such petty things that she really couldn't remember any specific one. She wanted them to be models people could look at and say, "I wish my children were as good." And they were good children, really. Yet, if they were noisy, she worried for fear they were too noisy; if they were quiet, she wondered if they were too quiet. No, she didn't get angry at them. They were good. But something was wrong that she should worry so much about them.

To questions about her husband, she admitted that she was sometimes upset that he gave so much of his time and energy to members of his church and so little to his family. But this was a part of his way of life, necessary to his work, and she wouldn't change it for anything. It was selfish of her even to have the thought. To questions about her childhood, she answered that she thought she had been a very unhappy child but she didn't know why. She had had as many advantages in life as had her friends. She didn't want to talk about her childhood. It had nothing to do with her present problems.

It was evident that she wished to deny a good deal of anger and resentment. Why was anger so threatening that she felt it could not be accepted? Her reasons were all phrased in religious terms. When asked her feelings about anger and hostility, she responded essentially with "Anger is evil." Her church preached and she believed that people who got angry were headed for eternal damnation. Her husband preached this with vigor and vehemence. One should oppose evil wherever he found it and oppose it openly and vigorously in an effort to vanquish it.

These statements gave the religious framework necessary to understand her wish to deny her anger. They also gave her physician material needed to make anger more acceptable to her. That her husband's vigor and vehemence were of themselves an expression of anger had not occurred to her. It was righteous indignation. That righteous indignation and anger had much in common, however, she could agree. After thoughtful consideration she decided the difference lay in what aroused the feeling and how it was expressed.

As she considered these matters at some length, she became less threatened by anger itself and was able to talk about some of the things which had aroused it. It soon became evident that she had greatly resented her father though she could not express this easily. Children should honor their parents. The love and respect this implied allowed no room in her mind for anger or resentment. But she had also said one should oppose injustice and evil wherever one found it. Suppose one found it in one's father, then what? The answer, in reverse, is in many books on child rearing. Parents should love the child while disapproving, even punishing if necessary, what he has done that is wrong. One can love and respect a person despite his mistakes. Should not the child as he grows older be allowed to disapprove of the mistakes which his parents have made? This was discussed within her religious frame of reference until she began to feel comfortable with the idea.

There was another block to discussion of these things. She believed that a person who had faith in God could not experience anxiety. Was her anxiety really related to the anger and resentment within her or was it lack of faith? If the latter, then discussion of her anger would not help, would it? She believed in a punitive God, however, and in eternal damnation for those who were evil. She considered herself evil insofar as she felt anger. Her anxiety therefore stemmed from her faith, not from her lack of it. The stronger her belief in her own responsibility for her thoughts and actions the more intense her feelings of guilt when these seemed wrong or bad. Through such a line of reasoning, anxiety was made more acceptable to her.

Working with these resistances was necessary before an adequate history could be obtained, but it was also a part of treatment. Much of her anxiety arose from her feelings of worthlessness because she was unable to live up to her ideals for herself. In the process of examining her beliefs more carefully and clarifying them in her own mind, she gained self-respect. By dealing with these resistances entirely within the framework of her own religious beliefs, her faith was not shaken. On the contrary, it was strengthened. Her moral code was clarified and became more realistic without being basically altered. The experience was beneficial and made it possible for her to enter into psychotherapy more fully, no longer fearful of what she might learn about herself.

Mrs. Brandvig's problem was not basically a religious one, but religious beliefs interfered with treatment. Many patients have similar resistances which are expressed in terms of beliefs about emotions and psychotherapy but without reference to religion. These may be approached in the same way, using contradictions present as a starting point for reevaluating the ideas blocking treatment or using motivations for health and happiness as forces to overcome these barriers.

A different but equally disturbing problem is presented when a patient is in doubt about his religious code or his system of values and is temporarily without a stable base from which to guide his behavior. Again the problem may be phrased in religious terms but it is not necessary to discuss religion as such. You seek instead to understand and deal with the reasons for the doubt, and the patient formulates his own value system once the conflicts have been resolved.

DEPENDENCE

The phrase "a dependent personality" is not a diagnosis, nor is it a very informative description. Everyone is more or less dependent upon those about him. The phrase is used for persons who seem more dependent than is usual and for those whose dependence is determined by emotional conflicts. There is no clear line of distinction. Dependence has many aspects which need to be explored in detail before the term has real meaning as applied to any one person.

Conflicts around dependency commonly have their origins in the relationship of the patient to his parents. The more fully this relationship is understood the better will physician and patient understand the development of the conflict and what needs to be done to resolve it. Early parent-child relationships therefore need to be explored in detail, relating this material to the situation currently facing the patient. Through this process the patient should gradually gain a better picture of himself and the influence of past events upon present behavior. More than this, however, can be done to help him overcome dependent patterns of behavior.

The two major aspects of dependence are physical and emotional —helplessness and the need for approval. Physical dependence is seen in the newborn, in people who are ill, and, symbolically, in those who are financially dependent on others. This state of dependence may be, but by no means invariably is, associated with a sense of helplessness, a feeling that one is devoid of personal power in the situation. A consideration of the meaning of power clarifies the problem and its treatment. Power has been defined as (1) the ability to introduce force, (2) the ability to influence the behavior of others, (3) the ability to carry out one's will despite resistance, and (4) the awareness of alternative lines of action.[95] All four aspects of power may be seen in the family setting. Parental discipline, whether by physical force or verbal persuasion, is a manifestation of power. Adolescent rebellion may give the developing adult a feeling of power over his own destiny. The relation of these patterns to the problem of dependence and independence is easily seen. Power and independence, helplessness and dependence, are closely allied concepts.

At times people find themselves in threatening situations where they can exert no physical force sufficient to alter it, have no hope of influencing the behavior of others concerned, and feel unable to carry out their own will. At such times, feelings of helplessness may be overwhelming and precipitate illness. Mrs. Winters (p. 19) was in such a situation. Her husband held her in contempt, gave her an inadequate allowance, was openly unfaithful to her, and tried to raise their children to hold her in contempt. She could not change him and felt totally inadequate to support herself. The situation seemed intolerable but there was no alternative but to stay with it. She was depressed and agitated and consulted her physician because of severe diarrhea.

Her treatment was essentially demonstrating to her that alternatives were available, that she did not have to remain in this situation if she did not want to. A volunteer job gave her confidence in her ability to support herself if the need arose. Her renewed self-esteem gave her an alternative pathway. She did not use it, choosing to remain with her husband instead, but the fact that an alternative existed removed her sense of helplessness, of being trapped in an intolerable situation, and her diarrhea subsided. Dependence, inadequacy, and powerlessness were intimately related to her symptoms; the realization that alternative solutions to her problem existed was sufficient to afford relief.

The emotional aspect of dependence, the need for approval can be equally disturbing. It is fostered by parents who give approval only for doing what they have requested. This may be used effectively in trying to socialize the child, though there is no need to apply it to all areas of activity. When continued through adolescence, maturity can be markedly delayed. You can use dependency of this sort to help the patient become independent. A strong doctor-patient relationship can usually be developed fairly readily, and you can then give approval for independent action.

It is not a long step from making one's own decisions in order to win approval from a physician to making them for oneself, if this is handled properly. The major portion of therapy is guiding the patient into making independent decisions which can be carried out and will bring satisfaction.

Patients who are accustomed to make decisions according to the likes and dislikes of others need help in a more logical approach to the problem of decision. It is not helpful to be told "It's your problem and you'll have to make your own decision" unless this is followed by guidance. Many steps are required and the patient needs to go through these slowly and thoughtfully. Physician and patient both may well heed the advice given executives: "The fine art of executive decision consists in not deciding questions that are not now pertinent, in not deciding prematurely, in not making decisions that cannot be made effective, and in not making decisions that others should make . . . Not to decide questions that are not pertinent at the time is uncommon good sense, though to raise them may be uncommon perspicacity. Not to decide questions prematurely is to refuse commitment of attitude or the development of prejudice. Not to make decisions that cannot be made effective is to refrain from destroying authority. Not to make decisions that others should make is to preserve morale, to develop competence, to fix responsibility, and to preserve authority." [96] The last sentence expresses well the gains to the patient when you allow him to make the decisions which he should make.

Though you may make decisions easily yourself, you may find it difficult to help your patients go through the necessary steps, or you may lose patience when it takes weeks or months for the patient to reach a decision you would make immediately. The actual decision is less important than the process and the attitude, however, except where life is endangered. The slow and laborious way may be far more productive in the long run, for in the process the patient is learning self-reliance and independence. This cannot be achieved quickly by one who has spent years dependent on the approval of others. Quick decisions should be viewed with suspicion.

What are the steps toward decision? First one must recognize that a decision is appropriate. Physician and patient may not agree that a decision is needed or on who should make that decision. Too often a physician is ahead of his patient and does not stop to consider this point with him. Mrs. Winters' physician at her first visit might have seen the problem as one requiring that she decide whether to remain with her husband or not and then leave or settle down and accept the situation. She would not have agreed since there seemed no possibility of leaving. No decision was appropriate until she had convinced herself that alternatives existed. Similarly Gladys' physician might have seen the situation at once as one in which she needed to decide whether her marriage meant more to her than being a little better than the neighbors. She would not have agreed with this at all. She saw no conflict there and felt that any decision rested with her husband. Was he going to act as a good husband should or not? It may take a good deal of discussion before the area of decision is clear to physician and patient.

Once the need for a decision has been agreed upon, the situation must be analyzed. This requires a consideration of the patient's assets and liabilities as they apply to the situation as well as the bare facts of what is happening. If other people are involved, and usually they are, their assets and liabilities and the relationships between the various participants need to be evaluated. In this way you get a picture of the forces at work and the meaning of the situation to everyone affected by it.

Following this the various alternatives need to be identified and the consequences of each considered. During this phase, alternatives which the patient cannot put into action are just as valid for discussion as are possible lines of action. Consideration of these personally "impossible" alternatives can illuminate basic deficiencies or emotional blocks and resistances more clearly than the possible alternatives. They help the patient see his place in the total picture, giving him a more objective view of what he contributes to it and what stands in the way of resolving the problem satisfactorily. For instance, a woman described her husband as totally unacceptable to her in every way but when asked why she didn't leave him answered "I can't. I need him." The physician knew this before asking the question and used it as a starting point for a discussion of the positive aspects of their marriage.

Only when the situation and the various potential lines of action have been discussed fully is the patient ready to make a decision. You should not be emotionally involved in this decision if you are to be sure that the patient makes the decision on the merits of the case and not to win approval for a specific decision. The decision must then be put into action. If there is trouble at this point, it is usually because analysis of the situation has not been complete—the blocks or resistances to action have not received sufficient consideration.

The other side of dependency also needs consideration. Fred (p. 56) seemed to develop a very independent attitude at the age of 4 when his father deserted the family. He could not trust others because this aroused feelings of insecurity and helplessness, since he felt that no one could really be depended on. In such a situation, only a superficial relationship is possible at first. The physician needs patience, a warm interest in the patient, and complete dependability so that the patient can learn that some people are dependable.

The 19 year old boy with a congenital heart lesion (p. 207), who even stipulated the length of his interview with the physician, was trying to prove his independence to avoid demands which to him were inherent in dependency, the demand to love and obey. Handling this problem also requires patience and a warm interest in the patient. The greatest threat to the doctor-patient relationship will be demands and restrictions imposed by the physician. A permissive relationship may eventually break down the generalizations this boy has formed about authority but the physician can hasten the process if the problem can be discussed openly. If power is expressed in the ability to influence the behavior of others, dependency in being influenced, one is as dependent when influenced to rebel as when influenced to conform.

The boy with congenital heart disease left school, though he said he would like to continue, in order to avoid unpleasant comments about his manner of dress, which could easily have been corrected. He felt this expressed independence, but if he really wanted the benefits of an education it did not. Repeated examples of this sort may give such a person a new outlook on dependence, decreasing the satisfactions he has obtained from so-called "independent" actions and increasing his capacity for more normal relationships.

Illness itself may arouse conflicts around adequacy and dependence. The conflicts are not different because illness has activated them, nor is treatment different. If the patient is able to do more than he thinks he can, he is encouraged to demonstrate this adequacy to himself. If he must be dependent and cannot return to former activities, you must help him find satisfactions at his new level of adjustment, altering his attitudes if necessary. This requires first an understanding of the patient's reaction to his illness and the reasons for it, then treatment directed at the emotional aspect and its underlying conflicts.

When you find a patient who has settled, apparently comfortably, into a dependent way of life you should suspect that dependency gives at least a partial mastery of the situation. Strong feelings of anxiety or hostility may be aroused by efforts to get such a patient to adjust at a level of greater independence. Your efforts may be directed at reducing the gains derived from being dependent or at increasing the satisfactions of being independent. But the whole situation needs to be evaluated carefully; sometimes it is best to leave the situation undisturbed.

It should be clear that social forces and intrapersonal conflicts are intimately related. You do not deal with one or the other individually but with the two simultaneously. A good social history clarifies the conflicts and indicates the direction in which treatment should proceed. But this is only true when you view the social forces through the eyes of the patient. The events of life and the forces impinging upon him can only be interpreted by him within the framework of his past experience. You must focus your attention upon his interpretation of these events and upon their emotional meaning to him if you are to gain understanding and be able to treat effectively.

Chapter 13

Course of Treatment

A$_N$ awareness of psychophysiologic phenomena is pertinent throughout the realm of medical and psychiatric practice. A psychophysiologic disorder may appear in a person whose general adjustment has been excellent despite many difficult circumstances or in one whose adjustment has been marked by severe personality disturbance. Treatment of two such dissimilar patients cannot be standardized in a single specific set of instructions. The physician must evaluate the person who is ill as well as diagnose the nature of his illness before he can outline a program of treatment. A few general principles have been offered from which such a program of treatment can be formulated. How the separate parts are put together in handling any one case depends on both patient and physician. But when the great diversity of patients and of situations is considered, it becomes evident that considerable flexibility in therapeutic approach is desirable.

APPROACH TO THERAPY

The approach to treatment of emotional disorders which has been presented is a more active one than that used in traditional psychotherapy but when used with judgment is applicable to most of the so-called functional complaints. It is not intended as a substitute for prolonged intensive psychotherapy in patients who need such treatment but as a method which can be used by internists and general practitioners in their daily practice. Most patients with functional psychoses, conversion hysterias, character disorders, or severe psychoneuroses should be treated by a trained psychiatrist. However, most psychosomatic complaints seen by the practitioner occur in patients with no psychiatric disorder or with a mild or moderate psychoneurosis. Hour-long interviews are often unnecessary. Much can be done with these patients in 15 or 20 minute discussions, if the time is used properly. Many of these patients, therefore, can be handled by the internist or general practitioner who is interested and willing to spend a little extra time early in the course of treatment in order to save much time later on.

Few rules of procedure are inviolable. Ordinarily when dealing with problems related to emotional disturbances the physician does not try to manipulate the situation but discusses it with the patient, allowing him to initiate any changes. Yet many physicians in practice can recall instances in which they took an active role in altering a situation to everyone's benefit. When emergencies arise in which prompt action seems necessary but the people involved are panic-stricken and unable to take action, the need for an outsider who can be decisive is obvious. Occasionally less dramatic circumstances may also be handled in a direct way.

Mrs. Hall, a woman in her late thirties, went to a medical clinic because of multiple aches and pains which were clearly related to stressful circumstances in her life. She had two children, a boy, 10, and a girl, 8. Her father-in-law, aging and partially deaf, lived in the home with them. He was careless in his habits and particularly so about dressing, which he might do any place in the house and in front of anyone. Mrs. Hall disliked this, especially because of her children. She had suggested that it would be better if he lived elsewhere, but her husband would not hear of it. He felt he owed it to his father to provide him with food and shelter in his old age, especially since he had no other place to go. Mrs. Hall tended to agree and accepted the situation as unpleasant but necessary. One day she heard giggling and unfamiliar noises from the bedroom. When she investigated she was horrified to find her father-in-law engaged in sexual play with her son. This she could not tolerate. Her husband, however, said he couldn't believe it, refused to speak to his father about it, and continued to insist that his father must remain in the household.

The medical student who saw this patient decided to visit at her home to talk with her husband and his father. He made the arrangements to do so, but when he arrived he found Mrs. Hall tearful and her husband gone. He had left for work in anger saying that no doctor from the clinic was going to tell him how to run his affairs. The student went to his place of work, and Mr. Hall was given an extra hour off before lunch so they could talk. For nearly 45 minutes they discussed his work and his recreations. During this time no mention was made of the situation at home, though both knew this was the reason for their meeting. Finally, Mr. Hall brought the subject up himself. Referring first to his wife's illness, he went on to say that if it was actually related to "nerves" he knew what the problem was. It was his father. But he didn't know what to do about it. His father had done much for him; he couldn't throw him out on the street and there was no place for him to go. He got a pension from the state which might pay for a room some place, but what about his meals? And he would be alone. The student suggested a home for elderly people, naming ones in the vicinity and stressing the positive features of such an arrangement. Mr. Hall was not sure how his father would react to such a suggestion; he might feel he was unwanted. So the student offered, with Mr. Hall's permission, to make the suggestion himself.

As they returned home, the student learned a little more about Mr. Hall's father and the sources of dissatisfaction to him in the current living arrangements. Thus he was able to talk to the father more easily, getting him to express the advantages in moving. He was actually pleased with the idea, contrary to expectations, and plans were made for him to look at homes near enough for the family to visit him easily.

When Mrs. Hall returned to the clinic, she was free of symptoms though her father-in-law had not yet moved. He had chosen a place, however, and all arrangements had been completed. On her following visit she seemed quite happy. Her father-in-law was no longer in the home; she and her husband were getting along better than they had in years; and she felt the home environment was a healthier one for the children.

In this instance, the medical student took very direct action to alter a situation, and everyone seemed to benefit from it. Since such a course is seldom recommended, some of the factors contributing to its success should be pointed out. Mr. and Mrs. Hall were people with good overall adjustment. The first potential block to success lay in Mr. Hall's relationship with his father. This needed to be evaluated before going further. A second block lay in his objection to having anyone tell him what to do. The student was careful to establish rapport first, avoiding any hint of trying to settle Mr. Hall's affairs for him without consideration for his desires. When the discussion turned to the immediate problem, Mr. Hall asked for the student's advice and indicated a willingness to alter the situation if an acceptable solution could be found. His father was also handled with respect for his interests. And, significantly, no action was taken which could not be reversed if anyone

o desired. All of these factors contributed to the success of this approach. A change in any one of them might have required alteration
in the way it was handled.

Manipulation of situations can easily lead to trouble. A person in
conflict who is ambivalent about the circumstances of his life may
emphasize how much he dislikes some aspect of it, giving little indication of its positive features. However, he both likes and dislikes it.
Altering such a situation only emphasizes the opposite side of the conflict, and the patient is no happier than before. If, in addition, the
change is permanent, he may feel he has lost the opportunity to decide
the issue for himself. The physician is then apt to be blamed for any
dissatisfactions. Such a situation requires treatment of the emotional
disturbance, not manipulation of the environment.

The prior level of adjustment of a patient is an important consideration in selecting the therapeutic approach. A patient with symptoms related to a situational reaction but with a good personality adjustment usually has sufficient inner resources and personal assets to
permit a fairly direct approach to his difficulty. In fact, explanation or
ventilation may be all that is necessary to make it possible for him to
handle the problem himself. The boy who had urticaria soon after a
critical supervisor checked his work (p. 66) needed only to be convinced of a relationship between the two to be able to handle the
situation effectively. The young man with headaches, filled with anger
because he felt his father-in-law had incestuous impulses toward his
wife (p. 222), needed only to express his anger so he could view the
situation more dispassionately to be able to take effective action. Both
patients achieved symptomatic relief through very simple therapeutic
devices which could be used by any practitioner.

As one moves from situational reactions to more generalized personality problems, the approach to therapy changes somewhat, and
the time required for it increases. But many of these problems can still
be handled fairly readily by the internist or general practitioner without fear of complications. As the emotional problems become more
complex, the approach of the physician should become more passive
and more cautious. This is only common sense; the more complex the
problem, the longer it will take to understand all its facets. Questioning may still be active, but the activity is directed toward increased
understanding, not toward definitive action. When doubt exists, a
passive, nondirective approach is the safest one.

When the somatic manifestations threaten life or limb, as they may in ulcerative colitis, Raynaud's disease, or angina pectoris, for example, you should proceed with caution. This does not mean that you should not encourage ventilation of strong emotions, if they are present, even during an acute exacerbation. Reducing the intensity of the emotion will be beneficial. It does mean that you should not arouse fresh anger or anxiety by your approach to the patient, since these are apt to increase the severity of the exacerbation. It also means that you should proceed cautiously in approaching central areas of conflict, since finding these under attack may also arouse anger or anxiety and thus intensify symptoms. The patient with ulcerative colitis, for instance, whose only significant interpersonal relationship is with his mother cannot tolerate a direct attack against this relationship no matter how obvious and serious the problem may be. One must begin by strengthening other relationships first—with you or with a spouse, if there is one. Not until another significant relationship exists is the patient ready to consider his relationship with his mother with any degree of objectivity or equanimity. To approach this subject first only arouses insecurity and anxiety whose intensity increases with the importance of the relationship. One can say that, in general, you should not try to weaken one relationship unless there is an adequate substitute, just as you do not try to remove a defense unless there is another one available or the need for the defense has been removed.

When drugs are available which are known to give symptomatic relief, they should be used. There is little justification for withholding treatment in the fear that relief of symptoms will remove motivation for dealing with emotional or personality problems. In giving such drugs, you should explain that the relief is temporary and give no assurance that the symptom will not return. If more than temporary relief is wanted, the emotional factors responsible for the symptoms need to be treated. How strongly you urge that these receive treatment will depend on how serious the disorder is and how effective you expect the treatment to be. This is similar to recommendations for surgery. If the operation is elective, the matter may be dropped as soon as the patient says he is not interested. If it is life-saving, it is urged despite strong resistance.

PSYCHIATRIC REFERRAL

When referral to a psychiatrist is indicated, it should be done in a matter-of-fact manner without camouflage and with no false promises.

Certain resistances to referral are common, and you should be prepared to meet these. If referral to a psychiatrist carries the implication for the patient that "it's all in your head," "it's imaginary," or "you're just putting on," explanation of psychophysiologic relationships may be sufficient to remove this block to referral. If the patient views symptoms related to stress as an evidence of inherent weakness, you may point out to him that it might just as well be viewed as the result of a strong personality pushing the body beyond its natural limitations, thus leading to symptoms, even as muscles become sore and painful after a day of unaccustomed labor. If the patient considers psychiatric referral to be tantamount to a diagnosis of "insanity," explanation coupled with reassurance may make the referral acceptable.

In making a referral it is most important to avoid any hint of rejection or abandonment. The patient who says in anger, "He couldn't diagnose my trouble so he sent me to Dr. Jones just to be rid of me," seldom plans to return to the referring physician nor is he in a favorable frame of mind to begin treatment with another physician. With psychiatric referral, the patient is not only faced with a new physician but also with a new technique of therapy, one about which there are many misconceptions. He needs the moral support of his regular physician.

Ordinarily the original visit should be presented as a consultation rather than as a change in therapists. This gives the psychiatrist freedom to accept the patient for treatment or not according to his evaluation of the problem. Not every patient with emotional problems can profit from psychiatric care. Not every patient who could profit can be fitted into a busy schedule. It is better to make no promises but to request a consultation, telling the patient that the decision concerning treatment will be made after the psychiatrist has had an opportunity to talk to him. It is well to discuss the case briefly with the psychiatrist before and after the consultation visit. The details of this discussion should not be given to the patient. Neither should letters giving psychiatric formulations be read to the patient or members of his family.

It is usually helpful to keep in touch with the patient during psychiatric care when this is possible. You will not discuss psychiatric material as such with the patient nor offer interpretations of your own. This is the psychiatrist's job and is left to him. However, many problems and questions arise that you can deal with more directly than the psychiatrist. Sometimes the patient feels offended by the psychiatrist's silence or becomes so uncomfortable because of it that he considers stopping treatment, or he may find comments of the psychiatrist tactless or embarrassing. Many patients feel that psychotherapy proceeds much too slowly and become discouraged before there has been any opportunity for improvement. Sometimes the patient feels he has achieved insight without a cure and sees no further advantage to therapy. What more can psychotherapy do than offer insight? At such times you can help by explaining psychiatric techniques and giving encouragement despite occasional barren plateaus during treatment. You should usually suggest to the patient that he bring these matters to the attention of the psychiatrist so they can discuss them together. Your support in addition, however, can smooth the course of therapy.

During this period you should be particularly careful to avoid being manipulated by the patient into saying or doing anything which will interfere with treatment. A patient may repeat comments of the psychiatrist, often out of context and colored by his own particular bias, and demand some reaction from you. The unwary physician can easily find himself entangled in the middle of the patient's emotional conflict, and his statements may be used in psychiatric sessions to block therapy. Thus the patient plays one physician against the other and avoids genuine personal involvement in treatment. Fortunately, this is not too common an occurrence; it can often be anticipated if you know your patients well. If anticipated, it may seem desirable to see the patient infrequently or not at all until psychiatric therapy is completed.

When psychotherapy is ended, you can help the patient and his family during the period of readjustment. This is particularly true when treatment was in a hospital and the patient and his family have not been able to make the adjustments gradually as the patient's status changed. Your help may also be useful in locating potential blocks to readjustment. One young man, after successful treatment for an acute schizophrenic episode, was discharged to his mother's care. No professional person visited the patient at home to see if an adequate readjustment was being made. Three months later both mother and son were institutionalized. A neighbor told the story. From the moment of her son's return the mother had gone about her household duties muttering to herself and to her son, "You'll never make it. You'll never make it." Even a casual observer would know that this was not an appropriate atmosphere for a convalescent patient.

PSYCHOTHERAPY BY THE PRACTITIONER

Psychiatric referral is necessary for only a small percentage of the patients seen in general practice. Many others have situational stresses and emotional problems which are pertinent to their physical symptoms, however. As one questions the patient about his symptoms and their relationship to eating, exercise, or other activities, he should also ask about the situation in which they arose. Identification of stressful situations, evaluation of the relative importance of different aspects of these situations, and full delineation of the patient's responses to them is usually not too difficult when these questions are posed in the context of the presenting complaints.

When stressful events have aroused intense feelings, treatment begins with ventilation of these emotions. Ventilation gives temporary relief; for more lasting benefit, something more is usually needed. When the situation cannot be altered, one may attempt to change the emotional reaction. This may be difficult to accomplish, but there are many ways of approaching the problem. An emotion is merely one expression of the meaning of a situation; change the meaning and the emotion automatically changes. And the meaning of an event, as indicated by our discussion of stress, is a composite formed from one's concept of himself, his past experiences with similar events, and his perception of the relationship between himself and the stressful stimulus. You can therefore attack the emotional reaction by changing the self-concept, so that the person feels adequate to handle the situation, or by changing the evaluation of past experience, so that the person sees that he is misjudging the situation because of a bias introduced by earlier experience. You can equally well try to alter the relationship perceived so that the patient, though in the same situation, no longer is threatened by it. Altering a person's system of values may do all three of these things simultaneously. Thus several routes are open and you can choose one or a combination, whichever best fits the circumstances.

Often, however, the patient is unaware that the events in his life have been stressful to him or that they are related in any way to his symptoms. It is then up to you to elicit information which will tell you what has been stressful and to learn the background material which will give him an understanding of why it has been stressful. Though some suggestions have been given on how to do this, it is time to put the material together and illustrate how the information is used to help the patient understand himself.

Mr. Camp affords a good example of how this can be accomplished. He was 28 years old when he came for treatment. His chief complaint was epigastric pain which usually began about 2 hours after a meal and was relieved by alkali or food. X-ray examination of his upper gastrointestinal tract had revealed a duodenal ulcer, and he was on a diet and receiving medications. He was aware of stressful situations in his life but saw no relationship between these and his symptoms. He was in business with his brother. Despite minor frictions, he felt they got along together better than most brothers. He was unmarried but "going steady" and this relationship was very satisfactory. He sometimes contemplated marriage but had not yet made up his mind. In general, life was busy and full but not unpleasant.

To the question "When did your pains first start?" Mr. Camp replied that his ulcer symptoms had first appeared when he was learning to fly. He enjoyed flying, however, and thought it unlikely that there was any connection between this and his ulcer. When asked why he took up flying, his answer was, "I don't know exactly why I took up flying—perhaps because my brother was learning to fly. But really there wasn't any good reason to do it." He then proceeded to give all the reasons why he should *not* have taken up flying. He had just completed formal training and was working 8 hours a day and Saturday mornings. He and his brother spent their evenings working on some ideas which they thought might eventually lead to a better income. He was studying for some special examinations. In addition to this he was reading philosophy in the hope of getting an understanding of his place in the world. He was dating occasionally. With all of this, his time was very well filled.

What does this tell us? He has given a catalog of reasons for not taking up flying. These are very good reasons. In addition we know that he has sufficient drive toward success in his work to spend 11 or 12 hours a day working at it and that he is sufficiently confused and uneasy about his position in the world to spend his hours after midnight reading. He has also said that flying was not of particular interest to him. He had started flying without any clear idea of why he did so. Obviously whatever that reason may have been, it was important enough to make him find time for flying in a schedule which was already overloaded.

In his answer, Mr. Camp gave a very good clue as to why he took up flying despite the cogent reasons for not doing so. When he said that he didn't know why, he meant only that flying itself was not of great interest to him. His catalog of reasons for not taking up flying was the basis for feelings of resentment which were beginning to become evident in his tone of voice. But what impelled him to take it up despite his resentment at doing so?

The clue he gave was in the very first sentence, "I don't know exactly why I took up flying—perhaps because my brother was learning to fly." Why should this impel him to do something of little interest to him personally? To find out, we need to know more about his brother and their relationship. This can be put to him as an open question: "Tell me what your brother is like" or "Have you always done everything your brother did?" There are many ways of asking this question. The main thing is to get the patient to talk freely. When this patient was asked to expand on his statement, he recounted an incident from his childhood. When he was about 4 years old a friend of the family asked him what he wanted to do when he grew up. He answered, "I want to do what my brudder do." This occasioned tremendous approval from his mother, and she repeated the remark to all members of the family and to most of the neighbors. Here in a simple sentence was proof that she had been a good mother and had two sons who loved each other. From her wholehearted approval of this comment we know that family cohesion and mutual affection among family members was extremely important to her. This piece of information is stored in the physician's mind, ready for future reference in understanding the relations between the two brothers and their parents. The episode is important not as an isolated incident but as an example which clearly states an attitude and relationship which must have been present throughout his childhood years. That it still influences his life is evident in his statement that it is one of the reasons he took up flying.

His brother was 2 years older than he and always a little ahead of him. When the older brother became interested in tennis, the younger boy was his playing partner. When the older boy began making model airplanes, the younger did likewise. When the older brother suddenly became very interested in classical music, the younger took this up too. In each of these endeavors he found that he was second best. His brother was older at a period of life when the differences in age meant a great deal in ability to perform. The patient's model airplanes were never quite as good as his brother's. His interest in music was strong but he did not feel that it was truly his interest in music because he had been led to it by his brother. During adolescence he found that he was a better tennis player than his brother, but this caused him to feel guilty, and he either avoided playing tennis with his brother or let him win.

During adolescence the two of them talked a great deal about their future plans. The older brother chose a career and they discussed its merits until the younger brother finally decided that it was exactly what he wanted too; so they decided to form a partnership. The older brother had made an outstanding record in school and had been asked to join the faculty, an honor which he had declined. The patient had had a hard time matching his brother's record but had managed to do so and, in addition, had taken a somewhat more active part in extracurricular activities. At the time that he came for treatment, Mr. Camp felt that his brother was better than he in technical details but lacked emotional warmth and originality.

What does this mean? First, the patient compares everything he does with what his brother does. He is in competition with his brother and judges himself by his brother's performance. He is acutely aware of exactly where he is inferior or superior to his brother. In the way he talks it is evident that he is proud of instances in which he betters his brother's performance. Yet, when he excels his brother he feels guilty and withdraws from the competition. At such times, he feels that he has not been true to some other standards. And these other standards are mutual friendliness and affection between brothers and a family cohesiveness which can be attained only by working together. He has given us a series of instances to demonstrate the potency of his initial statement that he wanted to do what his brother did, recalling a number of situations in which he has done exactly that. This supports the feeling that this attitude is extremely powerful in his life.

What gives this drive its power? He has given a partial explanation of this, too. It derives its power from the fact that it was approved by his mother. His relationship with his mother appears to be a very important one. He wants most to receive her approval. His brother is a focal point in this conflict because the two boys competed for this approval. The mother's insistence that they show mutual affection and work together might well have been the basis for his feelings of guilt when he excelled his brother. Therefore, one must know more about his relationship with his mother. In order to make this seem pertinent to him in terms of his ulcer, one might recall to his mind that the important part of his original statement "I want to do what my brudder do" was that his mother had approved of it heartily and told everybody about it.

When asked about his mother he described her as domineering. His father was easier to get along with, warm and affectionate, but not a person he really admired. His mother was the practical member of the family. She made all the major decisions. She was the one who repaired things which were broken about the house. She worked with her husband in their shop. She kept all of his books for him. She ran the household. She was not demanding of the patient but, being an extremely busy woman, had little time to spend with him. She gave her approval for excellent performances. In his school work she wanted him to be the best in the class. If he had the top grade, he was praised; anything less than this went without comment. At home she was particularly interested in having the two boys get along well together. She praised them for playing together in a friendly way. She was upset when they had arguments or fights.

He said that his mother was not demanding of him. Yet what can be more demanding than to expect a child always to be the best one in the class, not just to get an A but to get the best A? When he said that she was not demanding, he meant only that he accepted her demands as right and did not rebel against them. She did not tell him that he had to be best; she simply withheld her approval unless he *was* best. Consequently he never got the feeling that she was demanding it of him and never rebelled against it. His description of his childhood indicates that his mother fostered intense competition in her sons toward everyone outside the family. At the same time she demanded that they not compete with each other. This is a fine line of distinction, particularly in a household where one's activities are always being compared with what others in the household do.

In his brief description of his parents, he has also let it be known that his father did not amount to much in the household. It mattered little whether his father approved or didn't approve since he was not a very important figure. This more than doubles the significance of the mother's approval because it centers everything in one person. There was little division of responsibilities or of affection.

Some of the recurrences of his ulcer symptoms were in situations in which the conflict with his brother was very obvious. He was consciously irritated or resentful at something his brother had done. However, these were usually minor recurrences which subsided promptly.

More severe exacerbations not associated with any obvious difficulty with his brother had occurred. He thought it more likely that they were related to his feelings toward his girl, though he didn't understand how this could be since he was more apt to have pain from his ulcer when their relationship was good than when he was having trouble with her. Because of his competition with his brother, questions about the girl were followed closely by questions about his brother's wife. The answers to these two sets of questions gave a wealth of information. The essential points were these.

His brother had been married some years before to a girl from a lower middle-class family. She was very personable and a good housekeeper, but her family had no money. They had had difficulties from the very start. His brother wanted everything done in the most efficient manner and abhorred the slightest frustration or delay. When a decision had to be made, he wanted it settled immediately, she wanted to think it over at some length. If he pressed her too hard, she went to sleep. She could not have done anything which would have infuriated him more. He found her slow and methodical ways intolerable. Because of the tremendous difficulties in this marriage, the two brothers had discussed marriage at considerable length. The older brother had impressed on the younger one's mind the necessity of marrying somebody with wealth. Wealth was essential, not only to make living with a woman tolerable but for success in their partnership. To be successful in their work they had to know people with money. A woman with wealth would be able to introduce them to the right people and would be able to give them the money they needed to get started. They agreed that if one were going to fall in love it should be as easy to fall in love with a rich girl as with a poor one. The younger brother had therefore determined that he would marry a wealthy girl and improve the chances for the success of their partnership.

He had met girls of wealth, but with none of them did he feel at ease. He always wondered whether he went with them because he liked them personally or because they had money. He felt uneasy and insincere when with them. They were aware of this uneasiness and the dates never went quite as smoothly as he would wish. However, he had also met a girl of his own age who was a very competent secretary. She came, as he did, from a middle-class family. Her parents had no savings and no community prestige. He felt very much at ease with her, for her background and ambitions were similar to his. He liked her but had decided at the very outset that he was not going to become emotionally involved, since she had no money. He had not explained this to her, however, and she obviously saw in him a very charming young man whose company she enjoyed very much. He wanted to think that the friendship between them had been largely fostered by her, even though he knew that he had contributed a great deal to the steadiness of their relationship. When they had been going together for almost 3 years, both of them being of an age when marriage was prominently in their minds, he found himself in a situation where he felt that it was only decent of him to propose marriage or break off the affair entirely. Yet he was not sure which he wanted to do.

Attitudes of resentment were prominent in relation to his decision about marriage. He resented that she did not have wealth and was therefore not a suitable wife for him. He resented that he did not have money and had to make this a major factor in determining whom he would marry. He resented that he was in a field of work where money was of such importance. He resented that he had allowed himself to become so involved emotionally with this girl that the decision to marry or not to marry had become acute. He resented that he had never met a wealthy girl with whom he could feel at ease. He resented all the aims and goals which had got him into this dilemma. But he resented most of all his inability to reach a decision and thereby resolve the dilemma. There was no question about the intensity of these feelings of resentment though he did not emphasize them as he spoke. He had not really been aware of how strongly he felt until questions brought the feelings into the foreground.

This material forms a coherent mass of data which indicates some of the forces active in molding his behavior, establishing his goals, determining his attitudes, and contributing to his emotional reactions. Each statement raises new questions. One can follow whatever line of questioning seems most likely to be fruitful. But the physician is not the only one who has gained perspective in viewing the presenting complaints. The patient has also gained understanding of himself. He came complaining of epigastric pain, aware that it first arose when he began flying and aware that it had recurred in periods of indecision about marriage. Why flying was a stress he could not say even when asked directly, but with a little directed questioning he could give all the information necessary to understand why it was stressful. He could understand it too once the words had been spoken. None of this had been repressed. He simply had never seen the connection between these various facts before. It took the right sequence of questions to make it evident to him. In answering those questions, he obtained a new perspective on his problem and gained a new concept of himself. He gained "insight."

Many additional points about history taking are illustrated in this case. The patient wanted to discuss the petty irritations arising between him and his brother in their day-to-day activities. He was allowed to do this but with constant reminders that the specific episodes were not of major significance. They were related, however, to major problems: his need for approval from his mother, his dependence on his brother for decisions, and his resentment that his brother was making the decisions. Conversation was directed unobtrusively by questions related to the major areas of difficulty rather than by expressing disapproval of talking about trivia. In this way, the natural flow of conversation was not interrupted, but the problem was kept in clear focus.

This patient complained of indecisiveness. He had several problems which he wanted solved, and he asked for opinion and advice freely. It is a temptation at such a time to make decisions for the patient or, at least, to offer advice. The temptation must be resisted. A physician only entangles himself in the middle of the conflict if he tries to make decisions for the patient.

With Mr. Camp, discussion centered about his resentment at being trapped in his partnership with his brother. Discussion was directed each time to the same central core of attitudes and previous life experiences, emphasizing in his mind the importance of these things. Discussion of these matters went on for several weeks while he vacillated between one decision and another. Objectively, it was of little moment whether he stayed with his brother or not. He was well able to make his own living without his brother. There was no reason, either, why he should not work with his brother without being subjugated by him. The important thing was not whether he decided "yes" or "no" but that he decide something and decide it himself.

He considered at great length the possibilities of leaving the partnership entirely and striking out on his own. This was discussed with him in very concrete terms, exactly what he would do if he left his brother and what the chances were for success. This discussion was of considerable importance for it showed him that he was not trapped. If he wanted to leave, he could do so with good chances of being successful. There were disadvantages, however, and these were repeatedly emphasized because it was important that he remain undecided until he could make the decision calmly and logically. The ostile aspect of such a decision is clearly evident. Leaving his brother 'ould express his hostility toward him very trenchantly and proclaim is independence from both his brother and his mother. Such a ecision could very well be made purely in anger rather than logically. 'he ultimate decision rested upon his evaluation of the assets and the abilities in the alternative possibilities. The physician acted as a ioderating influence to keep him from deciding either way until he ad evaluated both adequately. He finally decided to stay with his rother.

This may sound like a poor decision. It certainly carried with it ome difficulties in adjustment. There was nothing dramatic in the ecision and it may seem a little disappointing in a person who prized idividuality and creativeness. What good has the physician done? Vhat value has the patient obtained from talking to a doctor when he ecides finally not to make any change?

There are a number of benefits from this decision. They would ave accrued whether the decision had been to leave or to stay. They re perhaps a little more interesting because they resulted from a ecision to stay in exactly the same situation. First of all, he made his decision himself, freely and after deliberation. He therefore need o longer feel that the partnership is imposed on him by someone else. Vorking with his brother has thus ceased to be a source of esentment. In making this decision he has increased his self-respect nd his feeling of capacity for decision. Energy previously bound up 1 feeling resentful is now free for use in work. In deciding to stay 'ith his brother he has reduced the competition between them and an therefore enter into the partnership with the feeling that they are eally working with each other toward a common goal.

In addition, this decision affected the other difficulties in his life.)ne of these was his difficulty in deciding whether to marry or not.)ne reason for not getting married was that the girl was poor and too iuch like his brother's wife. He would not be doing any better than is brother. His competition with his brother and his desire for pproval from his mother were both linked with this marital inde- ision. By coming to a decision about the partnership, he made the ecision to marry easier, even though no change had occurred in her ualifications as a wife. Their relationship had changed, however, ecause he felt able to make decisions. Ultimately he decided to iarry her. Thus his decision increased his work capacity, decreased he amount of resentment and irritation he felt in working with his brother, and made it possible for him to reach a decision abou marriage.

He had another problem—confusion about his place in the worle Part of this confusion arose from his relationship with his brother. H was expected to compete, to be the best, and yet never to be ahea of his brother. It was obviously impossible to be best and not b better than his brother. In coming to terms with this problem h partially clarified his confusion about his place in the world.

The relation between physician and patient was important in thi process. The physician was interested in the patient's problem respected his basic potentialities, accepted his indecision as unde standable under the circumstances, and yet did not interfere in hi personal life. Actually, the physician exerted a great deal of influenc but he did this by his questions, not by advice. He did not mak decisions, as the brother had, but left these for the patient to mak He did not condemn sibling rivalry but accepted it as normal. He di not disapprove of expressions of irritation and frustration in th fraternal relationship but permitted it free expression. All of thes attitudes were new in the patient's experience. While he was gainin intellectual insight into the origins of his problems through the proces of history taking, he was living a new type of relationship, learnin fresh attitudes, and establishing new orientations to people throug his relationship with the physician.

This patient did not come in complaining that he was angry o resentful. In fact he was not aware of resentment. Nevertheless hi treatment began with uncovering the sources of resentment in his lif and giving him ample opportunity to express resentment before help ing him to understand the reasons for it. To do this requires that physician be able to identify stresses the patient has not recognize as such. The initial statement of the patient cannot always be take at face value. Mr. Camp did not feel that flying had been stressful t him. Once one understands the circumstances surrounding learning t fly, however, there is little doubt as to its stressful nature. Identifyin such stresses is accomplished by talking with the patient about event and people in his life until their meaning is understood by the patien When the meaning is known the question whether the event wa stressful or not is solved.

Mr. Camp's story illustrates rather clearly that anger may b associated with symptoms and illness but not be immediately eviden The physician must be alert to statements which imply the presenc of anger even when dealing with a person whose surface relationships are friendly and warm. Once anger has been recognized it can be partially dissipated by expression.

Expression of anger may relieve the immediate pressures within the patient but does little to prevent its rearousal. More is needed. If the individual can remove himself from the situation, as did the patient with headaches who recognized incestuous desires between his father-in-law and his wife, the problem may be satisfactorily solved. Actually however, the solution is usually less simple. Similar situations will arise, and the person who tries to escape specific situations is only fooling himself. The man who cannot tolerate working under supervision because of its significance in terms of his feelings about authority, is not getting away from the problem by leaving one job for another. The problem recurs in any job in which he works for someone else. The physician's aim must then be to help the patient understand his reactions and their origins and to establish between himself and his patient a relationship in which new feelings can be learned about people in positions of authority.

In the process of learning to understand himself, Mr. Camp had to become aware of his conflicts and his defense mechanisms, since these were intimately related to his characteristic way of reacting to events in his life. His need to please others and his efforts to suppress his own drives and emotions in order to please were, of course, an expression of dependency, and the anger aroused was an outgrowth of his desire to be independent. The word "dependent" need never be used if it bears unpleasant connotations for the patient; but the effects of this conflict on his pattern of living must be given careful consideration.

Symptomatic relief was achieved early in the course of working with this patient, months before there was any consideration of terminating his visits to the doctor. The reasons for this are evident from what is known about anger and its relation to symptoms. Expression of anger dissipated it, and the physiologic changes were relieved, thus allowing his ulcer to heal. But expression of these feelings was only the first step toward recovery. Understanding the origins of these feelings was achieved later with considerable effort. Insight was not necessary for temporary symptomatic relief. It was necessary before more than temporary relief could be expected.

At times the goal of therapy may be limited to temporary symptomatic relief. In general, however, the aim of therapy should be to reach a state in which the patient may return to the stressful situation in which the symptoms arose without a recurrence of illness. Such a goal may or may not require fundamental changes in personality. It gives an end-point to therapy, however, which is practical and easily evaluated. If the patient wishes to make some alteration in the situation, it is ordinarily left to him but only after he has gained an understanding of his problem and the forces which have led to his illness. Mr. Camp, for example, should not be urged to leave his brother or to marry his girl friend without first understanding the conflicts which have blocked him from making these decisions himself. It would be far better to delay coming to these decisions until all aspects of the problem have become clear and the potential consequences of the alternatives have been carefully considered.

The physician should feel no pressure to change difficult situations for his patients. Stress is not inherently harmful nor can it be entirely eliminated. The physician is giving the patient lasting benefit when he helps him learn to cope effectively with stressful situations rather than to depend on someone else to handle them for him. This process begins in treatment itself. It is stressful to air resentments and impulses whose presence has been denied. It is stressful to face one's own limitations. Facing them is essential before one can deal with them objectively, however. Rather than a source of disability and illness, stress, properly met, can result in personal growth and development. A strong doctor-patient relationship and constructive guidance are potent supportive forces for patients who are threatened by events in their lives or impulses within their make-up.

What changes do you try to make during treatment of emotional problems? You do not expect to alter inherent capacities or basic constitutional traits. A person of superior intelligence will remain so; one who is subnormal in intelligence will continue to be. A person who is sensitive to the feelings of others will remain sensitive. One who is obtuse in his relationships with others is apt to continue to be obtuse. You cannot alter the nature of past events which have helped to mold these traits and capacities into the particular person who sits before you asking for help. These things have happened and have had their impact. If you can change neither the inherent capacities nor the nature of events which have shaped the way in which these capacities are used, what can you do?

There are a number of things which you attempt to do in psychotherapy. One of these is to decrease the intensity of emotional reactions so that the patient can deal with situations arousing these emotions without developing symptoms. This is a step in therapy even when, as with Mr. Camp, the emotion is not prominent on the surface. Another is to help the person understand the meaning of past events and his reactions to them so that their influence is not felt in situations where it is disadvantageous. Helping Mr. Camp understand the influence of his need for his mother's approval on his behavior in his partnership with his brother is an example of this type of activity. A third is to help a patient use his capacities effectively to meet problems without becoming ill. Changes of this nature happen frequently in the usual course of living. Growth and development is a process of learning ways of handling basic drives and traits in their interactions with the environment. The outcome of these interactions determines the person one is. In the process of growing into adulthood, many people of inconspicuous qualities and attainments in childhood and adolescence learn how to use their endowments more effectively to meet the problems of life. The physician meets people in times of stress and under circumstances which permit him to add his influence to remolding the patient's personality. The stronger the relationship with the patient, the more potent that influence can be. The changes which he is trying to effect are not really basic personality changes; yet, when successful, they may make the person seem to others to be a "new" person. This is accomplished by removing resistances to effective action, helping the person learn new ways to handle old problems, and releasing potential capacities so that they can become actual abilities.

If the goal of psychotherapy is increased understanding and learning to use one's basic capacities more effectively, why can't the patient do this for himself? For certain types of problems the patient can do much on his own; but it is always easier to view someone else's behavior objectively than one's own. The person who has spent his life denying that he has hostility is not apt to see hostility as a major problem. He needs the guidance of someone else in making an evaluation of himself.

More important than this, however, is the fact that many patients with psychophysiologic disorders have a major difficulty in their relationships with others. The crux of the need for another person in psychotherapy lies in relationship itself. No matter how well a man may understand himself or see the nature of his problems, he learns to change through action, Another person is needed for this. Since so many of the difficulties stem from childhood relationships with persons in authority, primarily the parents, this therapeutic relationship frequently needs to be with someone in authority. Other people can help, but the closer the tie of friendship or kinship the more difficult it is for the friend or family member to supply what is most needed. A physician can supply an authoritative relationship in which warmth and understanding predominate. This is the relationship most often needed and is something no patient can supply to himself.

Physicians affect the lives of their patients whether they wish to or not. If they use their influence to help others meet the stresses to which they are exposed effectively, much unnecessary suffering can be avoided. The influence spreads out in ever-widening circles as each of these alters his reactions to others. Physicians should be prepared to relieve mental anguish as well as the physical symptoms which may accompany it and should strive to help those who come to them become happier and more effective people. With these as their aims, physicians should have a rich and varied professional life of service to their patients.

REFERENCES

1. Gesell, A., and Ilg, F. L.: *Infant and Child in the Culture of Today* (New York: Harper & Brothers, 1943).
2. Sullivan, H. S.: *The Interpersonal Theory of Psychiatry* (New York: W. W. Norton & Company, Inc., 1953) .
3. Bergson, H.: *Creative Evolution* (reprint; New York: The Modern Library, 1944).
4. Cannon, W. B.: *Bodily Changes in Pain, Hunger, Fear, and Rage: An Account of Recent Researches Into the Function of Emotional Excitement* (2d ed.; reprint; Boston: C. T. Branford Company, 1953).
5. Grace, W. J., and Graham, D. T.: Relationship of specific attitudes and emotions to certain bodily diseases, Psychosom. Med. 14:243-251, 1952.
6. Darwin, C.: *The Expression of the Emotions in Man and Animals* (reprint; New York: Philosophical Library, 1955).
7. Ruesch, J., et al.: *Duodenal Ulcer* (Berkeley: University of California Press, 1948).
8. Magoun, H. W.: An ascending reticular activating system in the brain stem, Harvey Lect. 47:53-71, 1951-1952.
9. Hernandez-Peon, R., Scherrer, H., and Jouvet, M.: Modification of electric activity in cochlear nucleus during "attention" in unanesthetized cats, Science 123:331-332, 1956.
10. Lorente de No, R.: (a) Limits of variation of the synaptic delay of motoneurones, J. Neurophysiol. 1:187-194, 1938; (b) Synaptic stimulation of motoneurones as a local process, *ibid.*, pp. 195-206; (c) Analysis of the activity of the chains of internuncial neurones, *ibid.*, pp. 207-244.
11. Eccles, J. D., Fatt, P., and Landgren, S.: Central pathway for direct inhibitory action of impulses in largest afferent nerve fibers to muscle, J. Neurophysiol. 19:75-98, 1956.
12. Chapman, L. F., and Wolff, H.: Studies in human cerebral hemisphere function: adaptive capacity after loss of hemisphere tissue, Tr. Am. Neurol. A. 81:175-178, 1956.
13. Pavlov, I. P.: *Conditioned Reflexes* (New York: Oxford University Press, 1927).
14. Menzies, R.: Conditioned vasomotor response in human subjects, J. Psychol. 4:75, 1937.
15. Kaada, B. R.: Somatomotor, autonomic, and electrocortico-graphic responses to electrical stimulation of "rhinencephalic" and other structures in primates, cat, and dog: A study of responses from the limbia, subcallosal, arbito-insular, piriform, and temporal cortex, hippocampus—fornix and amygdala, Acta physiol. scandinav., Vol. 24 (supp. 83), 1951.
16. Delgado, J. M. R.: Emotional Behavior in Animals and Humans, in *Explorations in the Physiology of Emotions*, Psychiatric Research Reports 12, pp. 259-266, 1960.
17. Olds, J.: (a) Self-stimulation of the brain: Its use to study local effects of hunger, sex, and drugs, Science 127:315-324, 1958; (b) Positive Emotional Systems Studied by Techniques of Self-Stimulation, in *Explorations in the Physiology of Emotions*, Psychiatric Research Reports 12, pp. 238-258, 1960.
18. Brady, J. V.: Emotional behavior and the nervous system, Tr. New York Acad. Sc. 18:601-612, 1956.
19. French, J. D., et al.: Experimental gastroduodenal lesions induced by stimulation of the brain, Psychosom. Med. 19:209-220, 1957.
20. Funkenstein, D. H., King, S. H., and Drolette, M. E.: *Mastery of Stress* (Cambridge: Harvard University Press, 1957).

21. Selye, H.: *The Physiology and Pathology of Exposure to Stress* (Montreal: Acta Inc., Medical Publishers, 1950).
22. Hetzel, B. S., de la Haba, D. S., and Hinkle, L. E., Jr.: Rapid changes in plasma P.B.I. in euthyroid and hyperthyroid subjects, Tr. Am. Goiter A., pp. 242-249, 1952.
23. Hinkle, L. E., Jr., and Wolf, S.: Studies in Diabetes Mellitus: Changes in Glucose, Ketone, and Water Metabolism During Stress, in *Life Stress and Bodily Disease*, Proceedings of the Association for Research in Nervous and Mental Disease, vol. 29, pp. 338-389, 1950.
24. Gellhorn, E.: *Physiological Foundations of Neurology and Psychiatry* (Minneapolis: University of Minnesota Press, 1953).
25. Grossman, H. J., and Greenberg, N. H.: Psychosomatic differentiation in infancy: I. Autonomic activity in the newborn, Psychosom. Med. 19:293-306, 1957.
26. Richmond, J. B., and Lustman, S. L.: Autonomic function in the neonate: I. Implications for psychosomatic theory, Psychosom. Med. 17:269-275, 1955.
27. Wolf, S. G., and Wolff, H. G.: *Human Gastric Function: An Experimental Study of Man and His Stomach* (2d ed.; New York: Oxford University Press, 1947).
28. Grace, W. J., Wolf, S. G., and Wolff, H. G.: *The Human Colon: An Experimental Study Based on Direct Observation of Four Fistulous Subjects* (New York: Paul B. Hoeber, Inc., 1951).
29. Schneider, R. A., and Zangari, V. M.: Variations in clotting time, relative viscosity, and other physicochemical properties of the blood accompanying physical and emotional stress in the normotensive and hypertensive subject, Psychosom. Med. 13:289-303, 1951.
30. Schottstaedt, W. W., Grace, W. J., and Wolff, H. G.: Life situations, behavior, attitudes, emotions and renal excretion of fluid and electrolyte: (a) method of study, J. Psychosom. Res. 1:75-83, 1956; (b) Retention of water and sodium; diuresis of water, *ibid.*, pp. 147-159; (c) Diuresis of fluid and electrolyte, *ibid.*, pp. 203-211; (d) Retention of water, sodium and potassium, *ibid.*, pp. 289-291; (e) Variations in excretion of endogenous creatinine, *ibid.*, pp. 292-298.
31. Hinkle, L. E., Jr., Edwards, C. J., and Wolf, S. G.: Studies in diabetes mellitus: II. The occurrence of a diuresis in diabetic persons exposed to stressful life situations with experimental observations on its relation to the concentration of glucose in blood and urine, J. Clin. Invest. 30:819-839, 1951.
32. Holmes, T. H., and Wolff, H. G.: Life Situations, Emotions, and Backache, in *Life Stress and Bodily Disease*, Proceedings of the Association for Research in Nervous and Mental Disease, vol. 29, pp. 450-472, 1950.
33. Wolff, H. G.: *Stress and Disease* (Springfield, Ill.: Charles C Thomas, 1953).
34. Hardy, J. D., Wolff, H. G., and Goodell, H.: *Pain Sensations and Reactions* (Baltimore: Williams & Wilkins Company, 1952).
35. Freud, A.: *The Ego and the Mechanisms of Defense* (New York: International University Press, Inc., 1946).
36. Fenichel, O.: *The Psychoanalytic Theory of Neurosis* (New York: W. W. Norton & Company, Inc., 1945).
37. Breuer, J., and Freud, S.: *Studies on Hysteria* (New York: Basic Books, Inc., 1957).
38. Fromm-Reichman, F.: *Principles of Intensive Psychotherapy* (Chicago: University of Chicago Press, 1950).
39. Freud, S.: *A General Introduction to Psychoanalysis* (New York: Garden City Publishing Company, Inc., 1943).
40. Freud, S.: Instincts and Their Vicissitudes, in *Collected Papers*, Vol. IV, pp. 60-83 (London: Hogarth Press, 1949).
41. Nowlis, V., and Nowlis, H.: The description and analysis of mood, Ann. New York Acad. Sc. 65:345-355, 1956.

42. Betthelheim, B.: Individual and mass behavior in extreme situations, J. Abnorm. & Social Psychol. 38:417-452, 1943.
43. Lacey, J. I., Bateman, D. E., and von Lehn, R.: Autonomic response specificity: An experimental study, Psychosom. Med. 15:8-21, 1953.
44. Alexander, F., and French, T. M.: *Studies in Psychosomatic Medicine: An Approach to the Cause and Treatment of Vegetative Disturbances* (New York: Ronald Press Company, 1948).
45. Graham, D. T.: Cutaneous vascular reactions in Raynaud's disease and in states of hostility, anxiety, and depression, Psychosom. Med. 17:200-207, 1955.
46. Wolff, H. G.: *Headache and Other Head Pain* (New York: Oxford University Press, 1948).
47. Beecher, H. K.: Relationship of significance of wound to pain experienced, J.A.M.A. 161:1609-1613, 1956.
48. Zborowski, M.: Cultural components in responses to pain, J. Social Issues 4:16-30, 1952.
49. Diethelm, O., Fleetwood, M. F., and Milhorat, A. T.: The Predictable Association of Certain Emotions and Biochemical Changes in the Blood, in *Life Stress and Bodily Disease*, Proceedings of the Association for Research in Nervous and Mental Disease, vol. 29, pp. 262-278, 1950.
50. Barnes, R., and Schottstaedt, W. W.: The relation of emotional state to renal excretion of fluid and electrolytes in patients with congestive heart failure. In preparation.
51. Freud, S.: Mourning and Melancholia, in *Collected Papers*, Vol. IV, pp. 152-172 (London: Hogarth Press, 1949).
52. Wolf, S. G., personal communication.
53. Yamamoto, J., personal communication.
54. Malzberg, B., and Lee, E. S.: *Migration and Mental Disease* (New York: Social Science Research Council, 1956).
55. Foster, R. G.: Effect of mobility on the family, Am. J. Pub. Health 46:812-818, 1956.
56. Benedict, R.: *Patterns of Culture* (New York: Penguin Books, 1946).
57. Mead, M.: (a) *Sex and Temperament in Three Primitive Societies* (New York: William Morrow, 1934); (b) *Growing Up in New Guinea. A Comparative Study of Primitive Education* (New York: William Morrow, 1930).
58. Kardiner, A., and Ovsey, L.: *The Mark of Oppression. A Psychosocial Study of the American Negro* (New York: W. W. Norton & Company, Inc., 1951).
59. Parsons, T.: Certain primary sources and patterns of aggression in the social structure of the western world, Psychiatry 10:167-181, 1947.
60. Simmons, L. W.: The relation between the decline of anxiety-inducing and anxiety-resolving factors in a deteriorating culture and its relevance to bodily disease, A. Res. Nerv. & Ment. Dis., Proc. 29:127-136, 1950.
61. Plant, J. S.: *The Envelope: A Study of the Impact of the World Upon the Child* (New York: Commonwealth Fund, 1950).
62. Riesman, D.: *The Lonely Crowd* (New Haven: Yale University Press, 1950).
63. Whyte, W. H., Jr.: *The Organization Man* (New York: Simon and Schuster, 1956).
64. Mead, M.: *Male and Female* (New York: William Morrow, 1949).
65. Dynes, R. R., Clark, A. C., and Dinitz, S.: Levels of occupational aspiration: some aspects of family experience as a variable, Am. Sociol. Rev. 21:212-215, 1956.
66. Rosen, B. C.: The achievement syndrome: A psychocultural dimension of social stratification, Am. Sociol. Rev. 21:203-211, 1956.
67. Centers, R.: Motivational aspects of occupational stratification, J. Social Psychol. 28:187-217, 1948.

68. Warner, W. L., and Lunt, P. S.: *The Social Life of a Modern Community* (New Haven: Yale University Press, 1941).

69. Hollingshead, A. B.: Selected Characteristics of Classes in a Middle Western Community, in Bendix and Lipset (eds.), *Class, Status, and Power: A Reader in Social Stratification*, pp. 213-224 (Glencoe, Ill.: The Free Press, 1953).

70. Ruesch, J.: *Chronic Disease and Psychological Invalidism: A Psychosomatic Study* (Berkeley: University of California Press, 1951).

71. Rennie, T. A. C., and Srole, L.: Social class prevalence and distribution of psychosomatic conditions in an urban population, Psychosom. Med. 18:449-456, 1956.

72. King, S. H., and Cobb, S.: Psychosocial factors in the epidemiology of rheumatoid arthritis, J. Chronic Dis. 7:466-475, 1958.

73. Hyman, H. H.: The Value Systems of Different Classes: A Social Psychological Contribution to the Analysis of Stratification, in Bendix and Lipset (eds.), *Class, Status, and Power: A Reader in Social Stratification*, pp. 426-442 (Glencoe, Ill.: The Free Press, 1953).

74. Hooker, D.: Fetal reflexes and instinctual processes, Psychosom. Med. 4:199-205, 1942.

75. Sheldon, W. H.: *The Varieties of Human Physique: An Introduction to Constitutional Psychology* (New York: Harper & Brothers, 1940).

76. Sheldon, W. H.: *The Varieties of Temperament: A Psychology of Constitutional Differences* (New York: Harper & Brothers, 1942).

77. Ilg, F. L., and Ames, L. B.: *Child Behavior* (New York: Harper & Brothers, 1955).

78. Jones, M., and Bayley, N.: Physical maturing among boys as related to behavior, J. Educational Psychol. 41:129-148, 1950.

79. Barker, R. G.: *Adjustment to Physical Handicap and Illness: A Survey of the Social Psychology of Physique and Disability* (Bull. 55, revised; New York: Social Science Research Council, 1953).

80. Titchener, J. L., *et al.*: The problem of delay in seeking surgical care, J.A.M.A. 160:1187-1193, 1956.

81. Parsons, T.: Illness and the role of the physician: A sociological perspective, Am. J. Orthopsychiatry 21:452-460, 1951.

82. Sutherland, A.: Psychological impact of cancer surgery, Pub. Health Rep. 67:1139-1148, 1952.

83. Sheldon, H. D.: *The Older Population of the United States* (New York: John Wiley & Sons, Inc., 1958).

84. Kaplan, S. M.: Laboratory procedures as an emotional stress, J.A.M.A. 161:677-682, 1956.

85. Freeman, H. E., and Simmons, O. G.: Mental patients in the community: Family settings and performance levels, Am. Sociol. Rev. 23:147-154, 1958.

86. Dyk, R. B., and Sutherland, A. M.: Adaptation of the spouse and other family members to the colostomy patient, Cancer 8:123-138, 1956.

87. Greenspoon, J.: Unpublished doctoral dissertation, quoted in Verplanck, W. S., The operant from rat to man, Tr. New York Acad. Sc., Series II, 17:594-601, 1955.

88. Verplanck, William S.: The operant from rat to man: An introduction to some recent experiments on human behavior, Tr. New York Acad. Sc., Series II, 17:594-601, 1955.

89. Thaler, M., Weiner, H., and Reiser, M. F.: Exploration of the doctor-patient relationship through projective techniques, Psychosom. Med. 19:228-239, 1957.

90. Woods, J. W., *et al.*: The evaluation of "medical" therapy in essential hypertension, J. Psychosom. Res. 2:274-284, 1958.

91. Liddell, H.: Some specific factors that modify tolerance for environmental stress, A. Res. Nerv. & Ment. Dis., Proc. 29:155-171, 1950.

92. Malmo, R. B., Boag, T. J., and Smith, A. A.: Physiological study of personal interaction, Psychosom. Med. 19:105-119, 1957.
93. Dugan, J. B.: Psychotic response to attempted psychotherapy in a patient with hyperthyroidism, Psychosom. Med. 16:252-258, 1954.
94. James W.: *The Principles of Psychology* (New York: Henry Holt & Company, 1918).
95. Abramson, E., *et al.:* Social power and commitment: A theoretical statement, Am. Sociol. Rev. 23:15-22, 1958.
96. Barnard, C. I.: *The Functions of the Executive* (Cambridge: Harvard University Press, 1958).

Index